Therapeutic Potential of Natural Products in Internal Diseases

Therapeutic Potential of Natural Products in Internal Diseases

Guest Editors

Dorin Dragoş
Adelina Vlad

MDPI

Basel • Beijing • Wuhan • Barcelona • Belgrade • Novi Sad • Cluj • Manchester

Guest Editors
Dorin Dragoş
Department of Medical Semiology
Carol Davila University of Medicine and Pharmacy
Bucharest
Romania

Adelina Vlad
Department of Functional Sciences I/Physiology
Carol Davila University of Medicine and Pharmacy
Bucharest
Romania

Editorial Office
MDPI AG
Grosspeteranlage 5
4052 Basel, Switzerland

This is a reprint of the Special Issue, published open access by the journal *Pharmaceuticals* (ISSN 1424-8247), freely accessible at: https://www.mdpi.com/journal/pharmaceuticals/special_issues/9NUU2R8I5I.

For citation purposes, cite each article independently as indicated on the article page online and as indicated below:

Lastname, A.A.; Lastname, B.B. Article Title. *Journal Name* **Year**, *Volume Number*, Page Range.

ISBN 978-3-7258-6147-7 (Hbk)
ISBN 978-3-7258-6148-4 (PDF)
https://doi.org/10.3390/books978-3-7258-6148-4

Contents

pharmaceuticals

MDPI

Editorial

Editorial: Exploring the Therapeutic Potential of Natural Products in Internal Diseases

Dorin Dragos [1] and Adelina Vlad [2,*]

1 Department of Medical Semiology, Faculty of Medicine, Carol Davila University of Medicine and Pharmacy, 020021 Bucharest, Romania
2 Department of Functional Sciences I/Physiology and Neuroscience, Faculty of Medicine, Carol Davila University of Medicine and Pharmacy, 050474 Bucharest, Romania
* Correspondence: adelina.vlad@umfcd.ro

In recent decades, significant progress in drug development has transformed the treatment of internal diseases, improving both outcomes and prognosis [1]. However, these advances frequently come with a cost: serious, sometimes even life-threatening side effects [2]. Many clinicians acknowledge the need for alternatives but often lack the knowledge or confidence to use them. Meanwhile, an increasing number of people are resorting to complementary or alternative approaches, particularly herbal medicines [3,4]; these individuals have begun adopting healthier lifestyle changes alongside these treatments [5]. Despite this trend, skepticism toward natural products remains strong in mainstream medicine, largely due to the limited amount of high-quality evidence [3,4].

The Special Issue *"Therapeutic Potential of Natural Products in Internal Diseases"* was established to address the above challenges. It presents a collection of original research and critical reviews exploring how natural products might contribute to treating these conditions. Together, the studies included identify both the opportunities and the obstacles in translating traditional knowledge and early findings into evidence-based therapies.

With regard to metabolic disorders, several studies have illustrated the complexity of natural-product interventions. Bekheit et al. demonstrated that ferulic acid attenuated isoproterenol-induced myocardial infarction in diabetic rats, normalizing ECG patterns, lowering cardiac enzymes, and reducing oxidative stress and inflammatory cytokines by suppressing the AGE–RAGE axis [6]. Complementing this mechanistic insight, after conducting a before-and-after trial, Mantadaki et al. reported that quercetin supplementation (500 mg/day) over two 12-week periods increased the whole-blood absolute telomere length in type 2 diabetes patients, indicating potential anti-aging and cardiometabolic benefits [7]. A randomized, double-blind, placebo-controlled trial by Hariharan et al. examined carnosine supplementation (2 g/day) over 14 weeks in adults with prediabetes or well-controlled type 2 diabetes [8]. Although the intervention was safe and well-tolerated, it did not improve cognitive outcomes such as executive function or memory. The findings emphasize the importance of larger, longer trials targeting higher-risk or cognitively impaired populations to determine whether carnosine may offer benefit in metabolic disease.

Non-alcoholic fatty liver disease (NAFLD), especially in lean individuals, is being increasingly recognized as a distinct clinical challenge. Tang et al. investigated Ganjianglingzhu decoction, a traditional herbal formula, in a murine model of lean NAFLD [9]. The intervention ameliorated hepatic steatosis, inflammation, fibrosis, and oxidative stress, with metabolomics pointing to glycerophospholipid metabolism as a key mechanism. Specific metabolites such as sn-3-O-(geranylgeranyl)glycerol 1-phosphate emerged as potential biomarkers of effect, emphasizing how modern metabolomics can unlock new pathways in traditional medicine research.

Inflammation is a common thread in many chronic diseases, and plant-derived compounds demonstrate considerable promise as modulators of inflammatory processes. Du et al. revealed that the traditional Chinese medicine formula Qilianxiaopi reduced inflammation in models of chronic atrophic gastritis by targeting ADAM17 and lowering TNF-α secretion, with narirutin identified as a key active component [10]. Karinchai et al. reported that extracts from *Ficus lindsayana* roots and latex suppressed inflammation and improved adipocyte function in vitro, with effects on glucose uptake, lipolysis, and inflammatory cytokine expression [11]. These findings highlight the potential of herbal medicines to influence the intersection of inflammation and metabolic regulation.

Natural products are also garnering attention for their anticancer potential. Aziz et al. characterized methanol extracts of *Ammi visnaga* roots and seeds, showing antioxidant, antimicrobial, and cytotoxic activity against breast cancer cell lines, accompanied by an upregulation of pro-apoptotic genes and a downregulation of anti-apoptotic genes [12]. Pristimerin, a triterpenoid found in Celastraceae and Hippocrateaceae plants, has been highlighted by Prabhu et al. for its ability to inhibit cancer cell proliferation, induce apoptosis, and suppress metastasis through multiple signaling pathways [13]. Despite promising preclinical evidence, the authors recommend further clinical trials to confirm the therapeutic value of pristimerin.

Taken together, these contributions illustrate the therapeutic potential of natural products in addressing a wide spectrum of internal diseases, from metabolic and inflammatory disorders to liver disease and cancer. They underline the need for rigorous, mechanistic, and clinical investigations to transform traditional and preclinical insights into safe, effective, and evidence-based therapies. This Special Issue stands as a call to action for researchers and practitioners alike: let us continue to explore, validate, and integrate the immense potential of natural products in the future of internal medicine.

Conflicts of Interest: The authors declare no conflict of interest.

References

1. World Health Organization. *Global Report on Traditional and Complementary Medicine 2019*; WHO Press: Geneva, Switzerland, 2019.
2. Lazarou, J.; Pomeranz, B.H.; Corey, P.N. Incidence of adverse drug reactions in hospitalized patients: A meta-analysis of prospective studies. *JAMA* **1998**, *279*, 1200–1205. [CrossRef]
3. Posadzki, P.; Watson, L.K.; Alotaibi, A.; Ernst, E. Prevalence of complementary and alternative medicine (CAM) use by the general population: A systematic review and update. *Int. J. Clin. Pract.* **2013**, *67*, 928–939.
4. Barnes, P.M.; Bloom, B.; Nahin, R.L. Complementary and alternative medicine use among adults and children: United States, 2007. *Natl. Health Stat. Rep.* **2008**, *12*, 1–23. [PubMed]
5. Bishop, F.L.; Lewith, G.T. Who uses CAM? A narrative review of demographic characteristics and health factors associated with CAM use. *Evid. Based Complement. Alternat. Med.* **2010**, *7*, 11–28. [CrossRef] [PubMed]
6. Bekheit, S.O.; Kolieb, E.; El-Awady, E.-S.E.; Alwaili, M.A.; Alharthi, A.; Khodeer, D.M. Cardioprotective Effects of Ferulic Acid Through Inhibition of Advanced Glycation End Products in Diabetic Rats with Isoproterenol-Induced Myocardial Infarction. *Pharmaceuticals* **2025**, *18*, 319. [CrossRef] [PubMed]
7. Mantadaki, A.E.; Baliou, S.; Linardakis, M.; Vakonaki, E.; Tzatzarakis, M.N.; Tsatsakis, A.; Symvoulakis, E.K. Quercetin Intake and Absolute Telomere Length in Patients with Type 2 Diabetes Mellitus: Novel Findings from a Randomized Controlled Before-and-After Study. *Pharmaceuticals* **2024**, *17*, 1136. [CrossRef] [PubMed]
8. Hariharan, R.; Mousa, A.; Menon, K.; Feehan, J.; Ukropcová, B.; Ukropec, J.; Schön, M.; Majid, A.; Aldini, G.; de Courten, M.; et al. Effects of Carnosine Supplementation on Cognitive Outcomes in Prediabetes and Well-Controlled Type 2 Diabetes: A Randomised Placebo-Controlled Clinical Trial. *Pharmaceuticals* **2025**, *18*, 630. [CrossRef] [PubMed]
9. Tang, N.; Ji, L.; Shi, X.; Xiong, Y.; Xiong, X.; Zhao, H.; Song, H.; Wang, J.; Zhang, L.; You, S.; et al. Effects of Ganjianglingzhu Decoction on Lean Non-Alcoholic Fatty Liver Disease in Mice Based on Untargeted Metabolomics. *Pharmaceuticals* **2024**, *17*, 502. [CrossRef] [PubMed]

10. Du, S.; Wang, T.; Li, Z.; Li, T.; Miao, Z.; Chen, Y.; Zhu, S.; Wei, W.; Deng, H. Therapeutic Potential of Qilianxiaopi Formula: Targeting ADAM17-Mediated Chronic Inflammation in Atrophic Gastritis. *Pharmaceuticals* **2025**, *18*, 435. [CrossRef] [PubMed]
11. Karinchai, J.; Buacheen, P.; Rodthayoy, D.; Yodweerapong, T.; Imsumran, A.; Wongnoppavich, A.; Chantarasuwan, B.; Suttisansanee, U.; Temviriyanukul, P.; Pitchakarn, P. Anti-Inflammatory and Anti-Adipocyte Dysfunction Effects of *Ficus lindsayana* Latex and Root Extracts. *Pharmaceuticals* **2024**, *17*, 287. [CrossRef] [PubMed]
12. Aziz, I.M.; Alshalan, R.M.; Rizwana, H.; Alkhelaiwi, F.; Almuqrin, A.M.; Aljowaie, R.M.; Alkubaisi, N.A. Chemical Composition, Antioxidant, Anticancer, and Antibacterial Activities of Roots and Seeds of *Ammi visnaga* L. Methanol Extract. *Pharmaceuticals* **2024**, *17*, 121. [CrossRef] [PubMed]
13. Prabhu, K.S.; Jessy, S.; Kuttikrishnan, S.; Mujeeb, F.; Mariyam, Z.; Habeeba, U.; Ahmad, N.; Bhat, A.A.; Uddin, S. Anticancer Potential and Molecular Targets of Pristimerin in Human Malignancies. *Pharmaceuticals* **2024**, *17*, 578. [CrossRef] [PubMed]

pharmaceuticals

MDPI

Article

Cardioprotective Effects of Ferulic Acid Through Inhibition of Advanced Glycation End Products in Diabetic Rats with Isoproterenol-Induced Myocardial Infarction

Sarah Ouda Bekheit [1], Eman Kolieb [2], El-Sayed E. El-Awady [1], Maha Abdullah Alwaili [3], Afaf Alharthi [4] and Dina M. Khodeer [1,*]

1 Department of Pharmacology and Toxicology, Faculty of Pharmacy, Suez Canal University, Ismailia 41522, Egypt; saraouda97@gmail.com (S.O.B.); sayed.alawadi@pharm.suez.edu.eg (E.-S.E.E.-A.)
2 Department of Medical Physiology, Faculty of Medicine, Suez Canal University, Ismailia 41522, Egypt; eman.kolieb@med.suez.edu.eg
3 Department of Biology, College of Science, Princess Nourah bint Abdulrahman University, P.O. Box 84428, Riyadh 11671, Saudi Arabia; maalwaele@pnu.edu.sa
4 Department of Clinical Laboratory Sciences, College of Applied Medical Sciences, Taif University, P.O. Box 11099, Taif 21944, Saudi Arabia; a.awwadh@tu.edu.sa
* Correspondence: dina_khoudaer@pharm.suez.edu.eg

Abstract: Background/Objectives: Myocardial infarction (MI) and diabetes pose significant health challenges globally, necessitating the development of innovative medication strategies to improve outcomes in affected populations. This research aimed to determine the defensive impact of ferulic acid (FA) against isoproterenol-induced myocardial infarction (MI) in diabetic rats. Methods: A group of male rats was partitioned into five distinct groups: control group, diabetic group, diabetic + MI, diabetic + MI + 20 mg/kg FA, and diabetic + MI + 40 mg/kg FA. The experimental groups received isoproterenol (ISO) subcutaneously at a dosage of 50 mg/kg body weight for two consecutive days. Results: The outcome was severe cardiac toxicity, as shown by changes in electrocardiogram (ECG) rhythm and a substantial increase in blood cardiac enzymes such as creatinine kinase (CK-MB), cardiac troponin I (cTnI), and lactate dehydrogenase (LDH). Additionally, there was a surge in inflammatory cytokines, like tumor necrosis factor-alpha (TNF-α), and a disruption of the antioxidant system, evidenced by a rise in malondialdehyde (MDA) content. Moreover, there was a rise in cardiac receptor of advanced glycation end products (RAGE). Treatment with FA with escalating dosages of 20 and 40 mg/kg b.w. effectively mitigated changes in serum cardiac enzymes and improved the cellular architecture, which was evaluated by histopathological examination. Conclusions: In conclusion, in a dose-dependent manner, FA successfully showed a cardioprotective effect against ISO-induced cardiac toxicity in diabetic rats, as shown by the improvement in ECG findings, normalization of serum cardiac biomarkers, and augmentation of the endogenous antioxidant system. Therefore, the aforementioned data indicate that ferulic acid may potentially have a protective effect on MI patients who have diabetes mellitus.

Keywords: advanced glycation end products and their receptors; diabetes mellitus; ferulic acid; isoproterenol; myocardial infarction; oxidative stress

1. Introduction

Diabetes is a metabolic disease marked by prolonged high glucose levels in the bloodstream caused by insufficient insulin production or compromised insulin function, which can be attributed to poor pancreatic β-cell activity or insulin resistance. The two pathophysiologies are distinctive features of type 2 diabetes (T2D), the most prevalent form of diabetes [1]. This condition is a metabolic disease that disrupts the metabolic processes of large biological molecules [2]. Diabetes-related cardiovascular disease was the principal reason for the death of 17.9 million people globally in 2016, which affected 31% of all fatalities worldwide [3]. Moreover, the prevalence of CVDs, including stroke and myocardial infarction (MI), surged from 257 million cases in 1990 to 550 million cases in 2019 [4–6]. The pathophysiology of MI is complex and involves a combination of various mechanisms, for example, oxidative stress, contractile dysfunction, endothelial damage, and cell death by apoptosis or necrosis [7]. Patients with type 2 diabetes have a two to four times greater risk of CVD mortality than non-diabetic patients [8]. Myocardial infarction (MI) and diabetes are major contributors to global morbidity and mortality, presenting substantial challenges to healthcare systems worldwide [9]. These conditions frequently coexist, complicating patient management and prognosis. The interplay between diabetes and MI involves complex pathophysiological mechanisms, including impaired glucose metabolism, chronic inflammation, and increased thrombotic activity, which accelerate the progression of atherosclerosis and heighten the risk of cardiac events [10]. Current therapeutic approaches often fall short in fully addressing the needs of this patient demographic, highlighting an urgent need for innovative medication strategies. By focusing on the development of treatments that target specific pathological processes at the intersection of MI and diabetes, researchers aim to significantly improve clinical outcomes and enhance the quality of life for these patients [11].

Oxidative stress is the pivotal mediator in causing damage to the heart muscle secondary to ischemia and reperfusion in type 2 diabetes, distorting the diabetic myocardium structure and function [12]. The condition may be caused directly or indirectly by elevated blood sugar levels, high fats in the blood, and decreased insulin sensitivity. Reactive oxygen species (ROS) are highly reactive molecules resulting from their ability to accept electrons. In their higher concentrations, ROS cause many degenerative diseases. Several pharmaceutical compounds can generate ROS and induce oxidative stress [13]. For instance, isoproterenol (ISO) is known to be one of the agents that generate extremely cytotoxic ROS [14]. Moreover, isoproterenol stimulates the secretion of inflammatory cytokines, including TNF-α, IL-1β, and IL-6 [15].

Advanced glycation end products (AGEs) are potent oxidizing substances produced by a nonenzymatic glycation process involving nucleic acids, free amino acids, reducing sugars, and lipids. Multiple endogenous and exogenous sources can produce AGEs [16]. The production of AGEs is irreversible and generally slow in physiological conditions. In contrast, many factors may accelerate the formation of AGEs, such as oxidative stress, hypoxia, hyperglycemia, insulin resistance, obesity, and aging [17]. AGEs play a crucial role in triggering vascular complications of diabetes by inducing oxidative stress, inflammation, and thrombogenic and fibrotic reactions [18]. The next approach to preventing or postponing vascular problems in people with diabetes involves inhibiting the synthesis of AGEs. OPB-9195 and aminoguanidine, which are synthetic medications, can hinder the creation of AGEs. However, it is important to note that these drugs have a very high level of toxicity [19]. As a result, several studies have focused on natural products as sources of potential inhibitors of AGE development, prioritizing their high safety and low toxicity. Phenolic acids and flavonoids derived from plants have recently been shown to be effective glycation inhibitors [20].

Ferulic acid (FA), also known as 4-hydroxy-3-methoxy cinnamic acid ($C_{10}H_{10}O_4$), is a phenolic compound found in various plants and foods of plant origin. Some examples are tomatoes [21], sweet corn [22], and wheat [23]. FA is a bioactive compound with various functions, including antidiabetic, anti-inflammatory, and antioxidant functions. It can eliminate excessive ROS, function as a powerful scavenger of free radicals, such as hydroxyl and peroxyl radicals, and prevent lipid peroxidation [24]. Additionally, FA can inhibit platelet aggregation, reduce thrombosis [25], and prevent liver cholesterol synthesis by lowering blood lipid concentrations. Consequently, it can prevent coronary heart disease [26]. Ferulic acid, a natural phenolic compound found in various plants and foods, is beneficial in managing diabetes and cardiovascular diseases. Ferulic acid helps improve insulin sensitivity and reduce blood sugar levels by combating oxidative stress and inflammation, which are common complications in diabetic patients [27]. Ferulic acid exhibits strong antioxidant properties for cardiovascular diseases that can protect against heart tissue damage by reducing oxidative stress and inflammation. Additionally, it has been shown to help regulate blood pressure and cholesterol levels, further supporting heart health and preventing the progression of cardiovascular diseases [28]. While the general inhibitory effects of FA on AGEs have been reported in previous studies, our study provides new insights into the specific application of FA in a clinically relevant model of diabetic MI. By exploring FA's effects on AGE–RAGE-mediated oxidative stress and inflammation in this complex pathological setting, we aim to contribute to the growing body of evidence supporting FA's therapeutic potential in diabetic cardiovascular complications. Furthermore, this study assesses whether ferulic acid has a cardioprotective effect by improving ECG findings, normalizing serum cardiac biomarkers, and augmenting the endogenous antioxidant system. Consequently, these results may spotlight the benefits of natural products in preventing the complications of long-term disorders like diabetes.

2. Results

2.1. The Effect of Ferulic Acid on Body Weight, Left Ventricle Weight (LV), and Heart Weight (HtWt)-to-Body Weight (BWt) Ratios

Table 1 shows no significant difference between groups for body weight at baseline. At the same time, the end findings of the investigation revealed a substantial variation in body weight across the groups. The highest mean changes in body weight were recorded in the diabetic + MI group (34.27%), followed by the diabetic group (29.9%) and diabetic + MI + FA (20 mg/kg) group (22.0%), while the lowest mean was recorded in the diabetic + MI + FA (40 mg/kg) group (17.9%), followed by the control group (18.0%). Regarding the HtWt and LV weight ratios, the highest mean ratio was recorded in the diabetic + MI group, followed by the diabetic and diabetic + MI + FA (20 mg/kg) groups, while the lowest was recorded in the control group. Statistical analysis showed significant differences between groups for these variables.

Table 1. Impact of treatment with ferulic acid at doses of 20 or 40 mg/kg on body weight, left ventricular wet weight, and the ratio of heart weight to body weight (g/g) for different study groups.

Groups	Baseline BWt (g)	Final BWt (g)	% Change BWt	LV Weight to BWt (g/g) $\times 10^{-3}$	HtWt to BWt (g/g) $\times 10^{-3}$
Control	159.0 ± 3.6	187.7 ± 4.5 [c]	18.0 ± 0.8 [b]	1.1 ± 0.1 [b]	3.7 ± 0.6 [a]
Diabetic	159.0 ± 3.2	207.0 ± 3.7 [b]	29.9 ± 4.3 [ab]	1.3 ± 0.1 [a]	4.1 ± 0.3 [a]
Diabetic + MI	168.3 ± 2.1	226.0 ± 3.6 [a]	34.3 ± 27 [a]	1.3 ± 0.01 [a]	4.3 ± 0.2 [a]
Diabetic + MI + FA (20 mg/kg)	166.3 ± 2.7	202.7 ± 5.4 [bc]	22.0 ± 5.6 [b]	1.2 ± 0.1 [ab]	4.1 ± 0.2 [a]
Diabetic + MI + FA (40 mg/kg)	163.1 ± 4.4	191.7 ± 3.7 [bc]	17.9 ± 4.7 [b]	1.2 ± 0.1 [ab]	4.0 ± 0.1 [a]
F test	2.48	11.39	6.54	5.07	1.41
p-Value 0.05	0.111ns	0.0010 **	0.0075 **	0.017 **	0.29

** and different superscript letters indicate significant differences at $p < 0.05$.

The percentage change in body weight (BWt) was determined using the following formula: % change BWt = [(final BWt − baseline BWt)/baseline BWt] × 100. The initial body weight (BWt) was measured at the beginning of the trial, whereas the final BWt was measured after week 10. The data are shown as the mean value plus or minus the standard deviation (mean ± SD). They were analyzed using a one-way analysis of variance (ANOVA) followed by Bonferroni's post hoc test, with the significance level set at $p < 0.05$, n = 8. Significant differences were observed between the control group and all diabetic groups ($p < 0.05$). The diabetic + MI + FA 40 mg/kg group showed significant improvements compared to the diabetic + MI group ($p < 0.05$).

The effect of ferulic acid on fasting blood glucose:

Statistical analysis revealed significant differences between BGL, insulin, and HOMA-IR among the groups using one-way ANOVA at $p < 0.05$. For BGL, the highest mean values were recorded in the diabetic + MI group (10.60 ± 2.04), followed by the diabetic group (7.90 ± 0.52), diabetic + MI + FA (20 mg/kg) group (6.1 ± 0.10), and diabetic + MI + FA (40 mg/kg) group (6.0 ± 0.26), while the lowest value was recorded in the control group (5.13 ± 0.06). Regarding insulin, the highest mean values were recorded in the diabetic + MI group (37.20 ± 2.65), followed by the diabetic + MI + FA (20 mg/kg) group (20.60 ± 2.56), diabetic group (17.20 ± 0.20), and diabetic + MI + FA (40 mg/kg) group (9.47 ± 0.95), while the lowest value was recorded in the control group (4.90 ± 0.26). For HOMA-IR, the same trend as for insulin was found, where the highest mean values were recorded in the diabetic + MI group (17.60 ± 3.99), followed by the diabetic + MI + FA (20 mg/kg) group (6.43 ± 0.91), diabetic + MI + FA (20 mg/kg) group (5.70 ± 0.44), and diabetic + MI + FA (40 mg/kg) group (2.97 ± 0.60), while the lowest value was recorded in the control group (1.77 ± 0.06) (Table 2).

Table 2. The impact of administering ferulic acid at 20 or 40 mg/kg on fasting glucose levels, insulin concentration (unit/L), and insulin resistance in several groups was examined (n = 8 per group).

Groups	BGL (mM/L)	Insulin (μIU/mL)	HOMA-IR Index
Control	5.13 ± 0.06 ^{b}	4.90 ± 0.26 ^{e}	1.77 ± 0.06 ^{c}
Diabetic	7.90 ± 0.52 ^{b}	17.20 ± 0.20 ^{c}	5.70 ± 0.44 ^{bc}
Diabetic + MI	10.60 ± 2.04 ^{a}	37.20 ± 2.65 ^{a}	17.60 ± 3.99 ^{a}
Diabetic + MI + FA (20 mg/kg)	6.1 ± 0.10 ^{b}	20.60 ± 2.65 ^{b}	6.43 ± 0.91 ^{b}
Diabetic + MI + FA (40 mg/kg)	6.00 ± 0.26 ^{b}	9.47 ± 0.95 ^{d}	2.97 ± 0.60 ^{bc}
F test	6.32	155.49	34.16
p-Value 0.05	0.008 **	<0.0001 **	<0.0001 **

** and different superscript letters indicate significant differences at $p < 0.05$.

Data are presented as the mean ± SD and analyzed using a one-way analysis of variance (ANOVA) followed by Bonferroni's post hoc test at a significance level of $p < 0.05$, n = 8. The diabetic + MI group had significantly higher glucose levels compared to the control group ($p < 0.001$). FA treatment at 40 mg/kg significantly reduced glucose levels compared to the diabetic + MI group ($p < 0.05$).

a Compared to control group.

b Compared to diabetic group.

c Compared to diabetic + MI group.

2.2. The Effect of Ferulic Acid on ECG Patterns

After the examination, the control group displayed a standard electrocardiogram (ECG) pattern, which included a normal heart rate (H.R.), R-R interval, S.T. segment amplitude, and T wave amplitude. Both the diabetic group and the diabetic + MI group showed a statistically significant rise in H.R., S.T. segment amplitude, and T wave amplitude and a marked reduction in the R-R interval compared to the control group. Figure 1A,B demonstrate that compared to the control group, the H.R. of the diabetic and diabetic + MI groups increased significantly ($p < 0.001$). Rats administered FA (40 mg/kg), on the other hand, had a significantly lower H.R. than the diabetic and diabetic + MI groups ($p < 0.001$). Compared to a lower dose of FA (20 mg/kg), a higher dose of FA (40 mg/kg) significantly and much more greatly lowered H.R. ($p < 0.05$).

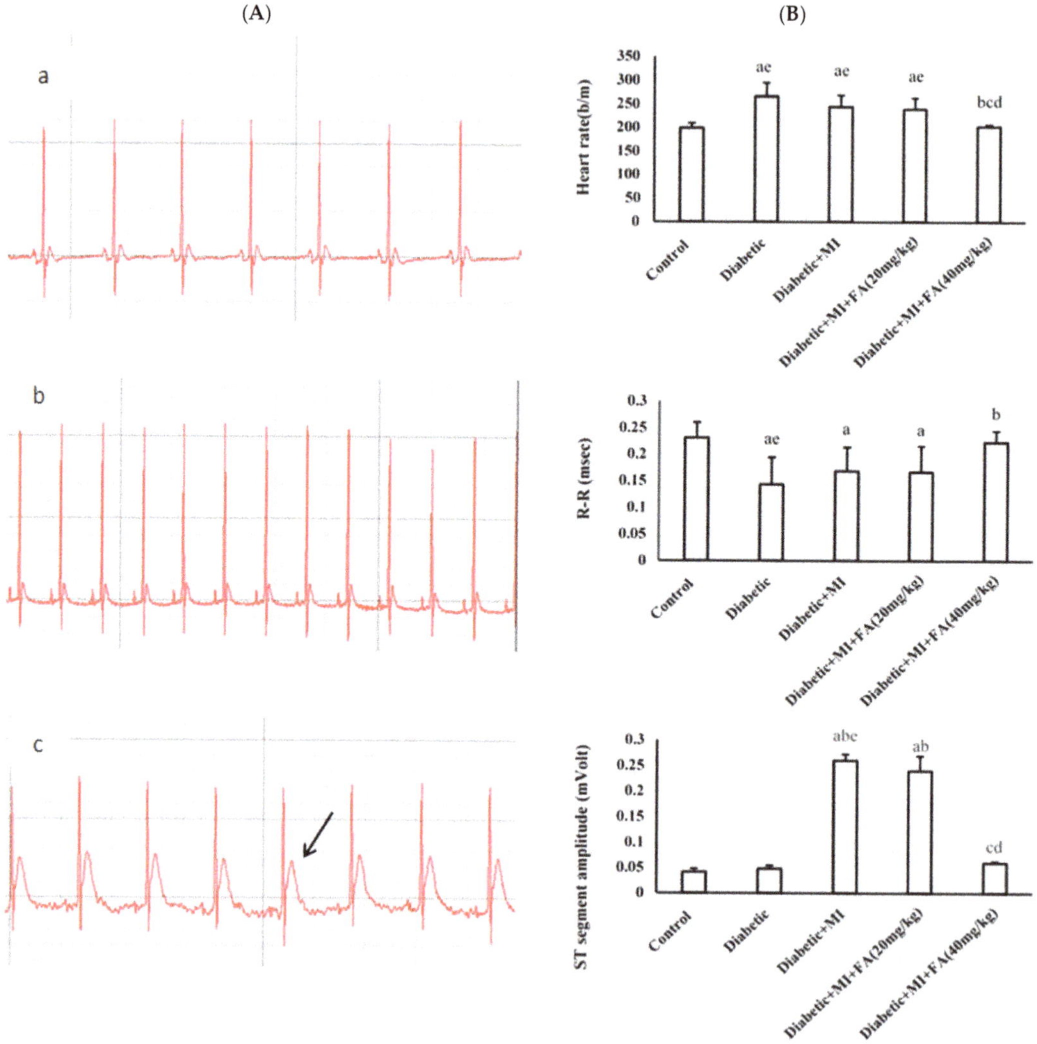

Figure 1. *Cont.*

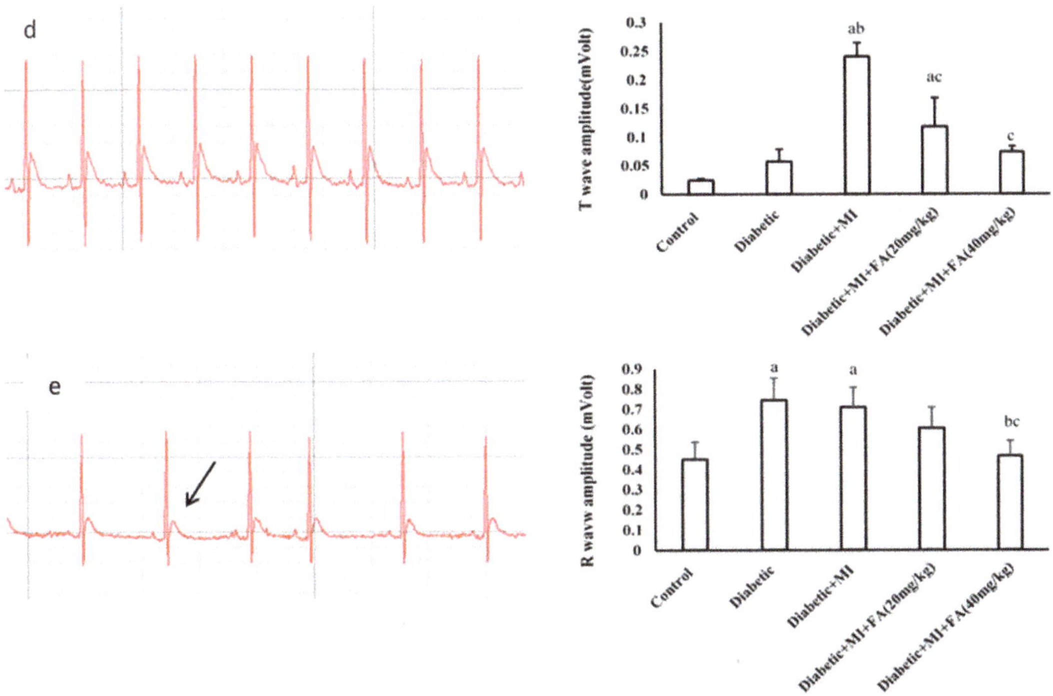

Figure 1. The ECG readings in the various treated groups. (**A**) The electrocardiographic impact of different FA dosages on ISO-induced MI in diabetic rats. (**B**) ECG parameters H.R., R-R interval, S.T. segment amplitude, T wave amplitude, and R wave amplitude in experimental rats pretreated with FA (20, 40 mg/kg) in an ISO-induced MI diabetic paradigm. (**a**) Control group, (**b**) diabetic group, (**c**) diabetic + MI group, (**d**) diabetic + MI + FA 20 mg/kg group, and (**e**) diabetic + MI + FA 40 mg/kg group, arrow shows reduced the T wave amplitude to a considerably greater extent than a lower dose (FA 20 mg/kg). Bars with various letters are significantly different according to Bonferroni's post hoc test at the $p < 0.001$ level (n = 8). Data are expressed as mean ± S.D. ECG: electrocardiogram; FA: ferulic acid; ISO: isoproterenol; MI: myocardial infarction; H.R.: heart rate.

Compared to the control group, the diabetic and diabetic + MI groups exhibited a significant reduction in the R-R interval ($p < 0.001$). When compared to the diabetic group ($p < 0.05$), the R-R interval was considerably enhanced by a larger dose of FA (40 mg/kg) compared to a lower dose of FA (20 mg/kg). This difference was also significant when compared to the diabetic + MI group. The S.T. segment amplitude of the diabetic + MI group was significantly higher than that of the control group ($p < 0.001$) and the diabetic group ($p < 0.001$). Rats administered 40 mg/kg of FA, in contrast to the diabetic + MI and FA (20 mg/kg) groups, exhibited a substantial decrease in the S.T. segment amplitude ($p < 0.001$). The T wave amplitude showed a significant increase in the diabetic + MI group compared to the control and diabetic groups ($p < 0.001$). When compared to the diabetic + MI group, a larger dose of FA (40 mg/kg) significantly reduced the T wave amplitude to a considerably greater extent than a lower dose (FA 20 mg/kg) ($p < 0.001$). The diabetic and diabetic + MI groups had a significantly larger R wave amplitude increase than the control group ($p < 0.001$). The administration of higher dosages of FA (40 mg/kg) resulted in a substantial decrease in the R wave amplitude, particularly when compared to the diabetic and diabetic + MI groups ($p < 0.001$).

2.3. The Effect of Ferulic Acid on Cardiac Enzymes

The administration of isoproterenol to diabetic rats significantly increased cardiac serum C.K., CK-MB, LDH, and cTnI levels compared to the diabetic rats that did not receive treatment and the control group that received the vehicle only. Ferulic acid administration at a dosage of 20 mg/kg did not result in noteworthy decreases in serum cardiac enzymes when compared to the group with both diabetes and myocardial infarction. However, the administration of a higher dosage of ferulic acid at 40 mg/kg led to a significant reduction ($p < 0.05$, as shown in Figure 2) in the levels of serum cardiac enzymes (C.K., CK-MB, LDH, and cTnI) when compared to the group with both diabetes and myocardial infarction.

2.4. Histopathological Examinations of the Cardiac Tissues in the Experimental Groups

The histological analysis of the cardiac tissues using hematoxylin and eosin (H&E) staining demonstrated that the control group had a typical arrangement of myocardial fibers with clear striations and no noticeable signs of degenerative alterations. The evaluation of myocardial tissue in the diabetic group showed that about 75% of cardiac tissue showed evidence of injury: edema (black arrow), splitting of myofibers, and mononuclear cell infiltrate (red arrow) (H&E, 10×). Also, its higher magnification picture shows myocyte edema (black arrow), mononuclear cell infiltrate (red arrow), and necrotic myocytes (black arrowhead) (H&E, 40×). However, about 75% of cardiac tissue in the diabetic + MI group showed evidence of injury: marked edema (black arrow), splitting of myofibers, and mononuclear cell infiltrate (red arrow) (H&E, 10×). The higher magnification shows myocyte edema (black arrow), mononuclear cell infiltrate (red arrow), necrotic myocytes (black arrowhead), and areas of hemorrhage (red arrowhead) (H&E, 40×). Regarding the diabetic + MI + FA (20 mg/kg) group, there was some reduction in the extent of injury in cardiac tissue, with a slight decrease in myocyte edema (black arrow) and mononuclear cell infiltrate (red arrow) (H&E, 10×). The higher magnification shows myocyte edema (black arrow), mononuclear cell infiltrate (red arrow), and necrotic myocytes (black arrowhead) (H&E, 40×). Administration of a greater dose of FA (40 mg/kg) resulted in a significant reduction in the extent of injury in cardiac tissue, with a marked decrease in myocyte edema (black arrow) and mononuclear cell infiltrate (red arrow) (H&E, 10×). Additionally, the higher magnification shows slight myocyte edema (black arrow), mononuclear cell infiltrate (red arrow), and no necrotic myocytes (H&E, 40×) (Figure 3).

2.5. The Effect of Treatment with Various Doses of Ferulic Acid (20 or 40 mg/kg) on Cardiac TNF-α as an Inflammatory Marker

Statistical analysis showed significant differences between groups for TNF-α using one-way ANOVA at $p < 0.05$ ($p < 0.001$). The highest mean values were recorded in the diabetic + MI group (79.87 ± 4.30), followed by the diabetic group (59.33 ± 2.53) and diabetic + MI + FA (20 mg/kg) group (40.55 ± 1.44), while the control group (26.10 ± 16.80) and diabetic + MI + FA (40 mg/kg) group (26.13 ± 2.25) had the lowest values (Figure 4A).

2.6. The Effect of Treatment with Diverse Doses of Ferulic Acid (20 or 40 mg/kg) on Cardiac MDA as an Oxidative Marker

Statistical analysis revealed notable differences in MDA levels among the groups, as determined by one-way ANOVA with a significance level of $p < 0.05$ ($p < 0.001$). The highest mean values were recorded in the diabetic + MI group (38.17 ± 3.55), followed by the diabetic group (25.67 ± 2.35) and diabetic + MI + FA (20 mg/kg) group (18.90 ± 1.30), while the control group (9.50 ± 0.02) and diabetic + MI + FA (40 mg/kg) group (13.57 ± 1.00) had the lowest values (Figure 4B).

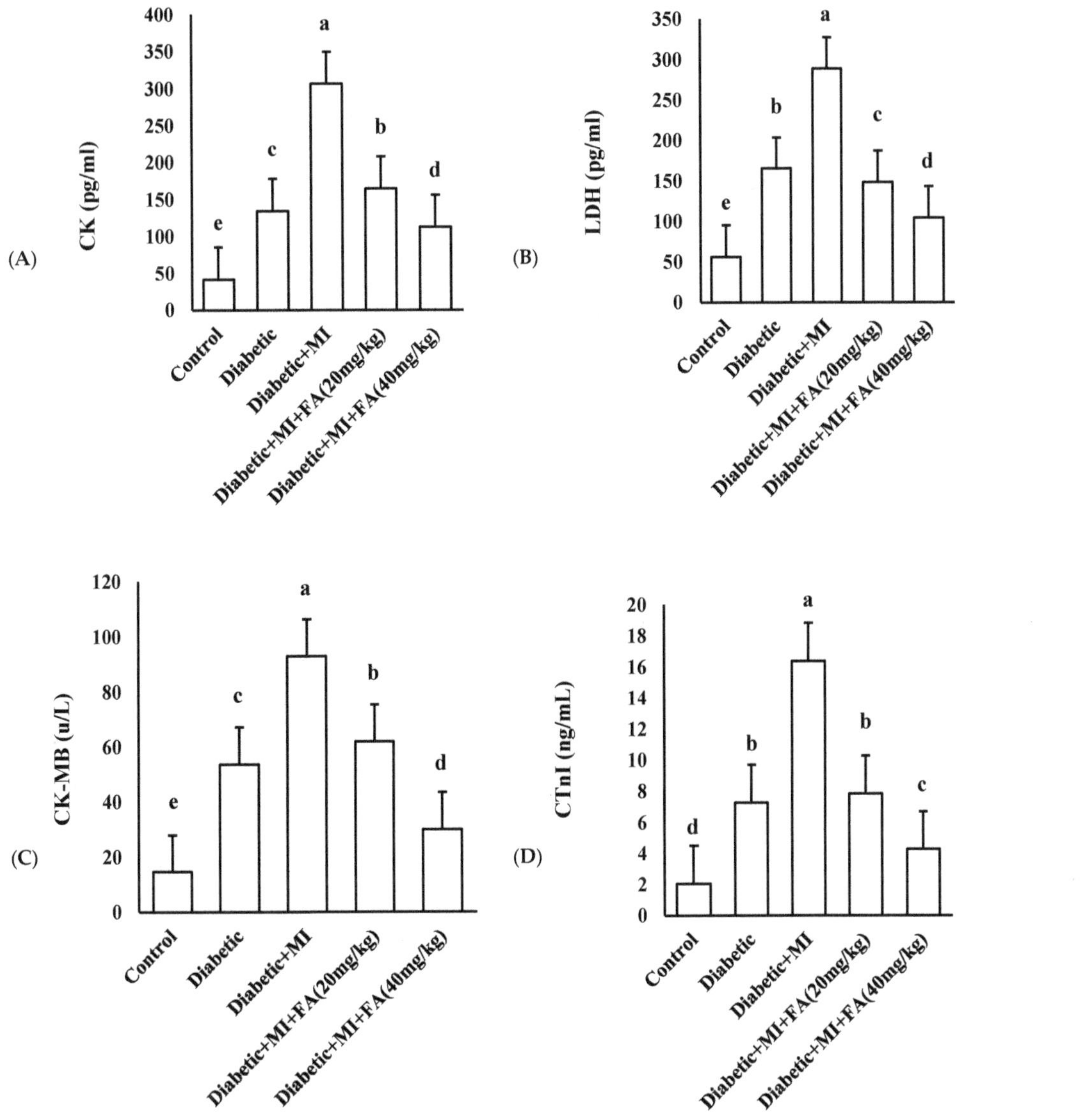

Figure 2. Serum levels of cardiac enzymes in the various groups. (**A**) CK, (**B**) LDH, (**C**) CK-MB, (**D**) CTnI. Data are presented as mean ± SD and analyzed using one-way ANOVA followed by Bonferroni's post hoc test at $p < 0.05$, n = 8. Bars with different letters are significantly different according to Bonferroni's post hoc test at a significance level of $p < 0.05$.

2.7. Effect of Treatment with Diverse Doses of Ferulic Acid (20 or 40 mg/kg) on Cardiac AGE–RAGE by PCR

Statistical analysis indicated a significant difference among the groups for AGEs and RAGE, as assessed by one-way ANOVA at $p < 0.05$ ($p < 0.001$). For AGEs, the highest mean values were recorded in the diabetic + MI group, diabetic + MI + FA (20 mg/kg) group, diabetic group, and diabetic + MI + FA (40 mg/kg) group, with values of 2.88 ± 0.07, 2.24 ± 0.12, 1.87 ± 0.15, and 1.66 ± 0.05, respectively, while the control group had the lowest value (0.80 ± 0.02). With regard to RAGE, the highest mean values were recorded in the diabetic + MI group (2.72 ± 0.10), followed by the diabetic + MI + FA (20 mg/kg) group (2.03 ± 0.15), diabetic group (1.62 ± 0.11), and diabetic + MI + FA (40 mg/kg) group (1.51 ± 0.09), while the control group had the lowest value (0.60 ± 0.01) (Figure 5).

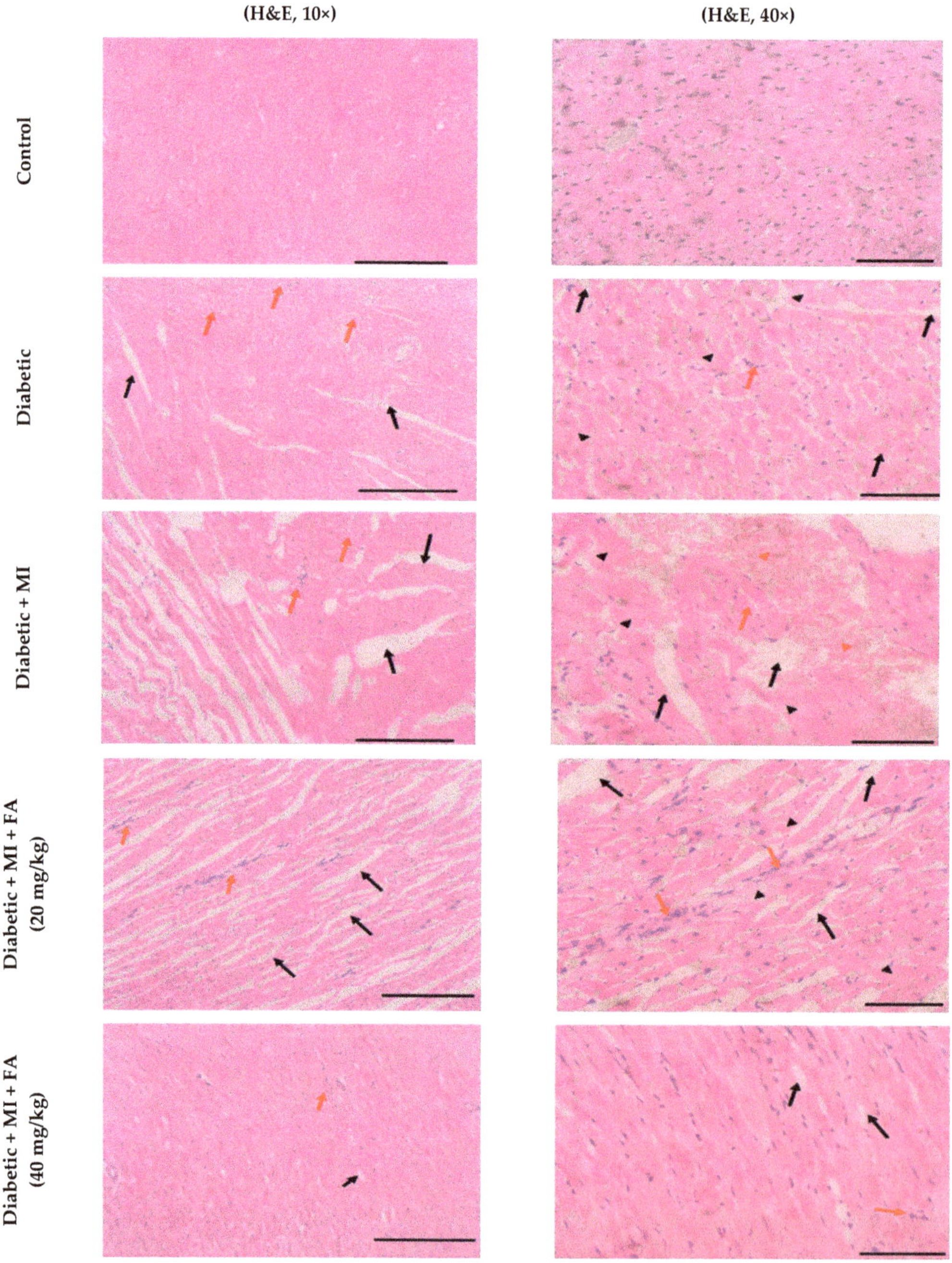

Figure 3. Histopathology images of hematoxylin and eosin-stained sections from the hearts of the experimental groups (×10 and ×40). MI: myocardial infarction. FA: ferulic acid. Black arrows indicate myocyte edema, and red arrows indicate mononuclear cell infiltration. Arrowhead indicate

necrotic myocytes with no detected nuclei. Control group: The section from the hearts of rats treated with saline (vehicle) has a typical and healthy appearance. Diabetic group: The images indicate histological alterations of a moderate degree. Diabetic + MI group: The images indicate a rise in the quantity of neutrophils and a decline in the size and condensation of nuclei. Additionally, the tissue exhibits a loss of striations, and the sarcoplasm displays a heavily eosinophilic appearance. The diabetic + MI + FA (20 mg/kg) group exhibits histopathological changes of moderate severity. The diabetic + MI + FA (40 mg/kg) group exhibits slight histological alterations.

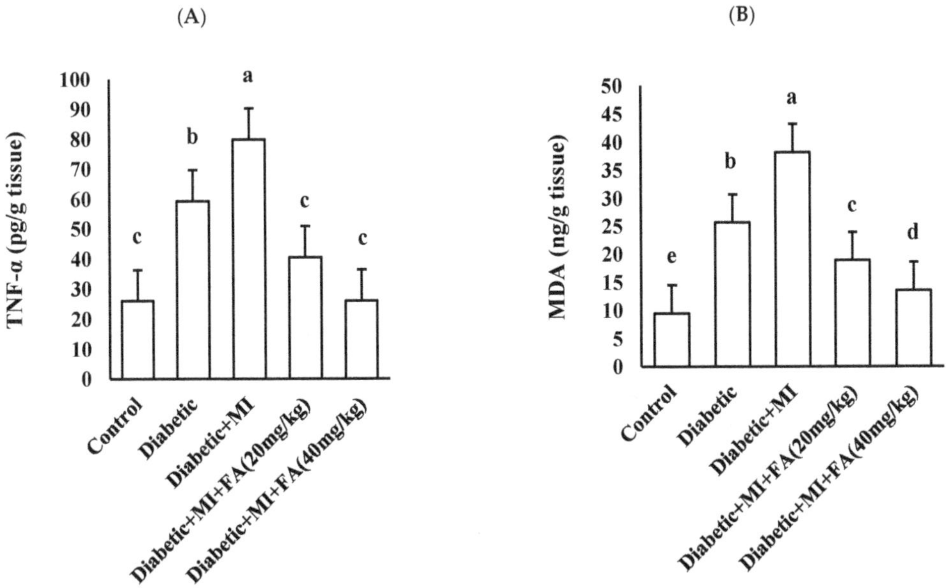

Figure 4. (**A**) Cardiac TNF-α and (**B**) cardiac MDA in different groups. Data are expressed as mean ± SD and analyzed using one-way ANOVA, n = 8. Bars with different letters are significantly different according to Bonferroni's post hoc test at a significance level of $p < 0.05$.

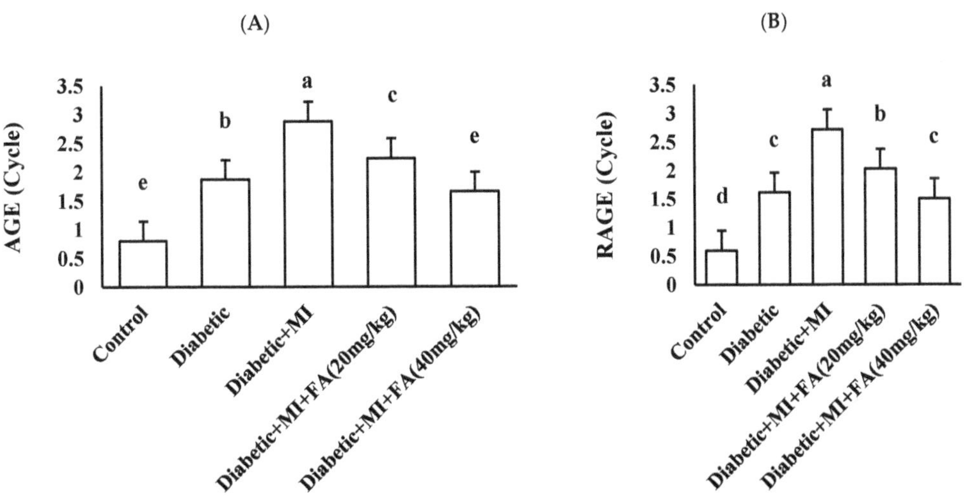

Figure 5. (**A**) Cardiac AGEs and (**B**) cardiac RAGE in different groups. Data are expressed as mean ± SD and analyzed using one-way ANOVA, n = 8. Bars with different letters are significantly different according to Bonferroni's post hoc test at a significance level of $p < 0.05$.

3. Discussion

The valuable outcomes of ferulic acid (FA) were evaluated against ISO-induced myocardial infarction (MI) in a diabetic rat model to determine whether these effects involve inhibiting the AGE–RAGE pathway. Induction of MI in diabetic rats resulted in various alterations in the electrocardiogram (ECG) patterns and histopathological characteristics of the heart, along with increased serum concentrations of insulin and cardiac enzymes and high levels of AGE and RAGE mRNA expression. The use of ISO to induce MI in diabetic rats is highly relevant to clinical comorbid conditions such as diabetic cardiomyopathy and stress-induced cardiac events. Diabetic patients often experience heightened sympathetic activity, which can exacerbate cardiac injury. The ISO model mimics this heightened sympathetic tone and oxidative stress, providing a valuable tool to study the effects of FA in a clinically relevant setting. Our findings demonstrate that FA mitigates ISO-induced cardiac injury, suggesting its potential to protect against stress-induced MI in diabetic patients. The present findings indicate that individuals diagnosed with type 2 diabetes face a heightened susceptibility to cardiovascular events than those without diabetes [29]. Isoproterenol (ISO) is a synthetic catecholamine molecule that is an agonist for β-adrenergic receptors. The administration of ISO through subcutaneous injection in rats results in permanent cellular damage and ultimately leads to MI [30].

Advanced glycation end products (AGEs) are a diverse group of chemicals that arise from the irreversible, nonenzymatic reactions between reducing sugars and various biomolecules, including lipids, proteins, or nucleic acids [31]. Also, AGEs can originate from external sources, such as food, or be internally produced within the body [32]. Vascular problems, particularly microvascular and cardiovascular complications, are the main causes of death and morbidity in people with diabetes [33]. AGEs can engage with their receptor (RAGE), resulting in a range of harmful consequences such as oxidative stress, apoptosis, inflammation, and the formation of what is commonly referred to as "hyperglycemia memory" [34]. The glycation and oxidative stress processes are closely interconnected, often called glycoxidation. It has been discovered that AGEs impair the activity of antioxidant systems and increase the formation of reactive oxygen species (ROS). However, it is important to highlight that some AGEs are naturally formed in oxidative conditions [35].

Based on the information presented in [36]'s model, the involvement of AGEs in different diabetic complications can be classified into two primary pathways. The first pathway involves a receptor-mediated signaling cascade, which entails the interaction between AGEs and the cell surface receptor for AGEs (RAGE). On the other hand, the second pathway involves extracellular matrix impairment caused by the cross-linking properties of AGEs.

Natural products are valuable sources of inhibitors that prevent the production of advanced glycation end products (AGEs). These inhibitors provide the benefits of being highly safe and having low toxicity levels. Recent research has demonstrated that phenolic acids and flavonoids derived from plants are potent glycation inhibitors [37]. Ferulic acid (FA) can mitigate the inflammatory response caused by AGEs by inhibiting the activation of the NF-κB and p38 MAPK signaling pathways [38]. The present findings align with previous reports indicating that FA can prevent and alleviate the progression of MI in individuals with diabetes.

Effective management of diabetes and monitoring of the glycemic index are necessary to prevent associated complications. As a result of hyperglycemia, excessive generation of free radicals occurred, subsequently inducing oxidative stress [39]. This study's findings revealed that delivering FA resulted in a reduction in blood glucose levels and insulin levels in diabetic rats in comparison to the control group. The observed outcome revealed a dependence on the dosage administered. The data presented align with a previous report by [40], which showed that FA therapy decreased blood glucose levels. In addition, the research conducted by [41] showed that FA treatment enhanced antioxidant capacity and reduced levels of reactive oxygen species (ROS). The intervention with FA demonstrated significant enhancements in blood glucose levels and improvements in insulin secretion and sensitivity. ROS and nitrogen–oxygen species can damage cellular constituents such as proteins, DNA, unsaturated fatty acids, and cell membranes [42]. According to [43], it was observed that ROS led to an elevation in protein glycation and the formation of AGEs.

The present study observed a decrease in serum MDA levels in MI-induced diabetic rats administered FA, which aligns with prior research indicating that low doses of FA can enhance the functioning of antioxidant enzymes. This enhancement leads to the scavenging of free radicals, recognized as the primary contributors to tissue damage [39]. The research conducted by [44] demonstrated that FA exhibited a protective effect against oxidative stress and photoaging. Also, Jung et al. [40] found that FA had hypoglycemic, hypolipidemic, and anti-inflammatory properties.

Furthermore, compared to the control group that did not receive any therapy, the group that received FA observed a decrease in the production of inflammatory markers, including IL-1β and TNFα. The anti-inflammatory impact of FA is explained by its ability to bind to AGEs and block their receptor (RAGE). This binding reduces pro-inflammatory cytokine production and prevents diabetic MI [18]. In line with the production of AGEs, it was shown that ISO-induced diabetic rats had a considerably higher expression of RAGE. However, this increase in RAGE expression was observed to be effectively blocked with the administration of FA.

According to earlier research, the delivery of an ISO injection causes a considerable rise in heart weight, heart rate, electrocardiographic changes, and cardiac marker enzyme levels (CK-MB, LDH), which provides strong evidence of the acute cardiotoxic effects of ISO injection [45]. According to the results of the present study, administering diabetic rats an ISO injection increased their heart weight, which in turn increased their heart weight-to-body weight ratio. There are several potential causes for the expansion of the heart's intravascular space and weight, including increased protein and water contents [46]. The ISO-treated rats exhibited a higher level of various cytokines, namely TNF-α, IL-1β, and IL-6. It is known that cardiac toxicity is associated with higher levels of these cytokines [47]. TNF-α, IL-6, and IL-1β levels were significantly reduced in the rats that received FA treatment. Nevertheless, diabetic rats were significantly protected against the harmful effects of the ISO injection when pretreated with a greater dosage of FA.

Changes in the electrocardiogram (ECG) pattern have been identified as a dependable indicator of MI [9]. ECG abnormalities were observed in the group that received an ISO injection. These anomalies suggest an increase in the S.T. segment, a sign of myocardial ischemia [48]. Nevertheless, these alterations were reversed following the administration of FA in rats. This research shows that FA positively affects the electrical waveforms of rats' hearts, which may indicate a protective effect.

The enzymes C.K., CK-MB, LDH, and CTnI are regarded as cardiac markers [49] and are therefore utilized as diagnostic markers for cellular injury. These enzymes most likely enter the circulation when myocytes sustain an injury that causes their cell membranes to burst or become more porous. Damaged myocytes are the main cause of these cardiac enzymes' high levels [50]. Our investigation found that C.K., CK-MB, LDH, and CTnI levels were significantly elevated, but these cardiac marker enzyme levels were successfully restored after FA treatment. FA administered at a modest dose of 20 mg/kg exhibited a minimal inhibitory impact on cardiac marker enzyme levels; however, when administered at 40 mg/kg, FA revealed notable and major suppression. The release of enzymes that indicate cellular damage from cardiac cells may be prevented by returning biochemical parameters to their normal levels. Therefore, FA contributes significantly to the avoidance of metabolic changes in MI.

The histopathological analysis demonstrated that the administration of ISO in diabetic rats resulted in cellular structural and architectural damage, along with an escalation in the presence of neutrophils and swelling in the heart tissue, as previously documented by [51]. In contrast, administration of FA at the full dosage level led to decreased inflammatory lesions, accompanied by edema and a remarkable reduction in the extent of neutrophil infiltration. The research findings showed that the injection of FA effectively alleviated the harmful effects of ISO in diabetic rats. The results of this research provide credence to the idea that FA may protect the heart by lowering levels of oxidative stress. The restoration of normal biochemical indicators, the normalization of histopathological damage, and the reduction in oxidative stress reveal the powerful antioxidant effect of ferulic acid.

While the current study evaluated two concentrations of ferulic acid (20 mg/kg and 40 mg/kg), future studies should include a broader range of doses to establish a more comprehensive dose–response relationship. Also, future studies should investigate FA discontinuation before MI induction and its potential impact on the findings. This would help to identify the optimal therapeutic dose and further validate the dose-dependent cardioprotective effects of FA.

4. Materials and Methods

4.1. Experimental Animals

Forty male Wistar albino rats (75 days old), with an average weight of 150 ± 20 gm, were acquired from Vacsera, which specializes in biological goods and vaccinations (Vacsera, Egypt). The rats were kept in standard housing with unrestricted access to tap water and standard rat chow food. Other standard circumstances included regular light and dark cycles, a relative humidity of 55%, and a temperature of 25 ± 3 °C. Each group had eight animals. The Suez Canal University Faculty of Pharmacy's Animal Care Committee approved all the experimental procedures (Ethical Number: 202205MA1).

4.2. Chemicals and Drugs

Streptozotocin (STZ) was obtained from Sigma-Aldrich (Munich, Germany) and freshly prepared using citrate buffer (0.1 M, pH = 4.5). Isoproterenol hydrochloride (ISO) was acquired from Sigma-Aldrich (Germany) and dissolved in a sterile saline solution. Ferulic acid (FA) was obtained from Career Henan Chemical Co., located in Zhengzhou, Henan Province, China. FA was suspended in a 0.2% carboxymethyl cellulose (CMC) aqueous solution. Ketamine hydrochloride was purchased from Egyptian International Pharmaceuticals Industries Company (EIPICO) (Cairo, Egypt), and xylazine hydrochloride was purchased from Adwia Pharmaceutical Company (Cairo, Egypt).

4.3. Induction of Type 2 Diabetes and Acute Myocardial Infarction

The rats were fed a diet high in fat for four weeks. After four weeks, the rats were fasted overnight and injected with freshly prepared streptozotocin at a dosage of 30 mg/kg, i.p. in a volume of 1 mL/kg [52]. Rats were fasted overnight (approximately 12 h) prior to STZ administration to ensure consistent fasting conditions across all animals. This fasting period aligns with the natural feeding cycle of rats, as they are nocturnal feeders and typically consume most of their food during the dark phase. Water was provided ad libitum during the fasting period to prevent dehydration. While the high-fat diet (HFD) was used to induce insulin resistance in the rats, glucose levels were not measured after the 4 weeks of HFD due to the focus of the study on the cardioprotective effects of ferulic acid in diabetic rats with isoproterenol-induced myocardial infarction. Diabetes was confirmed seven days after STZ administration by measuring fasting blood glucose levels, with levels exceeding 135 mg/dL considered indicative of diabetes. The blood glucose levels of each rat were measured using the One-Touch Ultra Mini glucometer seven days after STZ administration (USA). Rats with fasting blood glucose levels $\geq$ 135 mg/dL were considered diabetic, consistent with established protocols for STZ-induced type 2 diabetes models. This threshold reflects early-stage diabetes and aligns with clinical criteria for hyperglycemia in humans [5,9]. A dose of 50 mg/kg ISO was selected based on its ability to induce reproducible cardiac injury without excessive mortality. This dose is widely used in diabetic models to study the exacerbation of cardiac dysfunction due to heightened sympathetic activity [7,11]. The rationale behind this design was to evaluate the lasting effects of FA treatment after cessation, rather than its acute effects during the MI phase.

4.4. Experimental Design

For this investigation, 40 rats were randomly divided into five groups, with 8 in each group.

Group I (Control): Rats were given a regular, enjoyable diet. At the end of week 4, they were injected with citrate buffer (1 mL/kg, i.p.) as a control for STZ. In the tenth week, they received two doses of saline, the vehicle for isoproterenol.

Group II (Diabetic): Rats were administered a high-fat diet (HFD) for four weeks, after which they were given STZ at a specific dosage (30 mg/kg); then, rats were given two consecutive doses of saline, which served as the vehicle for isoproterenol at the tenth week.

Group III (Diabetic + MI): High-fat diet and STZ-induced diabetic rats were injected with two sequential subcutaneous dosages of isoproterenol (50 mg/kg/day) at the beginning of the tenth week.

Group IV (Diabetic + MI + low-dose FA): Rats received ferulic acid (20 mg/kg/day, P.O.).

Group V (Diabetic + MI + high-dose FA): Rats received ferulic acid (40 mg/kg/day, P.O.).

FA treatment (20 or 40 mg/kg/day) was initiated immediately after diabetes confirmation (week 4) and continued for 4 weeks until week 8. Isoproterenol (ISO, 50 mg/kg/day) was administered subcutaneously for two consecutive days at the beginning of week 10 to induce myocardial infarction (MI) [53].

4.5. Electrophysiology

Twenty-four hours after administering the second dosage of isoproterenol hydrochloride, the ECG was recorded from lead II for 2 min for each rat using the research Biopac Data Acquisition mp150 machine, ECG100 (BIOPAC system). The rats were administered thiopental sodium (20 mg/kg, I.P.) to induce anesthesia. Afterward, they were fastened to a board with adhesive tape to immobilize their legs, and the needle electrodes were inserted subcutaneously for the limb leads. The ground electrode was placed on the right leg. The negative (−ve) electrode was placed on the right arm. At the same time, the positive (+ve) electrode was placed on the left leg. The assessed ECG characteristics were heart rate (H.R.), R-R interval, S.T. segment amplitude, and T wave amplitude.

Blood Sampling

After the ECG recording, each rat had a 2 mL blood sample taken from its orbital vein for biochemical analysis. Immediate centrifugation at 2000$\times$ *g* for 15 min was performed on the blood samples following collection. The serum was chilled to −80 °C after separation until it was needed for various tests.

4.6. Processing of the Heart

At the termination of the research protocol, a surgical cut was performed in the abdomen, and the atria and great vessels were separated. Afterward, the hearts were extracted and washed using ice-cold phosphate-buffered saline. The hearts and left ventricles (LVs) were weighed to assess cardiac hypertrophy, and the ratio to body weight was estimated. Each ventricular myocardium was then separated into two distinct portions: The initial portion was reserved for the following biochemical assessments, while the second portion was subjected to overnight fixation at a concentration of 4% paraformaldehyde, followed by embedding in paraffin. The paraffin-embedded tissues were cut into sections with a thickness of 4 μm at the heart apex. These sections were then allowed to dry overnight at 37 °C. The sections were then treated to remove paraffin, rehydrated, and made ready for standard histological staining using hematoxylin and eosin (H&E).

4.7. Determination of Serum Cardiac Biomarkers

The measurement of blood cardiac enzymes was performed with pre-existing serum samples. The enzymatic kit developed by [54] was used to evaluate the activity of serum lactate dehydrogenase (LDH). The creatine phosphokinase (C.K.) activity was measured using a previously established technique [50]. An enzymatic approach was used to measure the activity of cardiac troponin I (cTnI) and serum creatine kinase-MB isoenzyme (CK-MB) [55]. An ultraviolet–visible spectrophotometer (UV-1601PC, Shimadzu, Tokyo, Japan) and commercial kits from Stanbio (Boerne, TX, USA) were used for all prior procedures.

4.8. Determination of TNF-α and MDA

After homogenizing, the cardiac samples were placed into the kits for the enzyme-linked immunosorbent assay (ELISA) for measuring malondialdehyde (MDA) and tumor necrosis factor-alpha (TNF-α). The assays were carried out using an automated ELISA reader (MyBioSource, San Diego, CA, USA) following the company's specifications. The samples were measured twice, and the mean was used to represent them.

4.9. Histopathological Examination of Heart Tissues

A pathologist who was not informed of the therapy conducted a histopathological evaluation using a light microscope. The heart portions were analyzed as previously reported [56]. Grades 1, 2, 3, and 4 were assigned to the histological changes, signifying mild, moderate, high, and intensive pathological abnormalities, respectively.

The histopathological evaluation focused on identifying and grading the following pathological abnormalities: myocyte edema, mononuclear cell infiltration, necrotic myocytes, splitting of myofibers, areas of hemorrhage, loss of striations, and eosinophilic appearance of the sarcoplasm. These abnormalities were graded on a scale of 1 to 4, where Grade 1 signifies mild pathological changes, Grade 2 signifies moderate pathological changes, Grade 3 signifies high pathological changes, and Grade 4 signifies intensive pathological changes.

4.10. Determination of AGEs and RAGE by Quantitative Real-Time PCR Analysis Using Heart Tissue

The expression of advanced glycation end products (AGEs) and their receptor (RAGE) in heart tissue was quantified using a real-time polymerase chain reaction (PCR). Total RNA was extracted from heart tissue samples using a standard RNA isolation kit. cDNA synthesis was performed using reverse transcription, followed by amplification using the GoTaq® 1-Step RT-qPCR System (https://worldwide.promega.com/products/pcr/qpcr-and-rt-qpcr/qpcr-kits/?tabset0=0&catNum=A6001 (accessed on 4 December 2024)). The following primer sequences were used for amplification:

- AGEs: Forward: GCT CTG ATA TCG GTG ACC CT; Reverse: TCG TAG TTG TGG TGG TCG AT.
- RAGE: Forward: GGA CAG TGT GGC TCG AAT CC; Reverse: CAA TTC CGA TAG CTG GAA GGA.
- β-actin (internal control): Forward: ACC CTA AGG CCA ACC GTG AA; Reverse: ACA GCC TGG ATG GCT ACG TAC A.

The PCR conditions included an initial reverse transcription step at 37 °C, followed by amplification cycles. The relative expression levels of AGEs and RAGE were normalized to β-actin and calculated using the $2^{(-\Delta\Delta Ct)}$ method. All reactions were performed in triplicate to ensure reproducibility.

Statistical Analysis

The data are presented as the mean values and the mean and standard deviation (S.D.). The results were evaluated using a one-way repeated measures analysis of variance (ANOVA), and pairwise comparisons were performed between all experimental groups using Bonferroni's post hoc test to identify significant differences in key parameters, including body weight, glucose levels, cardiac enzymes, and inflammatory markers. The non-parametric data underwent analysis using the Kruskal–Wallis analysis of variance (ANOVA) method. The data were analyzed using the Statistical Package for the Social Sciences, version 25 (SPSS Software, SPSS Inc., Chicago, IL, USA). For mean differences, statistical significance was established at a significance level of $p < 0.05$.

5. Conclusions

This study demonstrates that ferulic acid (FA) exhibits promising cardioprotective effects in a diabetic rat model of isoproterenol-induced myocardial infarction (MI). The observed improvements in cardiac structure and function, the normalization of serum cardiac enzymes, and the reduction in blood glucose and insulin levels suggest that FA may play a beneficial role in mitigating diabetic cardiovascular complications. Additionally, FA treatment reduced the expression of pro-inflammatory cytokines and suppressed the upregulation of advanced glycation end products (AGEs) and their receptor (RAGE), indicating its potential to attenuate the inflammatory and oxidative stress pathways associated with diabetic MI.

However, it is important to note that these findings are based on a preclinical animal model, and further research is needed to confirm the efficacy and safety of FA in human studies. Future investigations should focus on elucidating the molecular mechanisms underlying FA's cardioprotective effects and evaluating its long-term benefits in clinical settings. While our results are encouraging, they should be interpreted with caution, and FA should not yet be considered a definitive therapeutic option without further validation.

Author Contributions: Conceptualization, E.K., E.-S.E.E.-A. and D.M.K.; data curation, S.O.B.; formal analysis, S.O.B., E.K., M.A.A., A.A. and D.M.K.; investigation, E.K., E.-S.E.E.-A., M.A.A. and D.M.K.; methodology, S.O.B., M.A.A., A.A. and D.M.K.; project administration, D.M.K.; resources, E.-S.E.E.-A., M.A.A. and D.M.K.; software, S.O.B., M.A.A. and A.A.; supervision, E.K., E.-S.E.E.-A., A.A. and D.M.K.; validation, S.O.B., E.K., E.-S.E.E.-A., M.A.A., A.A. and D.M.K.; writing—original draft, S.O.B., E.K., E.-S.E.E.-A., M.A.A., A.A. and D.M.K.; writing—review and editing, S.O.B., E.K., E.-S.E.E.-A., M.A.A., A.A. and D.M.K. All authors have read and agreed to the published version of the manuscript.

Funding: This research received no external funding.

Institutional Review Board Statement: Not applicable.

Informed Consent Statement: Not applicable.

Data Availability Statement: The original contributions presented in this study are included in the article. Further inquiries can be directed to the corresponding author.

Acknowledgments: We want to thanks Princess Nourah bint Abdulrahman University Researchers Supporting Project number (PNURSP2025R227), Princess Nourah bint Abdulrahman University, Riyadh, Saudi Arabia. Also the authors extend their appreciation to Taif University, Saudi Arabia, for supporting this work through project number (TU-DSPP-2024-119).

Conflicts of Interest: The authors declare no conflicts of interest.

References

1. Khodeer, D.M. Beyond Glycemic Control: Cardiovascular, Renal, and Hepatic Benefits of GLP-1 Receptor Agonists. *Spectr. Sci. J.* **2024**, *1*, 15–26. [CrossRef]
2. Eltamany, E.E.; Nafie, M.S.; Khodeer, D.M.; El-Tanahy, A.H.H.; Abdel-Kader, M.S.; Badr, J.M.; Abdelhameed, R.F.A. Rubia Tinctorum Root Extracts: Chemical Profile and Management of Type II Diabetes Mellitus. *RSC Adv.* **2020**, *10*, 24159–24168. [CrossRef]
3. Al Hroob, A.M.; Abukhalil, M.H.; Hussein, O.E.; Mahmoud, A.M. Pathophysiological Mechanisms of Diabetic Cardiomyopathy and the Therapeutic Potential of Epigallocatechin-3-Gallate. *Biomed. Pharmacother.* **2019**, *109*, 2155–2172. [CrossRef] [PubMed]
4. Williams, R.; Colagiuri, S.; Chan, J.; Gregg, E.; Ke, C.; Lim, L.-L.; Yang, X. *IDF Atlas 9th Edition 2019*; IDF: Brussels, Belgium, 2019; ISBN 978-2-930229-87-4. Available online: https://diabetesatlas.org/upload/resources/material/20200302_133351_IDFATLAS9e-final-web.pdf (accessed on 4 December 2024).
5. Buettner, R.; Schunter, M. Efficient Machine Learning Based Detection of Heart Disease. In Proceedings of the 2019 IEEE International Conference on E-health Networking, Application & Services HealthCom, Bogota, Colombia, 14–16 October 2019; pp. 1–6. [CrossRef]
6. Abdelaziz, A.S.; Kamel, M.A.; Ahmed, A.I.; Shalaby, S.I.; El-Darier, S.M.; Beshbishy, A.M.; Batiha, G.E.-S.; Alomar, S.Y.; Khodeer, D.M. Chemotherapeutic Potential of Epimedium Brevicornum Extract: The CGMP-Specific Pde5 Inhibitor as Anti-Infertility Agent Following Long-Term Administration of Tramadol in Male Rats. *Antibiotics* **2020**, *9*, 318. [CrossRef] [PubMed]
7. Shin, S.Y.; Lee, J.; Park, J.; Lee, Y.; Ahn, S.; Lee, J.H.; Koh, D.; Lee, Y.H.; Lim, Y. Design, Synthesis, and Biological Activities of 1-Aryl-(3-(2-Styryl)Phenyl)Prop-2-En-1-Ones. *Bioorg. Chem.* **2019**, *83*, 438–449. [CrossRef]
8. Khodeer, D.M.; Bilasy, S.E.; Farag, N.E.; Mehana, A.E.; Elbaz, A.A. Sitagliptin Protects Diabetic Rats with Acute Myocardial Infarction through Induction of Angiogenesis: Role of IGF-1 and VEGF. *Can. J. Physiol. Pharmacol.* **2019**, *97*, 1053–1063. [CrossRef]
9. Anderson, J.L.; Morrow, D.A. Acute Myocardial Infarction. *N. Engl. J. Med.* **2017**, *376*, 2053–2064. [CrossRef]
10. Khodeer, D.M.; Nasr, A.M.; Swidan, S.A.; Shabayek, S.; Khinkar, R.M.; Aldurdunji, M.M.; Ramadan, M.A.; Badr, J.M. Characterization, Antibacterial, Antioxidant, Antidiabetic, and Anti-Inflammatory Activities of Green Synthesized Silver Nanoparticles Using *Phragmanthera austroarabica* A.G. Mill and J.A. Nyberg Extract. *Front. Microbiol.* **2023**, *13*, 1078061. [CrossRef]
11. Benetos, A.; Petrovic, M.; Strandberg, T. Hypertension Management in Older and Frail Older Patients. *Circ. Res.* **2019**, *124*, 1045–1060. [CrossRef]
12. Anderson, E.J.; Kypson, A.P.; Rodriguez, E.; Anderson, C.A.; Lehr, E.J.; Neufer, P.D. Substrate-Specific Derangements in Mitochondrial Metabolism and Redox Balance in the Atrium of the Type 2 Diabetic Human Heart. *J. Am. Coll. Cardiol.* **2009**, *54*, 1891–1898. [CrossRef]
13. Elkelish, A. New Plant Extracts toward Multidrug Resistance: The Convergence of Nanotechnology and Nanoscience. *Spectr. Sci. J.* **2024**, *1*, 396119. [CrossRef]
14. Sharma, M.; Kishore, K.; Gupta, S.K.; Joshi, S.; Arya, D.S. Cardioprotective Potential of Ocimum Sanctum in Isoproterenol Induced Myocardial Infarction in Rats. *Mol. Cell. Biochem.* **2001**, *225*, 75–83. [CrossRef] [PubMed]
15. Aihara, M.; Dobashi, K.; Iizuka, K.; Nakazawa, T.; Mori, M. Comparison of Effects of Y-27632 and Isoproterenol on Release of Cytokines from Human Peripheral T Cells. *Int. Immunopharmacol.* **2003**, *3*, 1619–1625. [CrossRef] [PubMed]
16. Silván, J.M.; Assar, S.H.; Srey, C.; Dolores del Castillo, M.; Ames, J.M. Control of the Maillard Reaction by Ferulic Acid. *Food Chem.* **2011**, *128*, 208–213. [CrossRef]
17. Yao, Q.; Liang, Y.; Shao, Y.; Bian, W.; Fu, H.; Xu, J.; Sui, L.; Yao, B.; Li, M. Advanced Glycation End Product Concentrations in Follicular Fluid of Women Undergoing IVF/ICSI with a GnRH Agonist Protocol. *Reprod. BioMed. Online* **2018**, *36*, 20–25. [CrossRef]
18. Matsui, T.; Nakamura, N.; Ojima, A.; Nishino, Y.; Yamagishi, S.-i. Sulforaphane Reduces Advanced Glycation End Products (AGEs)-Induced Inflammation in Endothelial Cells and Rat Aorta. *Nutr. Metab. Cardiovasc. Dis.* **2016**, *26*, 797–807. [CrossRef]
19. Sato, N.; Li, W.; Tsubaki, M.; Higai, K.; Takemoto, M.; Sasaki, T.; Onoda, T.; Suzuki, T.; Koike, K. Flavonoid Glycosides from Japanese Camellia Oil Cakes and Their Inhibitory Activity against Advanced Glycation End-Products Formation. *J. Funct. Foods* **2017**, *35*, 159–165. [CrossRef]

20. Mamdouh, A.M.; Khodeer, D.M.; Tantawy, M.A.; Moustafa, Y.M. In-Vitro and in-Vivo Investigation of Amygdalin, Metformin, and Combination of Both against Doxorubicin on Hepatocellular Carcinoma. *Life Sci.* **2021**, *285*, 119961. [CrossRef]
21. Navarrete, S.; Alarcón, M.; Palomo, I. Aqueous Extract of Tomato (*Solanum lycopersicum* L.) and Ferulic Acid Reduce the Expression of TNF-α and IL-1β in LPS-Activated Macrophages. *Molecules* **2015**, *20*, 15319–15329. [CrossRef]
22. Chaudhary, A.; Jaswal, V.S.; Choudhary, S.; Sonika; Sharma, A.; Beniwal, V.; Tuli, H.S.; Sharma, S. Ferulic Acid: A Promising Therapeutic Phytochemical and Recent Patents Advances. *Recent. Pat. Inflamm. Allergy Drug Discov.* **2019**, *13*, 115–123. [CrossRef]
23. Di Loreto, A.; Bosi, S.; Montero, L.; Bregola, V.; Marotti, I.; Sferrazza, R.E.; Dinelli, G.; Herrero, M.; Cifuentes, A. Determination of Phenolic Compounds in Ancient and Modern Durum Wheat Genotypes. *Electrophoresis* **2018**, *39*, 2001–2010. [CrossRef] [PubMed]
24. Zduńska, K.; Dana, A.; Kolodziejczak, A.; Rotsztejn, H. Antioxidant Properties of Ferulic Acid and Its Possible Application. *Ski. Pharmacol. Physiol.* **2018**, *31*, 332–336. [CrossRef] [PubMed]
25. Liu, H.; Chen, Z.; Shen, L.; Guo, X.; Ji, D. Well Modelling Methods in Thermal Reservoir Simulation. *Oil Gas Sci. Technol.—Rev. IFP Energies Nouv.* **2020**, *75*, 63. [CrossRef]
26. Chaikijurajai, T.; Tang, W.H.W. Myeloperoxidase: A Potential Therapeutic Target for Coronary Artery Disease. *Expert. Opin. Ther. Tar.* **2020**, *24*, 695–705. [CrossRef] [PubMed]
27. Li, X.; Wu, J.; Xu, F.; Chu, C.; Li, X.; Shi, X.; Zheng, W.; Wang, Z.; Jia, Y.; Xiao, W. Use of Ferulic Acid in the Management of Diabetes Mellitus and Its Complications. *Molecules* **2022**, *27*, 6010. [CrossRef]
28. Sun, S.; Ruan, Y.; Yan, M.; Xu, K.; Yang, Y.; Shen, T.; Jin, Z. Ferulic Acid Alleviates Oxidative Stress-Induced Cardiomyocyte Injury by the Regulation of miR-499-5p/P21 Signal Cascade. *Evid.-Based Complement. Altern. Med.* **2021**, *2021*, 1921457. [CrossRef]
29. Reasner, C.A. Reducing Cardiovascular Complications of Type 2 Diabetes by Targeting Multiple Risk Factors. *J. Cardiovasc. Pharmacol.* **2008**, *52*, 136–144. [CrossRef]
30. Elshourbagy, N. The Effects of Carvedilol and Q10 On Isoprenaline-Induced Cardiotoxicity: Electrocardiographic, Biochemical and Histopathological Evaluation in Rats. *Al-Azhar J. Pharm. Sci.* **2016**, *54*, 148–158. [CrossRef]
31. Perrone, A.; Giovino, A.; Benny, J.; Martinelli, F. Advanced Glycation End Products (AGEs): Biochemistry, Signaling, Analytical Methods, and Epigenetic Effects. *Oxid. Med. Cell. Longev.* **2020**, *2020*, 3818196. [CrossRef]
32. Vadakedath, S.; Kandi, V. Role of Advanced Glycation End Products (AGE) in Health and Disease: An Overview. *Biochem. Physiol.* **2018**, *7*, 1000246. [CrossRef]
33. Barrett, E.J.; Liu, Z.; Khamaisi, M.; King, G.L.; Klein, R.; Klein, B.E.K.; Hughes, T.M.; Craft, S.; Freedman, B.I.; Bowden, D.W.; et al. Diabetic Microvascular Disease: An Endocrine Society Scientific Statement. *J. Clin. Endocrinol. Metab.* **2017**, *102*, 4343–4410. [CrossRef] [PubMed]
34. Khalid, M.; Petroianu, G.; Adem, A. Advanced Glycation End Products and Diabetes Mellitus: Mechanisms and Perspectives. *Biomolecules* **2022**, *12*, 542. [CrossRef] [PubMed]
35. Nowotny, K.; Jung, T.; Höhn, A.; Weber, D.; Grune, T. Advanced Glycation End Products and Oxidative Stress in Type 2 Diabetes Mellitus. *Biomolecules* **2015**, *5*, 194–222. [CrossRef]
36. Singh, V.P.; Bali, A.; Singh, N.; Jaggi, A.S. Advanced Glycation End Products and Diabetic Complications. *Korean J. Physiol. Pharmacol.* **2014**, *18*, 1–14. [CrossRef] [PubMed]
37. Shen, Y.; Xu, Z.; Sheng, Z. Ability of Resveratrol to Inhibit Advanced Glycation End Product Formation and Carbohydrate-Hydrolyzing Enzyme Activity, and to Conjugate Methylglyoxal. *Food Chem.* **2017**, *216*, 153–160. [CrossRef]
38. Liu, J.; He, Y.; Wang, S.; He, Y.; Wang, W.; Li, Q.; Cao, X. Ferulic Acid Inhibits Advanced Glycation End Products (AGEs) Formation and Mitigates the AGEs-Induced Inflammatory Response in HUVEC Cells. *J. Funct. Foods* **2018**, *48*, 19–26. [CrossRef]
39. Srinivasan, M.; Sudheer, A.R.; Menon, V.P. Ferulic Acid: Therapeutic Potential Through Its Antioxidant Property. *J. Clin. Biochem. Nutr.* **2007**, *40*, 92–100. [CrossRef]
40. Jung, E.H.; Kim, S.R.; Hwang, I.K.; Ha, T.Y. Hypoglycemic Effects of a Phenolic Acid Fraction of Rice Bran and Ferulic Acid in C57BL/KsJ-Db/Db Mice. *J. Agric. Food Chem.* **2007**, *55*, 9800–9804. [CrossRef]
41. Sri Balasubashini, M.; Rukkumani, R.; Menon, V.P. Protective Effects of Ferulic Acid on Hyperlipidemic Diabetic Rats. *Acta Diabetol.* **2003**, *40*, 118–122. [CrossRef]
42. Ha, H.; Lee, H.B. Reactive Oxygen Species as Glucose Signaling Molecules in Mesangial Cells Cultured under High Glucose. *Kidney Int. Suppl.* **2000**, *77*, S19–S25. [CrossRef]
43. Ziyadeh, F.N. Mediators of Diabetic Renal Disease: The Case for Tgf-Beta as the Major Mediator. *J. Am. Soc. Nephrol.* **2004**, *15* (Suppl. S1), S55–S57. [CrossRef] [PubMed]
44. Lin, F.-H.; Lin, J.-Y.; Gupta, R.D.; Tournas, J.A.; Burch, J.A.; Selim, M.A.; Monteiro-Riviere, N.A.; Grichnik, J.M.; Zielinski, J.; Pinnell, S.R. Ferulic Acid Stabilizes a Solution of Vitamins C and E and Doubles Its Photoprotection of Skin. *J. Investig. Dermatol.* **2005**, *125*, 826–832. [CrossRef] [PubMed]
45. Nirmala, C.; Puvanakrishnan, R. Protective Role of Curcumin against Isoproterenol Induced Myocardial Infarction in Rats. *Mol. Cell. Biochem.* **1996**, *159*, 85–93. [CrossRef] [PubMed]

46. Patel, V.; Upaganlawar, A.; Zalawadia, R.; Balaraman, R. Cardioprotective Effect of Melatonin against Isoproterenol Induced Myocardial Infarction in Rats: A Biochemical, Electrocardiographic and Histoarchitectural Evaluation. *Eur. J. Pharmacol.* **2010**, *644*, 160–168. [CrossRef]
47. Nagoor Meeran, M.F.; Jagadeesh, G.S.; Selvaraj, P. Thymol Attenuates Inflammation in Isoproterenol Induced Myocardial Infarcted Rats by Inhibiting the Release of Lysosomal Enzymes and Downregulating the Expressions of Proinflammatory Cytokines. *Eur. J. Pharmacol.* **2015**, *754*, 153–161. [CrossRef]
48. Padmanabhan, M.; Mainzen Prince, P.S. S-Allylcysteine Ameliorates Isoproterenol-Induced Cardiac Toxicity in Rats by Stabilizing Cardiac Mitochondrial and Lysosomal Enzymes. *Life Sci.* **2007**, *80*, 972–978. [CrossRef]
49. Lim, K.H.; Ko, D.; Kim, J.-H. Cardioprotective Potential of Korean Red Ginseng Extract on Isoproterenol-Induced Cardiac Injury in Rats. *J. Ginseng Res.* **2013**, *37*, 273–282. [CrossRef]
50. Szasz. Proceedings of the Second International Symposium on Clinical Enzymology. San Diego, U.S.A., February 1979. *Clin. Biochem.* **1979**, *12*, 189–290.
51. Zhang, J.; Knapton, A.; Lipshultz, S.E.; Weaver, J.L.; Herman, E.H. Isoproterenol-Induced Cardiotoxicity in Sprague-Dawley Rats: Correlation of Reversible and Irreversible Myocardial Injury with Release of Cardiac Troponin T and Roles of iNOS in Myocardial Injury. *Toxicol. Pathol.* **2008**, *36*, 277–278. [CrossRef]
52. Vatandoust, N.; Rami, F.; Salehi, A.R.; Khosravi, S.; Dashti, G.; Eslami, G.; Momenzadeh, S.; Salehi, R. Novel High-Fat Diet Formulation and Streptozotocin Treatment for Induction of Prediabetes and Type 2 Diabetes in Rats. *Adv. Biomed. Res.* **2018**, *7*, 107. [CrossRef]
53. Jain, P.G.; Mahajan, U.B.; Shinde, S.D.; Surana, S.J. Cardioprotective Role of FA against Isoproterenol Induced Cardiac Toxicity. *Mol. Biol. Rep.* **2018**, *45*, 1357–1365. [CrossRef] [PubMed]
54. Buhl, S.N.; Jackson, K.Y. Optimal Conditions and Comparison of Lactate Dehydrogenase Catalysis of the Lactate-to-Pyruvate and Pyruvate-to-Lactate Reactions in Human Serum at 25, 30, and 37 Degrees C. *Clin. Chem.* **1978**, *24*, 828–831. [CrossRef] [PubMed]
55. Würzburg, U.; Hennrich, N.; Lang, H.; Prellwitz, W.; Neumeier, D.; Knedel, M. Bestimmung der Aktivität von Creatinkinase MB im Serum unter Verwendung inhibierender Antikörper. *Klin. Wochenschr.* **1976**, *54*, 357–360. [CrossRef] [PubMed]
56. Acikel, M.; Buyukokuroglu, M.E.; Erdogan, F.; Aksoy, H.; Bozkurt, E.; Senocak, H. Protective Effects of Dantrolene against Myocardial Injury Induced by Isoproterenol in Rats: Biochemical and Histological Findings. *Int. J. Cardiol.* **2005**, *98*, 389–394. [CrossRef]

pharmaceuticals MDPI

Article

Quercetin Intake and Absolute Telomere Length in Patients with Type 2 Diabetes Mellitus: Novel Findings from a Randomized Controlled Before-and-After Study

Aikaterini E. Mantadaki [1,*,†], Stella Baliou [2], Manolis Linardakis [1], Elena Vakonaki [2], Manolis N. Tzatzarakis [2], Aristides Tsatsakis [2] and Emmanouil K. Symvoulakis [1,†]

[1] Clinic of Social and Family Medicine, Department of Social Medicine, School of Medicine, University of Crete, 70013 Heraklion, Greece; linman@med.uoc.gr (M.L.); esymvoulakis@uoc.gr (E.K.S.)

[2] Laboratory of Toxicology, Medical School, University of Crete, 71003 Heraklion, Greece; s.baliou@med.uoc.gr or stellabaliou@gmail.com (S.B.); evakonaki@med.uoc.gr or evakonaki@gmail.com (E.V.); tzatzarakis@med.uoc.gr (M.N.T.); tsatsaka@uoc.gr (A.T.)

* Correspondence: medp2012012@med.uoc.gr or aikaterini.mantadaki@gmail.com; Tel.: +30-6977123064

† These authors contributed equally to this work.

Abstract: Telomeres, the protective chromosomal ends, progressively shorten and potentially are implicated in the pathogenesis of age-related diseases. In type 2 diabetes (T2DM), telomere shortening may play an important role, but the whole 'picture' remains limited. From a therapeutic perspective, the phytonutrient quercetin appears to be clinically effective and safe for patients with T2DM. Considering the above, we aimed to examine whether quercetin could interfere with telomere length (TL) dynamics. One hundred patients with T2DM on non-insulin medications registered within a primary healthcare facility were stratified by age and sex and randomly assigned to either standard care or standard care plus quercetin (500 mg/day) for 12 weeks, succeeded by an 8-week washout period and another 12 weeks of supplementation. Of the 88 patients completing the trial, 82 consented to blood sampling for TL measurements. Health assessments and whole blood absolute TL measurements using quantitative polymerase chain reaction (qPCR) were conducted at baseline and study end, and the findings of this subcohort are presented. Quercetin supplementation was associated with a significant increase in mean TL (odds ratio $\geq$ 2.44; $p < 0.05$) with a strengthened association after full adjustment for potential confounders through multiple logistic regression analysis (odds ratio = 3.48; $p = 0.026$), suggesting it as a potentially promising supplementation option. Further studies are needed to confirm this finding, elucidating the underlying molecular mechanisms of quercetin.

Keywords: type 2 diabetes mellitus; nutraceutical; quercetin; randomized trial; nutri-senotherapy; hypoglycemic effect; phytotherapy; integrated care; senolytic; telomere length

1. Introduction

Telomeres are nucleoprotein complexes capping the 23 pairs of linear chromosomes of each human cell. They contain tandem repeats of non-coding DNA motifs, specifically, in vertebrates, 5′-TTAGGG-3′ repeat units and their interacting protein partners, including a six-protein telomere-binding protective shelterin complex and a ribonucleoprotein (RNP), telomerase [1–4]. Importantly, the shelterin complex shields chromosomal ends of eukaryotic cells from recognition as double-stranded breaks (DSBs) [3]. The potential identification of telomeres as exposed DNA damage sites can lead to telomere fusion, degradation, recombination, or even telomere shortening (TS) [5], thereby compromising genomic stability [6].

More specifically, cellular proliferative rounds cause TS because of the end replication problem [7]. When telomeres reach a critically short length, they lose the protection of the shelterin protein complex, compromising their function. This leads to the triggering of the DNA damage response (DDR), inducing the activation of p53 transcription factor and the subsequent upregulation of cell-cycle inhibitors p16Ink4a and p21Cip1, resulting in cellular senescence, followed by apoptosis [8].

The most pronounced characteristic of senescent cells is their growth-arrested condition. In parallel, senescent cells are characterized by increased secretion of growth factors, cytokines, chemokines, proteases, and lipids, forming the senescence-associated secretory phenotype (SASP), thus sustaining low-grade inflammation [9]. On the other hand, uncapped telomeres can lead to numerous chromosome abnormalities and end-to-end fusion of chromosomes due to the absence of cell-cycle checkpoint mechanisms, resulting in genomic instability and widespread cell death [8].

Whereas TS is linked to aging and senescence, senescence does not always indicate cell aging [10]. Accordingly, a growing body of evidence proposes that the progression of age-related disorders may depend on the rate of TS [11–16]. Significantly, research has shown that telomere length (TL)—short, critically short, and critically long—is a recognized marker of biological aging and is considered a putative indicator of the cellular wellness of a person, with some predictive value for the risk of age-related illnesses like diabetes, osteoporosis, autoimmune diseases, neurodegenerative diseases, cardiovascular diseases, and some types of cancer [11–17]. For instance, TL has demonstrated utility in identifying patients with type 2 diabetes mellitus (T2DM) at risk of mortality [18]. The definitive role of TL in age-related diseases (ARDs) is still debated.

Relevant to this context, T2DM constitutes a global epidemic characterized by chronic dysglycemia, intertwined with heightened oxidative stress and inflammation [19], as elaborated elsewhere [20], a combination strongly correlated with accelerated TS. These interconnected processes may further contribute to genomic instability [21] and an increased vulnerability to vascular complications [22,23]. The interwoven relationship between telomere uncapping, senescence burden [23], and T2DM etiology underlines the necessity for innovative therapeutic interventions to preserve telomere integrity and mitigate disease progression in this population group.

Proceeding from this premise, emerging research suggests potential in targeting senescent cells and telomeres for the treatment and prevention of ARDs, and particularly T2DM [24]. Both senolytic and senomorphic therapies, designed to either eliminate senescent cells or mitigate their adverse effects, are being explored as possibly favorable interventions for age-associated morbidities [24,25].

The evolving field of telomere-targeted therapies, including senolytics, senomorphics, and potential telomerase activators, represents a promising research frontier in the pursuit of longevity and healthspan [26,27]. Nevertheless, telomerase activators have been implicated in oncogenesis concerns [27–29], hinting at a prerequisite for rigorous research and evaluation of the safety and regulatory efficacy of these interventions before their therapeutic potential in the context of healthy aging and age-related disease management can be fully understood.

The implications of telomere dysfunction and cellular senescence possibly associated with ARDs have instigated investigations into potential senotherapeutic interventions [8,30]. Quercetin, a flavonoid found ubiquitously in plant-derived dietary sources [31], has attracted considerable research interest as a potential therapeutic agent for mitigating cellular senescence [32–34]. This polyphenolic compound with potent antioxidant and anti-inflammatory properties [35–37] may exert a dual, pleiotropic action as both a senolytic and senomorphic [32–34]. The former indicates it can function by selectively inducing apoptosis of senescent cells and the latter implies the potential ability of modulating, particularly attenuating the SASP, possibly rendering it a promising candidate for mitigating the adverse consequences of cellular senescence and telomere dysfunction and potentially paving the way for innovative phytotherapeutic interventions in the supportive care management of ARDs.

The complex interplay between telomere dysfunction and T2DM pathophysiology generates mixed methodology hypotheses, justifying a combined laboratory and clinical approach to synchronically examine the variation of telomere status and disease progression in this vulnerable population group. Therefore, leveraging our prior work elucidating the safety and clinical efficacy aspects of quercetin nutritherapy [20,38], revealing a presumed improvement in standard risk factors, this randomized controlled before-and-after trial further delves into the potential of quercetin to modulate whole blood absolute TL in patients with T2DM, providing exploratory insights and putatively representing a novel nutritional senotherapeutic piece of knowledge to ARDs.

2. Results

Of the 88 patients concluding the trial [20], 82 voluntarily consented to blood sampling for absolute whole blood TL measurements by quantitative polymerase chain reaction (qPCR), as shown in the report-specific flowchart (Figure 1). This subsequent analysis was therefore confined to this subcohort of 42 control and 40 intervention participants. Aligning with the study design, adherence to the nutraceutical allocation was consistent within the treatment group.

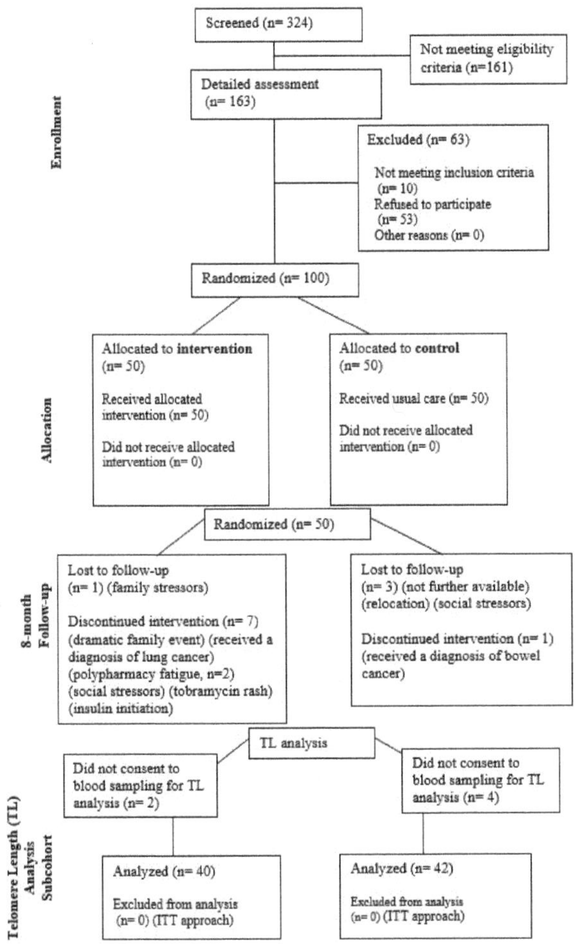

Figure 1. Flow diagram for the TL analysis subcohort, aligning with CONSORT standards.

The baseline characteristics of the 82 randomized patients with T2DM consenting to blood sampling for whole-blood TL measurements are displayed in Table 1 using chi-squared and Student's *t*-tests for comparison. The mean age of participants was 66.3 ± 7.4 for the intervention and 67.8 ± 6.2 years for the usual care group. The groups were well-balanced in sex, age, and nationality attributes ($p > 0.05$). Both groups were under treatment with oral antidiabetic pills (viz. metformin, SGLT-2 and DPP-4 inhibitors, sulfonylurea, or their combinations, $p > 0.05$), while eight in each group were additionally treated with GLP-1 agonists ($p = 0.913$). A balanced distribution of lifestyle risk factors between both groups was noted, without statistically significant intergroup differences in their prevalence (smoking, alcohol consumption, high body weight, physical inactivity, and lack of fruit consumption; $p > 0.05$). Also, no significant differences were discerned between the groups regarding the prevalence of multimorbidity, polypharmacy, or the mean duration since T2DM diagnosis ($p > 0.05$). Specifically, the occurrence of the most common age-related conditions (hypertension, dyslipidemia, chronic inflammatory airway diseases; CIADs, depression and anxiety disorder) was similar ($p > 0.05$) between the study groups of this subcohort.

Table 1. Baseline descriptive characteristics of the 82 patients with type II diabetes (T2DM) consenting to blood sampling for telomere length (TL) measurements and randomized to intervention and control groups.

		Groups	
		Intervention (n = 40)	**Control (n = 42)**
		n (%)	
Sex	male	22 (55.0)	23 (54.8)
	female	18 (45.0)	19 (45.2)
Age, years	mean ± stand. dev.	66.3 ± 7.4	67.8 ± 6.2
Nationality	Greek	36 (90.0)	42 (100.0)
Lifestyle Risk Factors	smoking	13 (32.5)	15 (35.7)
	alcohol consumption	28 (70.0)	28 (66.7)
	high body weight	35 (87.5)	39 (92.9)
	physical inactivity	16 (40.0)	21 (50.0)
	not consuming fruits	2 (5.0)	2 (4.8)
	3+ factors	16 (40.0)	23 (54.8)
Multimorbidity	3+ chronic conditions	32 (80.0)	28 (66.7)
Polypharmacy	4+ medications	28 (70.0)	29 (69.0)
Years diagnosed with T2DM	mean ± stand. dev.	11.0 ± 7.1	10.3 ± 6.6

Chi-square (χ^2) and Student's *t*-tests: * $p < 0.05$.

Overall, both groups were comparable at baseline, as demonstrated in Tables 1 and 2. The inter- and intra- group comparisons of health indicators of the 82 patients with T2DM randomized to intervention and control groups included in this analysis, from the starting point to the endpoint (8 months) of the study are presented in Table 2. The intervention group demonstrated a statistically significant improvement in night-time sleep duration, while the control group experienced a decrease (0.8 vs. −0.5 h, $p < 0.001$). Health self-assessment scores significantly improved in the intervention. In contrast, the control group experienced a decrease, yielding a statistically significant intergroup difference (1.5 vs. −0.6, $p < 0.001$). Between the two groups, no significant changes were observed in body mass index (BMI) values ($p > 0.05$). Systolic blood pressure significantly decreased in the intervention group, while it increased in the control group (−6.3 vs. 0.5 mmHg, $p = 0.02$). Neither inter- nor intra-group comparisons revealed significant alterations in diastolic blood pressure ($p > 0.05$). Between-group analyses showed no significant changes in total cholesterol, whereas the cholesterol ratio insignificantly decreased in the intervention group (p = 0.07). A statistically significant decrease in the glycated hemoglobin (HbA1c) measures of the intervention group was observed compared to the control group (−0.28 vs. 0.03%, p = 0.008). Average TL per chromosome end significantly increased in the intervention group (from 5.11 ± 1.35 to 5.63 ± 2.08 kb), while the control group experienced a decrease (5.19 ± 1.76 to 4.88 ± 1.19 kb; 0.52 vs. −0.31 kb, p = 0.048) over the eight-month supplementation period.

Table 2. Levels of and changes in health indicators of the 82 patients with T2DM consenting to blood sampling for whole-blood TL measurements and randomized to intervention (n = 40) and control (n = 42) groups from the starting point to the endpoint of the study.

		Groups			
		Intervention	**Control**		**Cohen's *d* Effect Size**
		Mean ± Stand. Dev.		***p*-Value**	
Night-time sleep (hours)	beginning	6.2 ± 1.7	6.6 ± 1.5		
	8 months	7.0 ± 1.3	6.1 ± 1.7		
	Δ-change	+0.8	−0.5	<0.001	0.93
	p-value	0.002	0.011		
Health self-assessment (scale 0 to 10, 10: excellent)	beginning	6.0 ± 2.1	5.9 ± 2.1		
	8 months	7.5 ± 1.7	5.3 ± 2.0		
	Δ-change	+1.5	−0.6	<0.001	1.56
	p-value	<0.001	0.005		
Body mass index (kg/m^2)	beginning	31.4 ± 5.1	30.6 ± 5.4		
	8 months	31.0 ± 5.1	30.3 ± 5.2		
	Δ-change	−0.4	−0.3	0.780	0.05
	p-value	0.012	0.089		
Systolic blood pressure (mmHg)	beginning	130.7 ± 14.2	128.4 ± 13.8		
	8 months	124.4 ± 13.8	128.9 ± 16.5		
	Δ-change	−6.3	+0.5	0.020	0.52
	p-value	0.003	0.804		
Diastolic blood pressure (mmHg)	beginning	76.0 ± 8.8	75.4 ± 10.7		
	8 months	77.4 ± 9.1	77.3 ± 8.8		
	Δ-change	+1.4	+1.9	0.822	0.05
	p-value	0.276	0.196		
Total cholesterol (mg/dL)	beginning	154.9 ± 35.9	163.7 ± 37.6		
	8 months	160.4 ± 36.4	163.9 ± 44.4		
	Δ-change	+5.5	+0.2	0.460	0.17
	p-value	0.122	0.966		
Glycosylated hemoglobin (HbA$_1$c) (%)	beginning	7.03 ± 1.12	6.71 ± 0.79		
	8 months	6.75 ± 0.89	6.74 ± 0.94		
	Δ-change	−0.28	+0.03	0.008	0.60
	p-value	0.005	0.655		
Cholesterol ratio	beginning	3.937 ± 1.962	3.567 ± 0.927		
	8 months	3.855 ± 1.403	4.109 ± 2.147		
	Δ-change	−0.072	+0.752	0.070	0.41
	p-value	0.802	0.035		
Telomere length (kb)	beginning	5.11 ± 1.35	5.19 ± 1.76		
	8 months	5.63 ± 2.08	4.88 ± 1.19		
	Δ-change	+0.52	−0.31	0.048	0.44
	p-value	0.120	0.235		

Student's t-tests in Δ-changes (in bold) and paired samples t-tests between the baseline and study endpoint for each group (in grey).

The percentage frequencies of TL changes, as increase or decrease, from baseline to the endpoint at 8 months for the 82 consenting patients analyzed in this report are illustrated in

Figure 2. A significant change in TL dynamics was observed between the two groups as the intervention group exhibited a higher frequency of TL increase compared to counterparts (57.5% vs. 35.7%) ($p = 0.048$).

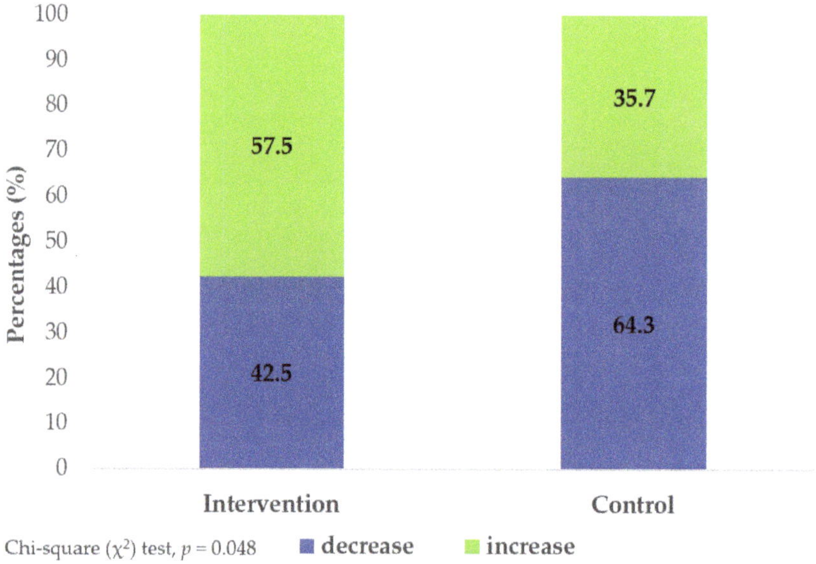

Figure 2. Frequency of telomere length (TL) changes (increase or decrease) in patients with type 2 diabetes mellitus (T2DM) consenting to blood sampling for whole-blood TL measurements, randomized to intervention (n = 40) and control (n = 42) groups over the 8-month study period.

The results of multiple logistic regression analyses examining the prognostic factors associated with an increase in average TL (versus decrease) over the 8-month subcohort-study period are delineated in Table 3. Except for the crude model, three more models were constructed, each incorporating a progressively comprehensive set of covariates. In the unadjusted model (crude), the intervention group exhibited a 2.44-fold higher odds of TL increase compared to the control group ($p = 0.05$). After adjusting for baseline TL through model 1, the intervention group maintained a 2.87-fold increased odds of TL increase ($p = 0.036$). Even after further accounting for sex and age attributes as additional confounders, the association was consistently statistically significant (model 2, odds ratio; OR = 2.90, $p = 0.04$). When the model included an expanded range of confounders, i.e., lifestyle risk factors, multimorbidity, polypharmacy, and years since T2DM diagnosis, an amplified effect was demonstrated (OR = 3.48, $p = 0.026$) (model 3). Furthermore, higher baseline TL was consistently related with a significantly decreased likelihood of telomere increase in patients with T2DM after controlling for multiple covariates (OR < 1.00, $p < 0.01$).

Table 3. Multiple logistic regression analysis of TL increase (versus decrease) over the 8-month study period among the 82 patients with T2DM consenting to blood sampling for whole-blood TL measurements and randomized to intervention (n = 40) and control (n = 42) groups.

			Telomere Length Changes over the 8-Month Study Period (Increase vs. Decrease)		
Model	**Prognostic Factors**		**Odds Ratio, OR**	**95% CIs**	**p-Value**
Crude	Groups	control	1.00 (ref.)		
		intervention	2.44	1.00, 5.93	0.050
1	Baseline Telomeres (per unit change)		0.52	0.35, 0.79	0.002
	Groups	control	1.00 (ref.)		
		intervention	2.87	1.07, 7.70	0.036
2	Sex	male	1.00 (ref.)		
		female	1.64	0.60, 4.52	0.336
	Age (per year change)		0.95	0.88, 1.02	0.167
	Baseline Telomeres (per unit change)		0.49	0.32, 0.76	0.002
	Groups	control	1.00 (ref.)		
		intervention	2.90	1.05, 8.00	0.040
3	Sex	male	1.00 (ref.)		
		female	1.99	0.66, 5.96	0.221
	Age (per year change)		0.94	0.86, 1.02	0.137
	Baseline Telomeres (per unit change)		0.48	0.30, 0.76	0.002
	Lifestyle Risk Factors	0–2 factors	1.00 (ref.)		
		3+	2.23	0.75, 6.63	0.148
	Multimorbidity	0–2 chronic conditions	1.00 (ref.)		
		3+	0.61	0.17, 2.20	0.453
	Polypharmacy	0–3 medications	1.00 (ref.)		
		4+	0.93	0.28, 3.10	0.909
	Years Diagnosed with T2DM (per year change)		1.06	0.97, 1.15	0.186
	Groups	control	1.00 (ref.)		
		intervention	3.48	1.16, 10.41	0.026

R^2 Nagelkerke estimations: Crude model $R^2 = 0.06$; 1st model $R^2 = 0.25$; 2nd model $R^2 = 0.30$; 3rd model $R^2 = 0.33$.

3. Discussion

The results deriving from this subcohort are in parallel with our prior clinical findings [20,38], further solidifying the promising potential of quercetin as an adjunct nutritional senotherapeutic intervention for T2DM. They also add a compelling layer of evidence, expanding previous knowledge on the overall health status, underscoring its role in disease progression and compelling further investigation of the translational senolytic potential of quercetin on diabetic sequalae. As a matter of fact, to the best of our knowledge, our study constitutes the first randomized controlled before-and-after trial to assess the impact of quercetin on absolute TL of an age-related disease while concurrently examining clinical features in primary care attendees.

Only one randomized controlled trial (RCT) on seniors with metabolic syndrome has evaluated the influence of quercetin supplementation on leukocyte TL (LTL) but found no changes post-supplementation [39]. Nevertheless, the limited 3-month study period, as well as the lower daily dosage of 240 mg, might have constrained the imprint of this intervention. Conversely, in our study, the intervention group received quercetin intermittently: for 12 weeks, followed by an 8-week washout period and another 12 weeks of supplementation. Another point for discussion within the limitations of the mentioned study includes its measurement of TL, which was based on a relative TL evaluation (T/S ratio) [40–44].

This analysis provides initial findings suggesting that quercetin could offer advantageous nutriprotective benefits in a population with T2DM. Specifically, within this subcohort of 82 patients who underwent TL blood sampling, significant positive effects were noted on TL and clinically relevant improvements, including nocturnal sleep duration and subjective health status. There was also a decrease in systolic blood pressure and glycated hemoglobin and a marginally insignificant decrease in the cholesterol ratio. BMI, diastolic blood pressure, and total cholesterol remained largely unchanged.

As the potential molecular mechanisms underlying these protective effects have been extensively explained in our prior publications [20,38] and the pre-defined primary endpoint of this study was the impact on TL [45], the current analysis will not reiterate previously explored mechanistic aspects. It will instead focus on a proof-of-concept approach.

Our results regarding the absolute TL of whole blood samples are consistent with previous research in the general population of similar age range [43,46–49]. Notably, our results lean towards the lower end of the observed TL distribution of healthy populations [50,51], aligning with the previous literature on the association between shorter telomeres and diabetes [52–55]. The observed increase in the absolute TL measurements within the intervention group, independent of potential confounders, suggests a potential reduction in the proportion of the senescence-inducing telomeres, potentially conferring beneficial effects on cellular health and longevity. While our methodology provides a measure of telomere length, it is also possible that the removal of cells with shorter telomeres could contribute to the observed net increase. Therefore, the detected increase in TL can only be discussed as a preliminary observation.

It is also important to highlight that when measuring TL in whole-blood samples, the absolute TL measurement primarily reflects the TL of the most abundant cells in blood, which are circulating immune cells, while other cell types present in blood typically do not contribute significantly to the overall measurement. The senolytic effects of quercetin have been investigated in endothelial and adipose tissue cells [56,57] to date, yet the evidence is less well-established regarding the circulating immune cells. Our exploratory results underline the necessity for further biological studies in this nascent field.

The existing literature on the consequences of different nutritive interventions on TL reveals divergent findings, with scant evidence from RCTs [58] demonstrating both beneficial and nuanced effects. Notably, the D-Health Trial, involving regular monthly vitamin D supplementation, did not provide a protective effect on telomere attrition in older individuals already possessing sufficient levels of vitamin D [59]. Similarly, in a subcohort of the double-blind, n-3 PUFA RCT of 106 subjects over 4 months, no significant differences in TL were observed between the intervention and control groups [60]. Conversely, a 6-month RCT including 33 adults over 65 years old with minor neurocognitive deficit suggested that omega-3 fatty acid intake may attenuate TS [61]. A two-year-long RCT with 162 participants examining LTL after walnut consumption indicated a potential trend towards LTL preservation in older adults, possibly associated with its alpha-linolenic acid and polyphenol-rich content [62]. Furthermore, a smaller, one year-long study with 65 individuals provided preliminary evidence of correlation between the supplementation with vitamins of the B-complex and the mitigation of telomere attrition [63].

Our findings add to the limited body of research on senescence-targeting interventions exploring telomere biology in humans [64]. Focusing on the available senolytic interventions, a prospective study investigated the use of hyperbaric oxygen therapy (HBOT) in 35 healthy adults over 64 years old. This study employed flow-fluorescence in situ hybridization (Flow-FISH) analysis of peripheral blood mononuclear cells (PBMCs) and reported a significant increase in TL across immune cell subsets, specifically, T helper cells, cytotoxic T cells, natural killer cells, and B cells, with the latter exhibiting a more pronounced effect [65]. In contrast, a longitudinal study evaluated the combination of dasatinib and quercetin (D + Q) for six months, followed by an identical six-month regimen plus fisetin one year later, in 19 participants utilizing a DNA methylation (DNAm)-based clock. Distinct effects on TL were revealed. The initial regimen resulted in a decrease in TL at the 3- and 6-month time points, whereas the subsequent addition of fisetin appeared to mitigate TS after one year of treatment [64].

An intriguing perspective unveiled from this analysis urges to be elucidated: the interconnection between favorable clinical and cellular homeostasis aspects following quercetin supplementation. These comprised ameliorated nocturnal sleep duration, well-being perception, blood pressure normalization and improved glycemic regulation. Interestingly, TS has been associated with poor sleep patterns [66–68], compromised psychophysiological health [69–71], hypertension [72,73], and impaired glycemic control [54,74].

The observed positive effects of quercetin on TL could be attributed to various, interrelated mechanistic reasons with yet unresolved intricacies and primarily to its capacity for mitigating oxidative stress and inflammation [35–37], both of which are known to accelerate TS [75,76]. This antioxidant protection potentially enables enhanced telomerase stability [3,77]. Furthermore, building upon the previously discussed contextualized rationale regarding its potential senolytic and senomorphic properties [32–34], quercetin may exert a preventive effect on TS by reducing the burden of senescent cells. Additionally, research suggests that quercetin could act as a regulator of key signaling pathways crucial for preserving cellular homeostasis, modulating sirtuins (especially activating SIRT1 and potentially dose-proportionally regulating SIRT6 [78–81]) and the AMP-activated protein kinase (AMPK) enzyme [82–84].

Remarkably, quercetin might exert intricate effects on telomerase activity, suggesting a potential for differential modulation in diverse cellular milieux and dose-dependent contexts, as bolstered by its polyphenolic property [85]. Although the relevant research is rapidly evolving, highlighting the necessity for further biological studies, the current literature proposes that in cancer cells, it inhibits telomerase activity [86–88], consistent with findings for other flavonoids [85,88], while concurrently selectively modulating the expression of POT1, TRF1, and TRF2 proteins [89]. This inhibitory effect in cancer cells, combined with an observed activation of hTERT in certain cell lines [90], raises the intriguing possibility that it may preferentially regulate telomerase activity in healthy human cells [91], potentially favoring the activation of hTERT or the expression of telomere-protective proteins and subsequent telomere elongation. Whether this proposed selective telomerase activation hypothesis is valid and translates to tangible benefits in telomeric elongation could initiate a pathway for ongoing investigation. Additionally, the literature supports its influence on epigenetic modifications, viz. DNA methylation, histone acetylation, and microRNA regulation [91,92], hinting at a broader role in regulating cellular processes involved in telomere maintenance.

Study Strengths and Limitations

A key strength of our study lies in its comprehensive assessment of telomere dynamics in T2DM, employing accurate, high-throughput absolute TL measurements by qPCR [40–44]. Considering our RCT prioritized the metabolic and clinical implications in a substantial population with T2DM, we opted for the more practical qPCR measurements through commercial kits, which are informative at the cell-population level. Even though qPCR provides an individual's average telomere data based on the specific amplification of telomere repeats, it is not considered a precise method [40]. The primary limitation of qPCR is its incapacity to offer details regarding the TL variations among cells and chromosomes [40]. For this reason, quantitative fluorescence in situ hybridization (qFISH) is the preferred technique for high-resolution evaluation of TL of cells in each chromosome at the single-cell level [93,94]. In addition, qFISH effectively captures even the extremely short telomeres [95], unveiling more precise TL alterations at the single-cell level [96,97] and could provide a more nuanced explanation of the observed effect on TL. While our study involved an open-label, non-placebo-controlled design, the primary outcome, TL, was directly measured using objective qPCR assays. Likewise, the staff conducting hematology tests for secondary outcomes were blinded to group allocations, further minimizing the risk of measurement bias. Furthermore, this study was prospectively registered within the International Standard Randomized Controlled Trial Number (ISRCTN) registry [45]. This work is the content of an ongoing PhD thesis, with no external funding, with permissions from all involved institutional bodies, after full protocol submission, and later performed in alignment with its protocol design requirements. Homogenous procedures across all study groups enabled for a standardized evaluation of the ascertained outcomes. Additionally, an intention-to-treat (ITT) approach was employed, which attenuates the potential for overestimation of intervention efficacy [98].

By incorporating absolute TL measurements from whole blood alongside relevant clinical biomarkers, we have attempted a deeper, integrative understanding of the intricate relationship between aging processes and T2DM. This approach provides unique, multilateral insights into how senotherapy may palpably influence telomere dynamics and interact with other cardiometabolic health parameters, potentially targeting disease progression and improving outcomes in patients with T2DM. Also, the 8-month rigorous RCT design, despite the availability of a subcohort of samples, equipped us with a power of detection of at least 80%, which should be mentioned. Moreover, the models fitted in the multiple logistic regression analysis were adjusted for several confounders. Another limitation is that we could not assess further biological variables which might have been proven helpful to explain the underlying mechanisms. Given the emerging role of cellular senescence in both the development of diabetes [99] and its complications [23], our study offers potentially relevant insights into promising therapeutic avenues for this disease. Nonetheless, our study design was not specifically tailored to address these elements. Future studies should include more extensive, larger-scale, blinded, placebo-controlled, dose-response assessment designs examining disease progression and complications so as to verify the senolytic results and to enable further decipherments.

4. Materials and Methods

4.1. Study Design, Participants, Phytonutrient

We conducted a prospective, randomized controlled before-and-after trial within a primary healthcare (PHC) facility in Heraklion, Crete, in the context of a PhD thesis of the Clinic of Social and Family Medicine, Department of Social Medicine, School of Medicine, University of Crete, with the aim to evaluate the clinical utility and potential of quercetin supplementation as an adjunct support for patients managing T2DM. Data were collected from registered patients within the 4th Local Health Unit of Heraklion (TOMY). Participants over 50 years old with an established diagnosis of T2DM and treated with non-insulin medications were enrolled in the trial between February and May 2023 after providing informed consent, as described in our previous report [20].

Of the 324 patients initially identified as candidates, 100 were ultimately randomized into two parallel groups after stratified randomization (1:1) ensuring balanced age and sex distribution: a control group (CTR, n = 50) receiving standard care and an intervention group (INT, n = 50) receiving quercetin dihydrate (500 mg/day) supplementation for two 12-week periods interspersed with an 8-week washout. Specifically, the INT received quercetin as an adjunctive treatment to their existing regimen and the control group did not, while both groups received uniform guidance. Further details on the phytonutrient supplement specifications and strategies to enhance participants' adherence to protocol requirements were formerly reported [20,38]. Participant flow throughout the randomized trial has also been delineated elsewhere [20], outlining reasons for attrition. Scheduled follow-up assessments were conducted in person: at baseline, at 3 months for a randomized subset, and at study endpoint. Participants underwent comprehensive health evaluations, and standardized fasting blood samples were collected at baseline and study conclusion, as mentioned in our previous work [20,38]. Participants self-rated their overall health status on a scale of 0 to 10, with 0 indicating extremely poor and 10 reflecting optimal health, for the needs of the health-self-assessment variable. TL was identified as the primary outcome of this study, as detailed in the study registry [45]. Of the 88 participants reaching the final study endpoint at 8 months, 82 consented to venipuncture for collection of blood samples in ethylenediaminetetraacetic acid (EDTA)-coated tubes.

Following gentle inversion to ensure thorough mixing, samples were securely stored at −20 °C, under strict quality and tracing control mandates, until genomic DNA extraction. Genomic DNA was subsequently isolated from the whole blood of these consenting patients. qPCR quantified absolute TL, and the resulting data are outlined in the current report.

Sample Size Estimation

Sample size estimates were determined at the clinical design stage as 45 participants per group using G*Power 3.1.9.7 [100,101], treating TL as a continuous variable, in consistency with calculations in methodologically comparable studies [60,102–106], and exceeding that of similar studies [107–109]. A post-hoc power analysis was conducted on the available sample, yielding a statistical power of at least 80%.

4.2. *Telomere Length Evaluation*

TL assessments were conducted at the Department of Morphology, Laboratory of Toxicology, School of Medicine, University of Crete, which has established expertise in this research field [110,111] under consistent experimental conditions.

4.2.1. DNA Extraction

Genomic DNA was extracted from human whole-blood samples using the NucleoSpin® Blood QuickPure kit (Macherey-Nagel, Düren, DE (Germany), catalog #740569.250, LOT no: 2311-003, exp.: 2026-02), as per manufacturer's recommendations. All samples were lysed with proteinase K and lysis buffer at 70 °C and to ensure optimal DNA yield, an extended lysis protocol was implemented, involving further incubation for 30 min with intermittent vortexing. Following lysis, DNA was bound to silica columns, washed, and eluted with pre-warmed elution buffer, according to the kit's instructions. DNA purity and integrity were evaluated utilizing a NanoDrop ND-1000 spectrophotometer (Thermo Fisher Scientific, Wilmington, DE, USA) and accompanying NanoDrop ND-1000 v.3.3 software (Coleman Technologies Inc., Langley, BC, Canada). Successfully extracted samples were then diluted to a working concentration of 5 ng/μL for downstream analysis and subsequently short-term stored at 4 °C.

4.2.2. Absolute Quantification of Telomere Length

qPCR quantified the absolute TL. Specifically, the Absolute Human Telomere Length Quantification qPCR Assay Kit (ScienCell, Carlsbad, CA, USA, Cat #8918) was used to quantify the average length of telomeric ends on each chromosome of pure genomic DNA (gDNA), isolated from human blood samples, as described previously. qPCR was performed on a Stratagene Mx3005P qPCR thermocycler (Agilent Technologies Inc., Santa Clara, CA, USA) through MxPro v.4.1.0.0 software. Following the manufacturer's protocol, two qPCR reactions were performed for each gDNA sample: one with telomere-specific (TEL) and one with single-copy reference (SCR) primers, targeting a 100 base-pair region on chromosome 17 for internal normalization. A reference gDNA sample of known TL (REF) provided in the kit served as a standard. Duplicate qPCR reactions were performed for each gDNA sample (4 qPCR reactions in total) on the same 96-well-plate, consistent with prior methodology [104,112], using water as the negative control and reference gDNA (REF) as the positive control in each run. In more detail, reactions contained 5 nanograms of gDNA template, combined with 2X GoldNStart TaqGreen qPCR Master Mix and either TEL or SCR primers. Samples from the intervention and control groups were run simultaneously on the same well plate. Additionally, minimal variation in Cq values was tolerated for all samples, while the entire experimental analysis was repeated in independent assays to ensure reliability and performance reproducibility [105,113–115]. The qPCR thermal cycling parameters consisted of a ten-minute preliminary denaturation at 95 °C, followed by 32 cycles of denaturation at 95 °C (20 s), a 20 s annealing at 52 °C, and a 45 s extension at 72 °C. Relative differences in TLs were calculated using the Livak comparative (ΔΔCq) method [116,117] through tabulation. Briefly, the difference in average quantification cycle

(Cq) values between the target and reference samples was calculated for both telomere (TEL) and single-copy reference (SCR) amplicons (ΔCq TEL and ΔCq SCR). The ΔΔCq value was then obtained by subtracting ΔCq SCR from ΔCq TEL. The fold change in TL relative to the reference was calculated as $2^{-\Delta\Delta Cq}$. Absolute TL per diploid genome was determined by multiplying the relative TL by the known TL of the reference gDNA sample. Average TL (in kb) per chromosome end was calculated by dividing the total TL per diploid genome by 92. Amplification plots derived from standard curves assessed the efficiency and specificity of the qPCR reactions.

4.3. Statistical Analysis

Statistical analyses were conducted using the SPSS software (IBM SPSS Statistics for Windows, Version 25.0. Armonk, NY, USA: IBM Corp). Data normality was assessed with Blom's method (Q-Q plot), and χ^2 and Student's *t*-test methods were implemented, respectively comparing categorical and continuous data between the two groups. Most of the results were presented with measures of location and dispersion or frequency distributions. Four multiple logistic regression models were constructed to assess the association between quercetin intake and the likelihood of TL increase, considering potential confounding factors, including established lifestyle-habit risk factors, previously associated with health outcomes [118–120]. The improvement in explained variance for TL changes was demonstrated by increasing Nagelkerke R^2 determination values across sequential models, indicating a progressively enhanced model fit [121].

4.4. Ethical Compliance and Approvals

This RCT was registered with ISRCTN [45] and received ethical approval from the University of Crete Research Ethics Committee (REC-UoC; 104/20-08-2021) and the 7th Health District of Crete, Heraklion (6380-14/02/2022), while aligning with international ethical and regulatory standards [122–127]. This RCT also adhered to the International Council for Harmonization (ICH) E18 guideline [128] on genomic sampling and data management, adopted by the European Medicines Agency [129].

5. Conclusions

Our study provides valuable insights through unifying hypotheses and integrating clinical parameters and telomere senescence pathways. We offer a deeper understanding of the relationship between aging processes and T2DM to assess the impact of quercetin intake in patients with T2DM. In this context, we highlight the potential of incorporating quercetin into PHC supportive interventions for T2DM. We report that quercetin, as a complementary phytonutritive senotherapy alongside standard pharmacological regimens, might propose an integrative care plan, as evidenced by its emerging potential to significantly increase the average telomere length of the intervention group, along with improvement of sleep, well-being perception, blood pressure and glycemic regulation. These findings create possibilities for targeting disease progression and improving patient outcomes, although future larger-scale, multi-center, placebo-controlled, dose-response assessment and blinded studies are needed for validation. Importantly, our work indirectly showcases how lifestyle choices might affect the progression of T2DM and underscores the value of implementing TL measurements into clinical assessments for T2DM populations. This opens avenues enabling specific, informed research initiatives, and early identification of aberrant telomere shortening before and after overt clinical manifestations, potentially paving the way for 'personalized medicine' and multi-omics approaches to learn more about disease trajectory and monitoring.

Author Contributions: Conceptualization, A.E.M. and E.K.S.; methodology, A.E.M. and E.K.S.; software, M.L.; validation, A.E.M., M.L., S.B., and E.V.; formal analysis, A.E.M. and M.L.; investigation, A.E.M., S.B., M.N.T., E.V., and A.T.; resources, A.E.M., S.B., M.N.T., and A.T.; data curation, A.E.M., M.L., and S.B.; writing—original draft preparation, A.E.M. and E.K.S.; writing—review and editing, A.E.M., M.L., S.B., E.V., M.N.T., A.T., and E.K.S.; visualization, A.E.M., M.L., S.B., and E.V.;

supervision, E.K.S.; project administration, A.E.M. and E.K.S. All authors have read and agreed to the published version of the manuscript.

Funding: This research received no external funding.

Institutional Review Board Statement: This randomized controlled trial, registered and curated in the International Standard Randomized Controlled Trial Number (ISRCTN) registry, aligned with the Declaration of Helsinki principles and received permission to conduct from the Research Ethics Committee of the University of Crete (REC-UoC) (protocol code 104; approval date 20 August 2021) and the 7th Health District of Crete, Heraklion (6380-14/02/2022).

Informed Consent Statement: Informed consent was obtained from all subjects involved in this study. Written informed consent was obtained from the patients to publish this paper.

Data Availability Statement: The principal investigators retained exclusive access to the trial dataset, which was maintained under stringent security protocols on protected servers housed at the University of Crete. External researchers may be permitted to access the de-identified dataset contingent upon submission of a reasonable request and execution of appropriate data sharing agreements. To safeguard participant confidentiality and anonymity, all personally identifiable information is expunged prior to data dissemination. Trial Registration Number: ISRCTN13131584.

Acknowledgments: The authors extend their sincere gratitude to the patients and staff of the 4th Local Health Unit (TOMY) of Heraklion for their participation in this research endeavor. Additionally, we genuinely appreciate the generous donation of quercetin supplements by Green Import, exclusive distributor of Lamberts Healthcare Ltd. in Greece, while affirming that the company had no involvement in the conception, implementation, or evaluation of this study. The presented data and their interpretations and insights described are independent of any external influence or conflicting interest and solely attributable to the authors. We would also like to thank Malakates, Neonaki, and Tsikandylakis for their invaluable contribution to the conclusion of this study. Finally, we gratefully acknowledge Baoussis for his indispensable assistance. Aikaterini E. Mantadaki and Emmanouil K. Symvoulakis contributed equally to this work.

Conflicts of Interest: The authors declare no conflicts of interest.

References

1. Gramatges, M.M.; Bertuch, A.A. Short Telomeres: From Dyskeratosis Congenita to Sporadic Aplastic Anemia and Malignancy. *Transl. Res.* **2013**, *162*, 353–363. [CrossRef]
2. Dhillon, V.; Bull, C.; Fenech, M. Chapter 10—Telomeres, Aging, and Nutrition. In *Molecular Basis of Nutrition and Aging*; Malavolta, M., Mocchegiani, E., Eds.; Academic Press: San Diego, CA, USA, 2016; pp. 129–140. ISBN 978-0-12-801816-3.
3. Maleki, M.; Khelghati, N.; Alemi, F.; Bazdar, M.; Asemi, Z.; Majidinia, M.; Sadeghpoor, A.; Mahmoodpoor, A.; Jadidi-Niaragh, F.; Targhazeh, N.; et al. Stabilization of Telomere by the Antioxidant Property of Polyphenols: Anti-Aging Potential. *Life Sci.* **2020**, *259*, 118341. [CrossRef]
4. Ruiz, A.; Flores-Gonzalez, J.; Buendia-Roldan, I.; Chavez-Galan, L. Telomere Shortening and Its Association with Cell Dysfunction in Lung Diseases. *Int. J. Mol. Sci.* **2022**, *23*, 425. [CrossRef] [PubMed]
5. Verdun, R.E.; Karlseder, J. Replication and Protection of Telomeres. *Nature* **2007**, *447*, 924–931. [CrossRef]
6. Shammas, M.A. Telomeres, Lifestyle, Cancer, and Aging. *Curr. Opin. Clin. Nutr. Metab. Care* **2011**, *14*, 28–34. [CrossRef]
7. Oeseburg, H.; de Boer, R.A.; van Gilst, W.H.; van der Harst, P. Telomere Biology in Healthy Aging and Disease. *Pflug. Arch.* **2010**, *459*, 259–268. [CrossRef] [PubMed]
8. Eppard, M.; Passos, J.F.; Victorelli, S. Telomeres, Cellular Senescence, and Aging: Past and Future. *Biogerontology* **2024**, *25*, 329–339. [CrossRef]
9. Coppé, J.-P.; Desprez, P.-Y.; Krtolica, A.; Campisi, J. The Senescence-Associated Secretory Phenotype: The Dark Side of Tumor Suppression. *Annu. Rev. Pathol.* **2010**, *5*, 99–118. [CrossRef]
10. Daniali, L.; Benetos, A.; Susser, E.; Kark, J.D.; Labat, C.; Kimura, M.; Desai, K.; Granick, M.; Aviv, A. Telomeres Shorten at Equivalent Rates in Somatic Tissues of Adults. *Nat. Commun.* **2013**, *4*, 1597. [CrossRef] [PubMed]
11. Fragkiadaki, P.; Renieri, E.; Kalliantasi, K.; Kouvidi, E.; Apalaki, E.; Vakonaki, E.; Mamoulakis, C.; Spandidos, D.A.; Tsatsakis, A. Telomerase Inhibitors and Activators in Aging and Cancer: A Systematic Review. *Mol. Med. Rep.* **2022**, *25*, 158. [CrossRef] [PubMed]
12. Kakridonis, F.; Pneumatikos, S.G.; Vakonaki, E.; Berdiaki, A.; Tzatzarakis, M.N.; Fragkiadaki, P.; Spandidos, D.A.; Baliou, S.; Ioannou, P.; Hatzidaki, E.; et al. Telomere Length as a Predictive Biomarker in Osteoporosis (Review). *Biomed. Rep.* **2023**, *19*, 87. [CrossRef]

13. Fragkiadaki, P.; Nikitovic, D.; Kalliantasi, K.; Sarandi, E.; Thanasoula, M.; Stivaktakis, P.; Nepka, C.; Spandidos, D.; Theodoros, T.; Tsatsakis, A. Telomere Length and Telomerase Activity in Osteoporosis and Osteoarthritis (Review). *Exp. Ther. Med.* **2019**, *19*, 1626–1632. [CrossRef] [PubMed]
14. Razgonova, M.P.; Zakharenko, A.M.; Golokhvast, K.S.; Thanasoula, M.; Sarandi, E.; Nikolouzakis, K.; Fragkiadaki, P.; Tsoukalas, D.; Spandidos, D.A.; Tsatsakis, A. Telomerase and Telomeres in Aging Theory and Chronographic Aging Theory (Review). *Mol. Med. Rep.* **2020**, *22*, 1679–1694. [CrossRef] [PubMed]
15. Vakonaki, E.; Tsiminikaki, K.; Plaitis, S.; Fragkiadaki, P.; Tsoukalas, D.; Katsikantami, I.; Vaki, G.; Tzatzarakis, M.N.; Spandidos, D.A.; Tsatsakis, A.M. Common Mental Disorders and Association with Telomere Length. *Biomed. Rep.* **2018**, *8*, 111–116. [CrossRef] [PubMed]
16. Fragkiadaki, P.; Tsoukalas, D.; Fragkiadoulaki, I.; Psycharakis, C.; Nikitovic, D.; Spandidos, D.A.; Tsatsakis, A.M. Telomerase Activity in Pregnancy Complications (Review). *Mol. Med. Rep.* **2016**, *14*, 16–21. [CrossRef]
17. Apetroaei, M.-M.; Fragkiadaki, P.; Velescu, B.Ș.; Baliou, S.; Renieri, E.; Dinu-Pirvu, C.E.; Drăgănescu, D.; Vlăsceanu, A.M.; Nedea, M.I.; Udeanu, D.I.; et al. Pharmacotherapeutic Considerations on Telomere Biology: The Positive Effect of Pharmacologically Active Substances on Telomere Length. *Int. J. Mol. Sci.* **2024**, *25*, 7694. [CrossRef]
18. Bonfigli, A.R.; Spazzafumo, L.; Prattichizzo, F.; Bonafè, M.; Mensà, E.; Micolucci, L.; Giuliani, A.; Fabbietti, P.; Testa, R.; Boemi, M.; et al. Leukocyte Telomere Length and Mortality Risk in Patients with Type 2 Diabetes. *Oncotarget* **2016**, *7*, 50835–50844. [CrossRef]
19. Palmer, A.K.; Tchkonia, T.; LeBrasseur, N.K.; Chini, E.N.; Xu, M.; Kirkland, J.L. Cellular Senescence in Type 2 Diabetes: A Therapeutic Opportunity. *Diabetes* **2015**, *64*, 2289–2298. [CrossRef]
20. Mantadaki, A.E.; Linardakis, M.; Tsakiri, M.; Baliou, S.; Fragkiadaki, P.; Vakonaki, E.; Tzatzarakis, M.N.; Tsatsakis, A.; Symvoulakis, E.K. Benefits of Quercetin on Glycated Hemoglobin, Blood Pressure, PiKo-6 Readings, Night-Time Sleep, Anxiety, and Quality of Life in Patients with Type 2 Diabetes Mellitus: A Randomized Controlled Trial. *J. Clin. Med.* **2024**, *13*, 3504. [CrossRef]
21. Palmer, A.K.; Gustafson, B.; Kirkland, J.L.; Smith, U. Cellular Senescence: At the Nexus between Ageing and Diabetes. *Diabetologia* **2019**, *62*, 1835–1841. [CrossRef]
22. Narasimhan, A.; Flores, R.R.; Robbins, P.D.; Niedernhofer, L.J. Role of Cellular Senescence in Type II Diabetes. *Endocrinology* **2021**, *162*, bqab136. [CrossRef] [PubMed]
23. Prattichizzo, F.; de Candia, P.; Ceriello, A. Diabetes and Kidney Disease: Emphasis on Treatment with SGLT-2 Inhibitors and GLP-1 Receptor Agonists. *Metabolism* **2021**, *120*, 154799. [CrossRef] [PubMed]
24. Murakami, T.; Inagaki, N.; Kondoh, H. Cellular Senescence in Diabetes Mellitus: Distinct Senotherapeutic Strategies for Adipose Tissue and Pancreatic β Cells. *Front. Endocrinol.* **2022**, *13*, 869414. [CrossRef]
25. Iwasaki, K.; Abarca, C.; Aguayo-Mazzucato, C. Regulation of Cellular Senescence in Type 2 Diabetes Mellitus: From Mechanisms to Clinical Applications. *Diabetes Metab. J.* **2023**, *47*, 441–453. [CrossRef] [PubMed]
26. Martel, J.; Ojcius, D.M.; Wu, C.-Y.; Peng, H.-H.; Voisin, L.; Perfettini, J.-L.; Ko, Y.-F.; Young, J.D. Emerging Use of Senolytics and Senomorphics against Aging and Chronic Diseases. *Med. Res. Rev.* **2020**, *40*, 2114–2131. [CrossRef]
27. Boccardi, V.; Paolisso, G. Telomerase Activation: A Potential Key Modulator for Human Healthspan and Longevity. *Ageing Res. Rev.* **2014**, *15*, 1–5. [CrossRef]
28. Jafri, M.A.; Ansari, S.A.; Alqahtani, M.H.; Shay, J.W. Roles of Telomeres and Telomerase in Cancer, and Advances in Telomerase-Targeted Therapies. *Genome Med.* **2016**, *8*, 69. [CrossRef]
29. Yuan, X.; Larsson, C.; Xu, D. Mechanisms Underlying the Activation of TERT Transcription and Telomerase Activity in Human Cancer: Old Actors and New Players. *Oncogene* **2019**, *38*, 6172–6183. [CrossRef]
30. Zhang, L.; Pitcher, L.E.; Yousefzadeh, M.J.; Niedernhofer, L.J.; Robbins, P.D.; Zhu, Y. Cellular Senescence: A Key Therapeutic Target in Aging and Diseases. *J. Clin. Investig.* **2022**, *132*, e158450. [CrossRef]
31. D'Andrea, G. Quercetin: A Flavonol with Multifaceted Therapeutic Applications? *Fitoterapia* **2015**, *106*, 256–271. [CrossRef]
32. Mbara, K.C.; Devnarain, N.; Owira, P.M.O. Potential Role of Polyphenolic Flavonoids as Senotherapeutic Agents in Degenerative Diseases and Geroprotection. *Pharm. Med.* **2022**, *36*, 331–352. [CrossRef]
33. Shao, Z.; Wang, B.; Shi, Y.; Xie, C.; Huang, C.; Chen, B.; Zhang, H.; Zeng, G.; Liang, H.; Wu, Y.; et al. Senolytic Agent Quercetin Ameliorates Intervertebral Disc Degeneration *via* the Nrf2/NF-κB Axis. *Osteoarthr. Cartil.* **2021**, *29*, 413–422. [CrossRef]
34. Kim, S.R.; Jiang, K.; Ogrodnik, M.; Chen, X.; Zhu, X.-Y.; Lohmeier, H.; Ahmed, L.; Tang, H.; Tchkonia, T.; Hickson, L.J.; et al. Increased Renal Cellular Senescence in Murine High-Fat Diet: Effect of the Senolytic Drug Quercetin. *Transl. Res.* **2019**, *213*, 112–123. [CrossRef] [PubMed]
35. Aghababaei, F.; Hadidi, M. Recent Advances in Potential Health Benefits of Quercetin. *Pharmaceuticals* **2023**, *16*, 1020. [CrossRef] [PubMed]
36. Chiang, M.-C.; Tsai, T.-Y.; Wang, C.-J. The Potential Benefits of Quercetin for Brain Health: A Review of Anti-Inflammatory and Neuroprotective Mechanisms. *Int. J. Mol. Sci.* **2023**, *24*, 6328. [CrossRef]
37. Ioannou, P.; Baliou, S. The Molecular Mechanisms and Therapeutic Potential of Cranberry, D-Mannose, and Flavonoids against Infectious Diseases: The Example of Urinary Tract Infections. *Antibiotics* **2024**, *13*, 593. [CrossRef]
38. Mantadaki, A.E.; Linardakis, M.; Vafeiadi, M.; Anastasiou, F.; Tsatsakis, A.; Symvoulakis, E.K. The Impact of Three-Month Quercetin Intake on Quality of Life and Anxiety in Patients with Type II Diabetes Mellitus: An Early Data Analysis from a Randomized Controlled Trial. *Cureus* **2024**, *16*, e58219. [CrossRef] [PubMed]

39. Shatylo, V.; Antoniuk-Shcheglova, I.; Naskalova, S.; Bondarenko, O.; Havalko, A.; Krasnienkov, D.; Zabuga, O.; Kukharskyy, V.; Guryanov, V.; Vaiserman, A. Cardio-Metabolic Benefits of Quercetin in Elderly Patients with Metabolic Syndrome. *PharmaNutrition* **2021**, *15*, 100250. [CrossRef]
40. O'Callaghan, N.J.; Fenech, M. A Quantitative PCR Method for Measuring Absolute Telomere Length. *Biol. Proced. Online* **2011**, *13*, 3. [CrossRef]
41. Lai, T.-P.; Wright, W.E.; Shay, J.W. Comparison of Telomere Length Measurement Methods. *Philos. Trans. R. Soc. B Biol. Sci.* **2018**, *373*, 20160451. [CrossRef]
42. O'Callaghan, N.J.; Dhillon, V.S.; Thomas, P.; Fenech, M. A Quantitative Real-Time PCR Method for Absolute Telomere Length. *BioTechniques* **2008**, *44*, 807–809. [CrossRef]
43. Kahl, V.F.S.; Allen, J.A.M.; Nelson, C.B.; Sobinoff, A.P.; Lee, M.; Kilo, T.; Vasireddy, R.S.; Pickett, H.A. Telomere Length Measurement by Molecular Combing. *Front. Cell Dev. Biol.* **2020**, *8*, 493. [CrossRef] [PubMed]
44. Lindrose, A.R.; McLester-Davis, L.W.Y.; Tristano, R.I.; Kataria, L.; Gadalla, S.M.; Eisenberg, D.T.A.; Verhulst, S.; Drury, S. Method Comparison Studies of Telomere Length Measurement Using qPCR Approaches: A Critical Appraisal of the Literature. *PLoS ONE* **2021**, *16*, e0245582. [CrossRef] [PubMed]
45. ISRCTN—ISRCTN13131584: Study on the Benefit of Quercetin Intake in Diabetic Patients Treated with Antidiabetic Tablets. Available online: https://www.isrctn.com/ISRCTN13131584 (accessed on 14 July 2024).
46. Behrens, Y.L.; Thomay, K.; Hagedorn, M.; Ebersold, J.; Henrich, L.; Nustede, R.; Schlegelberger, B.; Göhring, G. Comparison of Different Methods for Telomere Length Measurement in Whole Blood and Blood Cell Subsets: Recommendations for Telomere Length Measurement in Hematological Diseases. *Genes Chromosomes Cancer* **2017**, *56*, 700–708. [CrossRef] [PubMed]
47. Butler, M.G.; Tilburt, J.; DeVries, A.; Muralidhar, B.; Aue, G.; Hedges, L.; Atkinson, J.; Schwartz, H. Comparison of Chromosome Telomere Integrity in Multiple Tissues from Subjects at Different Ages. *Cancer Genet. Cytogenet.* **1998**, *105*, 138–144. [CrossRef]
48. Arai, Y.; Martin-Ruiz, C.M.; Takayama, M.; Abe, Y.; Takebayashi, T.; Koyasu, S.; Suematsu, M.; Hirose, N.; von Zglinicki, T. Inflammation, But Not Telomere Length, Predicts Successful Ageing at Extreme Old Age: A Longitudinal Study of Semi-Supercentenarians. *EBioMedicine* **2015**, *2*, 1549–1558. [CrossRef]
49. Vaiserman, A.; Krasnienkov, D. Telomere Length as a Marker of Biological Age: State-of-the-Art, Open Issues, and Future Perspectives. *Front. Genet.* **2021**, *11*, 630186. [CrossRef]
50. Shin, D.-Y.; Lim, K.M.; Park, H.S.; Kwon, S.; Yoon, S.-S.; Lee, D.-S. The Importance of Critically Short Telomere in Myelodysplastic Syndrome. *Biomark. Res.* **2022**, *10*, 79. [CrossRef]
51. Whittemore, K.; Vera, E.; Martínez-Nevado, E.; Sanpera, C.; Blasco, M.A. Telomere Shortening Rate Predicts Species Life Span. *Proc. Natl. Acad. Sci. USA* **2019**, *116*, 15122–15127. [CrossRef]
52. Yan, X.; Yang, P.; Li, Y.; Liu, T.; Zha, Y.; Wang, T.; Zhang, J.; Feng, Z.; Li, M. New Insights from Bidirectional Mendelian Randomization: Causal Relationships between Telomere Length and Mitochondrial DNA Copy Number in Aging Biomarkers. *Aging* **2024**, *16*, 7387. [CrossRef]
53. Cheng, F.; Carroll, L.; Joglekar, M.V.; Januszewski, A.S.; Wong, K.K.; Hardikar, A.A.; Jenkins, A.J.; Ma, R.C.W. Diabetes, Metabolic Disease, and Telomere Length. *Lancet Diabetes Endocrinol.* **2021**, *9*, 117–126. [CrossRef] [PubMed]
54. Cheng, F.; Luk, A.O.; Shi, M.; Huang, C.; Jiang, G.; Yang, A.; Wu, H.; Lim, C.K.P.; Tam, C.H.T.; Fan, B.; et al. Shortened Leukocyte Telomere Length Is Associated With Glycemic Progression in Type 2 Diabetes: A Prospective and Mendelian Randomization Analysis. *Diabetes Care* **2022**, *45*, 701–709. [CrossRef] [PubMed]
55. Salpea, K.D.; Humphries, S.E. Telomere Length in Atherosclerosis and Diabetes. *Atherosclerosis* **2010**, *209*, 35–38. [CrossRef] [PubMed]
56. Hickson, L.J.; Langhi Prata, L.G.P.; Bobart, S.A.; Evans, T.K.; Giorgadze, N.; Hashmi, S.K.; Herrmann, S.M.; Jensen, M.D.; Jia, Q.; Jordan, K.L.; et al. Senolytics Decrease Senescent Cells in Humans: Preliminary Report from a Clinical Trial of Dasatinib plus Quercetin in Individuals with Diabetic Kidney Disease. *EBioMedicine* **2019**, *47*, 446–456. [CrossRef] [PubMed]
57. Zhu, Y.; Tchkonia, T.; Pirtskhalava, T.; Gower, A.C.; Ding, H.; Giorgadze, N.; Palmer, A.K.; Ikeno, Y.; Hubbard, G.B.; Lenburg, M.; et al. The Achilles' Heel of Senescent Cells: From Transcriptome to Senolytic Drugs. *Aging Cell* **2015**, *14*, 644–658. [CrossRef]
58. Crous-Bou, M.; Molinuevo, J.-L.; Sala-Vila, A. Plant-Rich Dietary Patterns, Plant Foods and Nutrients, and Telomere Length. *Adv. Nutr.* **2019**, *10*, S296–S303. [CrossRef]
59. Rahman, S.T.; Waterhouse, M.; Pham, H.; Romero, B.D.; Baxter, C.; McLeod, D.S.A.; English, D.R.; Ebeling, P.R.; Hartel, G.; Armstrong, B.K.; et al. Effects of Vitamin D Supplementation on Telomere Length: An Analysis of Data from the Randomised Controlled D-Health Trial. *J. Nutr. Health Aging* **2023**, *27*, 609–616. Available online: https://link.springer.com/article/10.1007/s12603-023-1948-3 (accessed on 18 July 2024). [CrossRef]
60. Kiecolt-Glaser, J.K.; Epel, E.S.; Belury, M.A.; Andridge, R.; Lin, J.; Glaser, R.; Malarkey, W.B.; Hwang, B.S.; Blackburn, E. Omega-3 Fatty Acids, Oxidative Stress, and Leukocyte Telomere Length: A Randomized Controlled Trial. *Brain Behav. Immun.* **2013**, *28*, 16–24. [CrossRef]
61. O'Callaghan, N.; Parletta, N.; Milte, C.M.; Benassi-Evans, B.; Fenech, M.; Howe, P.R.C. Telomere Shortening in Elderly Individuals with Mild Cognitive Impairment May Be Attenuated with ω-3 Fatty Acid Supplementation: A Randomized Controlled Pilot Study. *Nutrition* **2014**, *30*, 489–491. [CrossRef]

62. Freitas-Simoes, T.-M.; Cofán, M.; Blasco, M.A.; Soberón, N.; Foronda, M.; Serra-Mir, M.; Roth, I.; Valls-Pedret, C.; Doménech, M.; Ponferrada-Ariza, E.; et al. Walnut Consumption for Two Years and Leukocyte Telomere Attrition in Mediterranean Elders: Results of a Randomized Controlled Trial. *Nutrients* **2018**, *10*, 1907. [CrossRef]
63. Pusceddu, I.; Herrmann, M.; Kirsch, S.H.; Werner, C.; Hübner, U.; Bodis, M.; Laufs, U.; Widmann, T.; Wagenpfeil, S.; Geisel, J.; et al. One-Carbon Metabolites and Telomere Length in a Prospective and Randomized Study of B- and/or D-Vitamin Supplementation. *Eur. J. Nutr.* **2017**, *56*, 1887–1898. [CrossRef]
64. Exploring the Effects of Dasatinib, Quercetin, and Fisetin on DNA Methylation Clocks: A Longitudinal Study on Senolytic Interventions—PMC. Available online: https://www.ncbi.nlm.nih.gov/pmc/articles/PMC10929829/ (accessed on 20 July 2024).
65. Hachmo, Y.; Hadanny, A.; Hamed, R.A.; Daniel-Kotovsky, M.; Catalogna, M.; Fishlev, G.; Lang, E.; Polak, N.; Doenyas, K.; Friedman, M.; et al. Hyperbaric Oxygen Therapy Increases Telomere Length and Decreases Immunosenescence in Isolated Blood Cells: A Prospective Trial. *Aging* **2020**, *12*, 22445–22456. [CrossRef] [PubMed]
66. Carroll, J.E.; Esquivel, S.; Goldberg, A.; Seeman, T.E.; Effros, R.B.; Dock, J.; Olmstead, R.; Breen, E.C.; Irwin, M.R. Insomnia and Telomere Length in Older Adults. *Sleep* **2016**, *39*, 559–564. [CrossRef] [PubMed]
67. Tempaku, P.; Hirotsu, C.; Mazzotti, D.; Xavier, G.; Maurya, P.; Brietzke, E.; Belangero, S.; Poyares, D.; Bittencourt, L.; Tufik, S. Long Sleep Duration, Insomnia, and Insomnia with Short Objective Sleep Duration Are Independently Associated With Short Telomere Length. *J. Clin. Sleep Med.* **2018**, *14*, 2037–2045. [CrossRef]
68. Jin, J.-H.; Kwon, H.S.; Choi, S.H.; Koh, S.-H.; Lee, E.-H.; Jeong, J.H.; Jang, J.-W.; Park, K.W.; Kim, E.-J.; Kim, H.J.; et al. Association between Sleep Parameters and Longitudinal Shortening of Telomere Length. *Aging* **2022**, *14*, 2930–2944. [CrossRef] [PubMed]
69. Choi, E.S.; Chang, Y.K.; Lee, D.H.; Ko, J.-H.; Lim, I.; Bang, H.; Kim, J.-H. Gender-Specific Associations between Quality of Life and Leukocyte Telomere Length. *Maturitas* **2018**, *107*, 68–70. [CrossRef] [PubMed]
70. Huzen, J.; van der Harst, P.; de Boer, R.A.; Lesman-Leegte, I.; Voors, A.A.; van Gilst, W.H.; Samani, N.J.; Jaarsma, T.; van Veldhuisen, D.J. Telomere Length and Psychological Well-Being in Patients with Chronic Heart Failure. *Age Ageing* **2010**, *39*, 223–227. [CrossRef]
71. Tsur, N.; Levin, Y.; Abumock, H.; Solomon, Z. One 'Knows': Self-Rated Health and Telomere Length among Ex-Prisoners of War. *Psychol. Health* **2018**, *33*, 1503–1518. [CrossRef]
72. Tellechea, M.L.; Pirola, C.J. The Impact of Hypertension on Leukocyte Telomere Length: A Systematic Review and Meta-Analysis of Human Studies. *J. Hum. Hypertens.* **2017**, *31*, 99–105. [CrossRef]
73. Lung, F.-W.; Ku, C.-S.; Kao, W.-T. Telomere Length May Be Associated with Hypertension. *J. Hum. Hypertens.* **2008**, *22*, 230–232. [CrossRef]
74. Monickaraj, F.; Aravind, S.; Gokulakrishnan, K.; Sathishkumar, C.; Prabu, P.; Prabu, D.; Mohan, V.; Balasubramanyam, M. Accelerated Aging as Evidenced by Increased Telomere Shortening and Mitochondrial DNA Depletion in Patients with Type 2 Diabetes. *Mol. Cell. Biochem.* **2012**, *365*, 343–350. [CrossRef] [PubMed]
75. Ojeda-Rodriguez, A.; Morell-Azanza, L.; Alonso-Pedrero, L.; del Moral, A.M. Chapter 12—Aging, Telomere Integrity, and Antioxidant Food. In *Obesity*; del Moral, A.M., Aguilera García, C.M., Eds.; Academic Press: Cambridge, MA, USA, 2018; pp. 241–261. ISBN 978-0-12-812504-5. [CrossRef]
76. Prasad, K.N.; Wu, M.; Bondy, S.C. Telomere Shortening during Aging: Attenuation by Antioxidants and Anti-Inflammatory Agents. *Mech. Ageing Dev.* **2017**, *164*, 61–66. [CrossRef] [PubMed]
77. D'Angelo, S. Diet and Aging: The Role of Polyphenol-Rich Diets in Slow Down the Shortening of Telomeres: A Review. *Antioxidants* **2023**, *12*, 2086. [CrossRef] [PubMed]
78. Heger, V.; Tyni, J.; Hunyadi, A.; Horáková, L.; Lahtela-Kakkonen, M.; Rahnasto-Rilla, M. Quercetin Based Derivatives as Sirtuin Inhibitors. *Biomed. Pharmacother.* **2019**, *111*, 1326–1333. [CrossRef]
79. Ungurianu, A.; Zanfirescu, A.; Margină, D. Exploring the Therapeutic Potential of Quercetin: A Focus on Its Sirtuin-Mediated Benefits. *Phytother. Res.* **2024**, *38*, 2361–2387. [CrossRef] [PubMed]
80. Cui, Z.; Zhao, X.; Amevor, F.K.; Du, X.; Wang, Y.; Li, D.; Shu, G.; Tian, Y.; Zhao, X. Therapeutic Application of Quercetin in Aging-Related Diseases: SIRT1 as a Potential Mechanism. *Front. Immunol.* **2022**, *13*, 943321. [CrossRef] [PubMed]
81. Rahnasto-Rilla, M.; Tyni, J.; Huovinen, M.; Jarho, E.; Kulikowicz, T.; Ravichandran, S.; Bohr, V.A.; Ferrucci, L.; Lahtela-Kakkonen, M.; Moaddel, R. Natural Polyphenols as Sirtuin 6 Modulators. *Sci. Rep.* **2018**, *8*, 4163. [CrossRef] [PubMed]
82. Su, Q.; Peng, M.; Zhang, Y.; Xu, W.; Darko, K.O.; Tao, T.; Huang, Y.; Tao, X.; Yang, X. Quercetin Induces Bladder Cancer Cells Apoptosis by Activation of AMPK Signaling Pathway. *Am. J. Cancer Res.* **2016**, *6*, 498–508.
83. Guo, H.; Ding, H.; Tang, X.; Liang, M.; Li, S.; Zhang, J.; Cao, J. Quercetin Induces Pro-Apoptotic Autophagy via SIRT1/AMPK Signaling Pathway in Human Lung Cancer Cell Lines A549 and H1299 In Vitro. *Thorac. Cancer* **2021**, *12*, 1415–1422. [CrossRef]
84. Shen, Y.; Croft, K.D.; Hodgson, J.M.; Kyle, R.; Lee, I.-L.E.; Wang, Y.; Stocker, R.; Ward, N.C. Quercetin and Its Metabolites Improve Vessel Function by Inducing eNOS Activity via Phosphorylation of AMPK. *Biochem. Pharmacol.* **2012**, *84*, 1036–1044. [CrossRef]
85. Jacczak, B.; Rubiś, B.; Totoń, E. Potential of Naturally Derived Compounds in Telomerase and Telomere Modulation in Skin Senescence and Aging. *Int. J. Mol. Sci.* **2021**, *22*, 6381. [CrossRef] [PubMed]
86. Khan, F.; Niaz, K.; Maqbool, F.; Ismail Hassan, F.; Abdollahi, M.; Nagulapalli Venkata, K.C.; Nabavi, S.M.; Bishayee, A. Molecular Targets Underlying the Anticancer Effects of Quercetin: An Update. *Nutrients* **2016**, *8*, 529. [CrossRef] [PubMed]
87. Ganesan, K.; Xu, B. Telomerase Inhibitors from Natural Products and Their Anticancer Potential. *Int. J. Mol. Sci.* **2018**, *19*, 13. [CrossRef]

88. Parekh, N.; Garg, A.; Choudhary, R.; Gupta, M.; Kaur, G.; Ramniwas, S.; Shahwan, M.; Tuli, H.S.; Sethi, G. The Role of Natural Flavonoids as Telomerase Inhibitors in Suppressing Cancer Growth. *Pharmaceuticals* **2023**, *16*, 605. [CrossRef] [PubMed]
89. Cui, S.; Wu, X.; Wang, Z.; Guo, Y.; Xu, R. Quercetin Regulates Telomere-Binding Proteins Expression of POT1, TRF1, TRF2 TO Inhibit Proliferation and Induce Apoptosis in AML THP-1 Cells. Available online: https://library.ehaweb.org/eha/2017/22nd/182385/ruirong.xu.quercetin.regulates.telomere-binding.proteins.expression.of.pot1.html (accessed on 22 July 2024).
90. Avci, C.B.; Yilmaz, S.; Dogan, Z.O.; Saydam, G.; Dodurga, Y.; Ekiz, H.A.; Kartal, M.; Sahin, F.; Baran, Y.; Gunduz, C. Quercetin-Induced Apoptosis Involves Increased hTERT Enzyme Activity of Leukemic Cells. *Hematology* **2011**, *16*, 303–307. [CrossRef]
91. Bhatiya, M.; Pathak, S.; Jothimani, G.; Duttaroy, A.K.; Banerjee, A. A Comprehensive Study on the Anti-Cancer Effects of Quercetin and Its Epigenetic Modifications in Arresting Progression of Colon Cancer Cell Proliferation. *Arch. Immunol. Ther. Exp.* **2023**, *71*, 6. [CrossRef]
92. Zhu, J.; Cheng, X.; Naumovski, N.; Hu, L.; Wang, K. Epigenetic Regulation by Quercetin: A Comprehensive Review Focused on Its Biological Mechanisms. *Crit. Rev. Food Sci. Nutr.* **2023**, 1–20. [CrossRef]
93. Canela, A.; Vera, E.; Klatt, P.; Blasco, M.A. High-Throughput Telomere Length Quantification by FISH and Its Application to Human Population Studies. *Proc. Natl. Acad. Sci. USA* **2007**, *104*, 5300–5305. [CrossRef]
94. Tsatsakis, A.; Tsoukalas, D.; Fragkiadaki, P.; Vakonaki, E.; Tzatzarakis, M.; Sarandi, E.; Nikitovic, D.; Tsilimidos, G.; Alegakis, A.K. Developing BIOTEL: A Semi-Automated Spreadsheet for Estimating Telomere Length and Biological Age. *Front. Genet.* **2019**, *10*, 84. [CrossRef]
95. Dweck, A.; Maitra, R. The Advancement of Telomere Quantification Methods. *Mol. Biol. Rep.* **2021**, *48*, 5621–5627. [CrossRef]
96. Vera, E.; Blasco, M.A. Beyond Average: Potential for Measurement of Short Telomeres. *Aging* **2012**, *4*, 379–392. [CrossRef] [PubMed]
97. Joksic, G.; Joksic, I.; Filipović, J.; Liehr, T. Telomere Length Measurement by FISH. In *Fluorescence In Situ Hybridization (FISH): Application Guide*; Liehr, T., Ed.; Springer: Berlin/Heidelberg, Germany, 2017; pp. 147–152. ISBN 978-3-662-52959-1.
98. Heritier, S.R.; Gebski, V.J.; Keech, A.C. Inclusion of Patients in Clinical Trial Analysis: The Intention-to-Treat Principle. *Med. J. Aust.* **2003**, *179*, 438–440. [CrossRef] [PubMed]
99. Matacchione, G.; Perugini, J.; Di Mercurio, E.; Sabbatinelli, J.; Prattichizzo, F.; Senzacqua, M.; Storci, G.; Dani, C.; Lezoche, G.; Guerrieri, M.; et al. Senescent Macrophages in the Human Adipose Tissue as a Source of Inflammaging. *Geroscience* **2022**, *44*, 1941–1960. [CrossRef] [PubMed]
100. Faul, F.; Erdfelder, E.; Lang, A.-G.; Buchner, A. G*Power 3: A Flexible Statistical Power Analysis Program for the Social, Behavioral, and Biomedical Sciences. *Behav. Res. Methods* **2007**, *39*, 175–191. [CrossRef] [PubMed]
101. Faul, F.; Erdfelder, E.; Buchner, A.; Lang, A.-G. Statistical Power Analyses Using G*Power 3.1: Tests for Correlation and Regression Analyses. *Behav. Res. Methods* **2009**, *41*, 1149–1160. [CrossRef]
102. Kiecolt-Glaser, J.K.; Belury, M.A.; Andridge, R.; Malarkey, W.B.; Hwang, B.S.; Glaser, R. Omega-3 Supplementation Lowers Inflammation in Healthy Middle-Aged and Older Adults: A Randomized Controlled Trial. *Brain Behav. Immun.* **2012**, *26*, 988–995. [CrossRef]
103. Harrigan, M.; Cartmel, B.; Loftfield, E.; Sanft, T.; Chagpar, A.B.; Zhou, Y.; Playdon, M.; Li, F.; Irwin, M.L. Randomized Trial Comparing Telephone Versus In-Person Weight Loss Counseling on Body Composition and Circulating Biomarkers in Women Treated for Breast Cancer: The Lifestyle, Exercise, and Nutrition (LEAN) Study. *J. Clin. Oncol.* **2016**, *34*, 669–676. [CrossRef]
104. Sanft, T.; Usiskin, I.; Harrigan, M.; Cartmel, B.; Lu, L.; Li, F.-Y.; Zhou, Y.; Chagpar, A.; Ferrucci, L.M.; Pusztai, L.; et al. Randomized Controlled Trial of Weight Loss versus Usual Care on Telomere Length in Women with Breast Cancer: The Lifestyle, Exercise, and Nutrition (LEAN) Study. *Breast Cancer Res. Treat.* **2018**, *172*, 105–112. [CrossRef]
105. Opstad, T.B.; Alexander, J.; Aaseth, J.O.; Larsson, A.; Seljeflot, I.; Alehagen, U. Selenium and Coenzyme Q10 Intervention Prevents Telomere Attrition, with Association to Reduced Cardiovascular Mortality—Sub-Study of a Randomized Clinical Trial. *Nutrients* **2022**, *14*, 3346. [CrossRef]
106. Ward, S.J.; Hill, A.M.; Buckley, J.D.; Banks, S.; Dhillon, V.S.; Holman, S.L.; Morrison, J.L.; Coates, A.M. Minimal Changes in Telomere Length after a 12-Week Dietary Intervention with Almonds in Mid-Age to Older, Overweight and Obese Australians: Results of a Randomised Clinical Trial. *Br. J. Nutr.* **2022**, *127*, 872–884. [CrossRef]
107. Denham, J.; O'Brien, B.J.; Prestes, P.R.; Brown, N.J.; Charchar, F.J. Increased Expression of Telomere-Regulating Genes in Endurance Athletes with Long Leukocyte Telomeres. *J. Appl. Physiol.* **2016**, *120*, 148–158. [CrossRef] [PubMed]
108. Manchia, M.; Paribello, P.; Arzedi, C.; Bocchetta, A.; Caria, P.; Cocco, C.; Congiu, D.; Cossu, E.; Dettori, T.; Frau, D.V.; et al. A Multidisciplinary Approach to Mental Illness: Do Inflammation, Telomere Length and Microbiota Form a Loop? A Protocol for a Cross-Sectional Study on the Complex Relationship between Inflammation, Telomere Length, Gut Microbiota and Psychiatric Disorders. *BMJ Open* **2020**, *10*, e032513. [CrossRef]
109. Franzoni, L.T.; Garcia, E.L.; Motta, S.B.; Ahner, M.M.; Bertoletti, O.A.; Saffi, M.A.L.; da Silveira, A.D.; Pereira, A.A.; Pereira, A.H.; Danzmann, L.C.; et al. Aerobic Exercise and Telomere Length in Patients with Systolic Heart Failure: Protocol Study for a Randomized Controlled Trial. *Trials* **2022**, *23*, 283. [CrossRef] [PubMed]
110. Tsoukalas, D.; Fragkiadaki, P.; Docea, A.O.; Alegakis, A.K.; Sarandi, E.; Vakonaki, E.; Salataj, E.; Kouvidi, E.; Nikitovic, D.; Kovatsi, L.; et al. Association of Nutraceutical Supplements with Longer Telomere Length. *Int. J. Mol. Med.* **2019**, *44*, 218–226. [CrossRef] [PubMed]

111. Tsatsakis, A.; Renieri, E.; Tsoukalas, D.; Buga, A.M.; Sarandi, E.; Vakonaki, E.; Fragkiadaki, P.; Alegakis, A.; Nikitovic, D.; Calina, D.; et al. A Novel Nutraceutical Formulation Increases Telomere Length and Activates Telomerase Activity in Middle-aged Rats. *Mol. Med. Rep.* **2023**, *28*, 1–11. [CrossRef]
112. Chung, S.S.; Dutta, P.; Chard, N.; Wu, Y.; Chen, Q.-H.; Chen, G.; Vadgama, J. A Novel Curcumin Analog Inhibits Canonical and Non-Canonical Functions of Telomerase through STAT3 and NF-κB Inactivation in Colorectal Cancer Cells. *Oncotarget* **2019**, *10*, 4516–4531. [CrossRef]
113. Precision in qPCR—GR. Available online: https://www.thermofisher.com/tr/en/home/life-science/pcr/real-time-pcr/real-time-pcr-learning-center/gene-expression-analysis-real-time-pcr-information/precision-qpcr.html (accessed on 20 July 2024).
114. Taylor, S.; Wakem, M.; Dijkman, G.; Alsarraj, M.; Nguyen, M. A Practical Approach to RT-qPCR—Publishing Data That Conform to the MIQE Guidelines. *Methods* **2010**, *50*, S1–S5. [CrossRef]
115. Kitchen, R.R.; Kubista, M.; Tichopad, A. Statistical Aspects of Quantitative Real-Time PCR Experiment Design. *Methods* **2010**, *50*, 231–236. [CrossRef]
116. Livak, K.J.; Schmittgen, T.D. Analysis of Relative Gene Expression Data Using Real-Time Quantitative PCR and the $2-\Delta\Delta CT$ Method. *Methods* **2001**, *25*, 402–408. [CrossRef]
117. Schmittgen, T.D.; Livak, K.J. Analyzing Real-Time PCR Data by the Comparative CT Method. *Nat. Protoc.* **2008**, *3*, 1101–1108. [CrossRef]
118. Linardakis, M.; Papadaki, A.; Smpokos, E.; Kafatos, A.; Lionis, C. Prevalence of Multiple Behavioral Risk Factors for Chronic Diseases in Medical Students and Associations with Their Academic Performance. *J. Public Health* **2020**, *28*, 383–392. [CrossRef]
119. Linardakis, M.; Papadaki, A.; Smpokos, E.; Micheli, K.; Vozikaki, M.; Philalithis, A. Relationship of Behavioral Risk Factors for Chronic Diseases and Preventive Health Services Utilization among Adults, Aged 50+, from Eleven European Countries. *J. Public Health* **2015**, *23*, 257–265. [CrossRef]
120. Symvoulakis, E.K.; Stachteas, P.; Smyrnakis, E.; Volkos, P.; Mantadaki, A.E.; Karelis, A.; Petraki, C.; Nioti, K.; Mastronikolis, S.; Antoniou, A.M.; et al. Multiple Behavioral Risk Factors As Assets for Chronic Disease Prevention: Observations From Urban Primary Care Settings in Crete, Greece. *Cureus* **2024**, *16*, e56711. [CrossRef]
121. Nagelkerke, N.J.D. A Note on a General Definition of the Coefficient of Determination. *Biometrika* **1991**, *78*, 691–692. [CrossRef]
122. ICH Harmonised Guideline Integrated Addendum to ICH E6(R1): Guideline for Good Clinical Practice ICH E6(R2) ICH Consensus Guideline. Available online: https://ichgcp.net/home (accessed on 25 April 2024).
123. European Medicines Agency Guideline for Good Clinical Practice E6 (R2). Available online: https://www.ema.europa.eu/en/documents/scientific-guideline/ich-guideline-good-clinical-practice-e6r2-4-step-2b_en.pdf (accessed on 22 March 2024).
124. European Parliament and the Council of the European Union Regulation (EU) No 536/2014 of the European Parliament and of the Council of 16 April 2014 on Clinical Trials on Medicinal Products for Human Use, and Repealing Directive 2001/20/EC. Available online: https://health.ec.europa.eu/document/download/f724d198-9ec8-4cad-9ce7-b6d2ac1ec44e_en (accessed on 22 March 2024).
125. World Medical Association. World Medical Association Declaration of Helsinki: Ethical Principles for Medical Research Involving Human Subjects. *JAMA* **2013**, *310*, 2191–2194. [CrossRef] [PubMed]
126. Moher, D.; Hopewell, S.; Schulz, K.F.; Montori, V.; Gøtzsche, P.C.; Devereaux, P.J.; Elbourne, D.; Egger, M.; Altman, D.G. CONSORT 2010 Explanation and Elaboration: Updated Guidelines for Reporting Parallel Group Randomised Trials. *BMJ* **2010**, *340*, c869. [CrossRef]
127. World Health Organization. *Handbook for Good Clinical Research Practice (GCP): Guidance for Implementation*; World Health Organization: Geneva, Switzerland, 2005; Available online: https://iris.who.int/bitstream/handle/10665/43392/924159392X_eng.pdf (accessed on 14 July 2024).
128. International Council For Harmonisation (ICH). Harmonised Guideline on Genomic Sampling and Management of Genomic Data E18. Available online: https://database.ich.org/sites/default/files/E18_Guideline.pdf (accessed on 14 July 2024).
129. European Medicines Agency (EMA). ICH Guideline E18 on Genomic Sampling and Management of Genomic Data. Available online: https://www.ema.europa.eu/en/documents/scientific-guideline/ich-guideline-e18-genomic-sampling-and-management-genomic-data-step-3_en.pdf (accessed on 14 July 2024).

pharmaceuticals

MDPI

Article

Effects of Carnosine Supplementation on Cognitive Outcomes in Prediabetes and Well-Controlled Type 2 Diabetes: A Randomised Placebo-Controlled Clinical Trial

Rohit Hariharan [1,2], Aya Mousa [1,*], Kirthi Menon [1], Jack Feehan [3], Barbara Ukropcová [4], Jozef Ukropec [4], Martin Schön [5,6,7], Arshad Majid [8], Giancarlo Aldini [9], Maximilian de Courten [10], James Cameron [2], Simon M. Bell [8,11,12] and Barbora de Courten [2,3,*]

1 Monash Centre for Health Research Implementation, Faculty of Medicine, Nursing and Health Sciences, Monash University, 43–51 Kanooka Grove, Clayton, VIC 3168, Australia; rohit.hariharan@monash.edu (R.H.); kirthimenon7@gmail.com (K.M.)
2 Department of Medicine, School of Clinical Sciences, Faculty of Medicine, Nursing and Health Sciences, Monash University, 246 Clayton Road, Clayton, VIC 3168, Australia; james.cameron@monash.edu
3 School of Health and Biomedical Sciences, STEM College, RMIT University, 30 Janefield Drive, Bundoora, VIC 3083, Australia; jack.feehan@rmit.edu.au
4 Department of Metabolic Disease Research, Institute of Experimental Endocrinology, Biomedical Research Centre, Slovak Academy of Sciences, Dúbravská Cesta 9, 845 05 Bratislava, Slovakia; barbara.ukropcova@gmail.com (B.U.); jozef.ukropec@savba.sk (J.U.)
5 Division of Endocrinology and Diabetology, Medical Faculty and University Hospital Düsseldorf, Heinrich Heine University, Moorenstraße 5 Universitätsklinikum, 40225 Düsseldorf, Germany; martin.schoen@ddz.de
6 Institute for Clinical Diabetology, German Diabetes Center, Leibniz Center for Diabetes Research at Heinrich Heine University, Auf'm Hennekamp 65, 40225 Düsseldorf, Germany
7 German Center for Diabetes Research (DZD), Ingolstädter Landstraße 1, 85764 Neuherberg, Germany
8 Sheffield Institute for Translational Neuroscience, School of Medicine and Population Health, University of Sheffield, 385a Glossop Rd, Sheffield S10 2HQ, UK; arshad.majid@sheffield.ac.uk (A.M.); s.m.bell@sheffield.ac.uk (S.M.B.)
9 Department of Pharmaceutical Sciences, University of Milan, Via Luigi Mangiagalli, 25, 20133 Milan, Italy; giancarlo.aldini@unimi.it
10 Institute of Health and Sport, Victoria University, 70/104 Ballarat Rd, Footscray, VIC 3011, Australia; maximilian.decourten@vu.edu.au
11 NIHR Sheffield Biomedical Research Centre, University of Sheffield and Sheffield Teaching Hospitals NHS Foundation Trust, Glossop Rd, Broomhall, Sheffield S10 2JF, UK
12 Neuroscience Institute, University of Sheffield, Firth Court, 385a Glossop Rd, Broomhall, Sheffield S10 2TN, UK
* Correspondence: aya.mousa@monash.edu (A.M.); barbora.decourten@monash.edu (B.d.C.)

Abstract: Background: Trends in global ageing underscore the rising burden of age-related cognitive decline and concomitant cardiometabolic diseases, including type 2 diabetes mellitus (T2DM). Carnosine, a naturally occurring dipeptide with anti-inflammatory, antioxidant and anti-glycating properties, has shown promise in animal models and limited human studies for improving cognitive function, insulin resistance and T2DM, but its therapeutic effects on cognition remain unclear. The aim of this study is to assess the effects of carnosine on cognitive function in individuals with prediabetes or well-controlled T2DM. **Methods:** This is a secondary analysis of a double-blind randomised controlled trial (RCT), whereby 49 adults with prediabetes or early-stage well-controlled T2DM were randomised to receive 2 g of carnosine or identical placebo daily for 14 weeks. At baseline and follow-up, cognitive function was assessed as a secondary outcome using the Digit-Symbol Substitution Test, Stroop test, Trail Making Tests A & B, and the Cambridge Automated Neuropsychological Test Battery (CANTAB). **Results:** In total, 42 adults (23 males and 19 females) completed the trial. There were no differences in participant anthropometry or cognitive functioning between carnosine and placebo groups at baseline (all $p > 0.1$). After the 14-week supplementation period, there were no differences between carnosine and placebo groups in change and follow-up values for any cognitive measures including Stroop, Digit Symbol Substitution Sest, Trail Making A/B or CANTAB (all $p > 0.05$). Adjustments for baseline cognitive scores, diabetic status, level of education, age or interaction effects with participants' sex did not change the results. **Conclusions:** Carnosine supplementation did not improve cognitive measures in individuals with prediabetes or T2DM in this study. While larger trials may provide further insights, alternative factors—such as the relatively young and healthy profile of our cohort—may have contributed to the lack of observed effect. Future research should examine individuals with existing cognitive impairment or those at higher risk of cognitive decline to better define the therapeutic potential of carnosine in this context.

Keywords: carnosine supplementation; cognition and diabetes; cognitive function; prediabetes and cognition; type 2 diabetes; neurocognitive outcomes; randomised controlled trial (RCT); neuropsychological assessment; metabolic health and cognition; diabetes and neurodegeneration; antioxidants and cognitive function; insulin resistance and cognition; CANTAB cognitive testing; executive function and diabetes; inflammation and cognitive decline

1. Introduction

Type 2 diabetes (T2DM) is a major contributor to global mortality and morbidity and has steadily increased in prevalence over the past decade, from 366 million individuals in 2011 to 536.6 million individuals living with T2DM globally in 2021 [1,2]. These estimates are projected to rise to 783.3 million (11.2% of the global population) by 2045 [2]. Obesity and overweight are key risk factors for T2DM [3], caused by an imbalance between energy consumption and energy expenditure. This imbalance is often driven by a combination of sedentary lifestyles and excessive consumption of highly processed, energy-dense and nutrient-deficient diets, which are often more palatable and less expensive than healthier diets [4]. As of 2022, there were 2.5 billion adults with overweight or obesity, representing a staggering 43% of the global population and an increase from 25% in 1990 [5].

Both obesity and T2DM contribute to neurodegenerative diseases, including Alzheimer's dementia [6] and Parkinson's disease [7]. Insulin resistance, the central pathophysiological mechanism of T2DM and a common feature in obesity [8] has been identified as an important risk factor for cognitive impairment [9,10]. Ageing compounds the risk of cognitive impairment, with older individuals with T2DM more likely to have cognitive impairment compared with younger populations. However, interconnected mechanisms underpinning these cognitive changes can promote the development of early cognitive decline even in younger individuals with obesity and T2DM [11–13]. In the clinical setting, T2DM and cognitive impairment are treated independently [14], an approach that may be insufficient to address the syndromic nature of either condition. Therefore, investigating new treatments that can act synergistically to improve both neurocognitive function and glucose metabolism in T2DM and at-risk populations is warranted.

Carnosine, a dipeptide consisting of beta-alanine and L-histidine, has well-documented anti-glycating, anti-inflammatory and antioxidant abilities [15], processes which impact both glycaemia and cognitive function [16]. Carnosine is naturally abundant in skeletal muscle tissue and brain tissue in vivo [15] and can be derived through diet, mainly via the consumption of beef, chicken and turkey, as well as prawn, mackerel and tuna meat [17]. Carnosine is also available in supplements [18], where it has been shown to improve exercise performance by boosting the buffering capacity of skeletal muscle and delaying fatigue during intense physical activity [19]. In the context of cognition, the anti-inflammatory properties of carnosine are of particular relevance since inflammation is correlated with increased oxidative stress, and both are associated with low cognitive performance [20]. Indeed, antioxidant and anti-inflammatory agents which reduce oxidative stress and neuroinflammation, including endogenous histidine-containing dipeptides (HCDs) [15], vitamin K2 [21], polyphenols from olive trees [22], isoamericanin A [23], and ellagitannin [24], have been shown to reduce cognitive decline in preclinical models [20].

However, studies examining the effects of carnosine on cognition and metabolism to date have been largely based on animal and experimental models, with limited human data [25]. In our recent meta-analysis, we identified 10 RCTs examining the impact of HCDs on cognitive function, eight of which supplemented carnosine combined with anserine, with none using carnosine alone. Although we reported improved memory in elderly populations and improved delayed recall following supplementation among individuals with and without mild cognitive impairment assessed using the Wechsler Memory Test (WMS-2), these effects could not be attributed solely to carnosine. The same systematic review identified other key gaps in the evidence, namely the reliance on relatively brief global tests of cognition following carnosine supplementation [16,26]. Additionally, no studies have examined whether carnosine supplementation may affect cognitive measures in prediabetes or T2DM, despite the reported neurocognitive benefits of carnosine and the higher prevalence of cognitive impairment—often uncurable, in T2DM [27].

To address this critical evidence gap, the aim of the present study was to examine the effects of carnosine supplementation on cognitive function using RCT data with comprehensive neuropsychological and cognitive assessments in individuals with prediabetes or early-stage well-controlled T2DM.

2. Results

A total of 49 participants were randomised, with 24 assigned to the carnosine intervention (1 g orally twice daily) and 25 to the placebo group. Baseline characteristics did not differ between groups (Tables 1 and S1). The modified intention-to-treat (mITT) analysis included all participants with a follow-up assessment. A total of seven participants were excluded from the analysis: five due to the absence of follow-up data and two due to incorrectly collected cognitive data. Consequently, 42 participants (21 per group) were included in the final mITT analysis (Figure 1). Data were collected between 2016 and 2020.

Table 1. Sample characteristics at baseline.

Variable	**Placebo (21)**	**Carnosine (21)**	
	Mean ± SD	**Mean ± SD**	
Demographics			
Age	50.17 ± 10.64	51.7 ± 10.19	
Sex (males), *n* (%)	15 (75%)	14 (67%)	
Prediabetes/diabetes proportions, *n* (%)	15 (71%)/6 (29%)	10 (47.6%)/11 (52.4%)	
Metformin: yes/no, *n* (%)	9 (43%)/12 (57%)	8 (38%)/13 (62%)	
	Digit symbol test		Performance Range
Score: (Number of correct responses)	70.5 ± 9.987	64.89 ± 17.62	1–93

Table 1. *Cont.*

Variable	Placebo (21)	Carnosine (21)	
	Mean ± SD	Mean ± SD	
	Stroop tests		
Off Time	66.81 ± 7.9	70.14 ± 13.62	1–125.84
Off Time + On Time	142.62 ± 15.48	153.52 ± 28.9	1–274.9
On Time	75.81 ± 8.74	83.38 ± 16.19	1–148.7
On Time–Off Time	9 ± 6.19	13.25 ± 7.73	1–29.8
Successful times ×attempts (Off)	380.31 ± 74.61	389.67 ± 97.76	NA
Successful times × attempts (On)	440 ± 112.74	470.05 ± 98.02	NA
	Trail making Tests		
Trail making Test A (s)	17.05 ± 5.13	16.75 ± 4.90	1–300
Trail making Test B (s)	58.38 ± 31.07	63.18 ± 39.56	1–300
TMT ratio (B/A)	3.59 ± 1.6	3.76 ± 1.90	NA
Cambridge Neuropsychological Test Automated Battery			
	Delayed Match to Sample (DMS)		
DMS Percent correct (all delays)	87.00 (13.00)	87.00 (13.00)	0–100
DMS Probability of error given correct	0.12 (0.12)	0.12 (0.13)	−1 to 1
DMS Probability of error given error	0 (0)	0 (0)	−1 to 1
DMS Total correct (simultaneous)	18.00 (2.00)	18.00 (2.00)	0–20
	Paired Associates Learning (PAL)		
PAL First-attempt memory score	12.20 (3.00)	12.70 (4.05)	0–20
PAL Mean errors to success	2.05 (1.43)	1.50 (1.54)	0–4
PAL Number of patterns reached	8.00 (0)	8.00 (0)	2–8
PAL Total attempts	8.00 (1.50)	7.50 (3.00)	0–4
PAL Total errors	12.00 (11.00)	13.00 (9.00)	0–80
PAL Total errors (adjusted)	15.00 (13.00)	14.50 (16.75)	0–70
	Pattern Recognition Memory (PRM)		
Pattern Recognition Memory Median correct latency–Delayed	1978.25 (458.13)	1778.75 (390.25)	100–∞
Pattern Recognition Memory median correct latency–Immediate	1618.25 (281.75)	1612.00 (440)	100–∞
PRM Percent Correct Delayed	100 (8.33)	91.67 (8.34)	0–100
PRM Percent Correct Immediate	95.84 (8.33)	100 (8.33)	0–100
	Reaction time index (RTI)		
RTI Five-choice error score (all)	0 (0)	0 (1.00)	0–30
RTI Simple error score (all)	2.00 (3.00)	1.00 (2.00)	0–30
RTI Simple movement time	203.00 (107.50)	193.50 (42.50)	100–5100
RTI Simple reaction time	39.24 (25.45)	38.20 (23.76)	100–5100

Table 1. *Cont.*

Variable	Placebo (21)	Carnosine (21)	
	Mean ± SD	**Mean ± SD**	
	Rapid visual processing (RVP)		
RVP A Prime	0.89 (0.06)	0.91 (0.06)	0–1
RVP Response latency	192.66 (81.68)	149.65 (96.14)	100–1900
RVP Total false alarms	5.00 (8.00)	1.00 (3.00)	0–546
RVP Total hits	31.00 (10.25)	36.00 (13.00)	0–54
RVP Total misses	23.00 (10.25)	18.00 (13.00)	0–54
	Spatial working memory (SWM)		
SWM Between errors	10 (21.25)	12.00 (11.00)	0–90
SWM Strategy	8.00 (6.00)	8.00 (4.00)	2–14

Results are presented as mean ± standard deviation or median (interquartile range) unless otherwise specified.

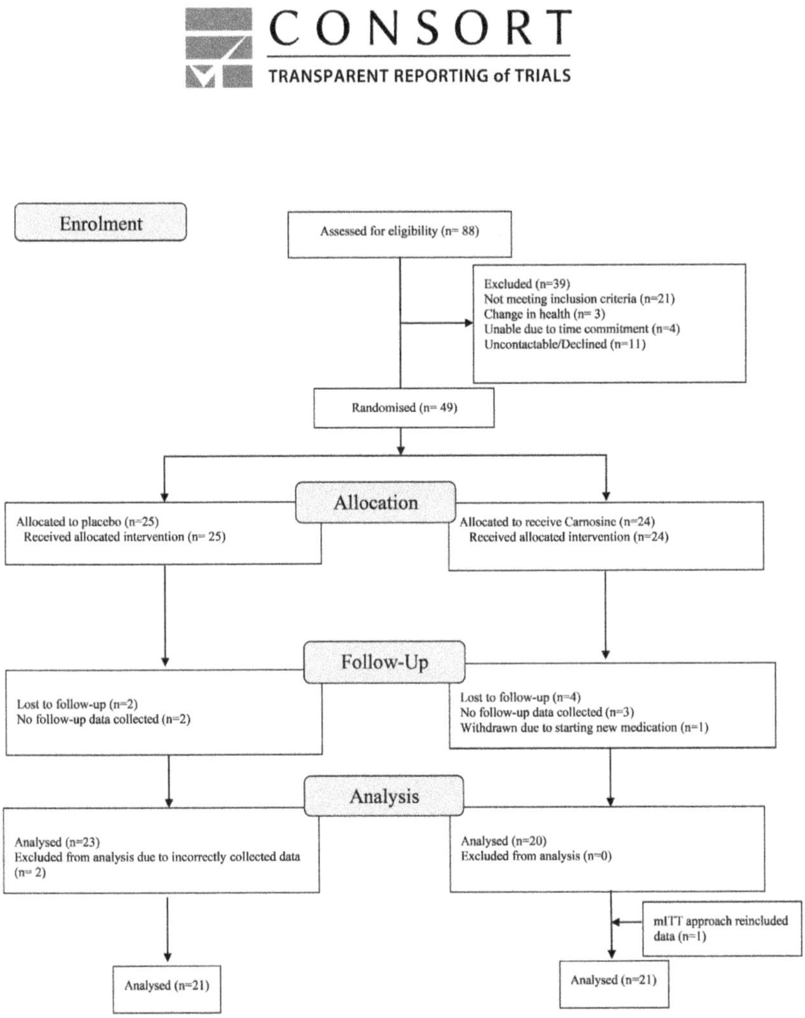

Figure 1. CONSORT flow diagram.

Among these 42 participants, the mean age was 52.0 ± 10.2 years (range 28–66 years), and 19 were female. There were 25 (60%) individuals with prediabetes, while the remaining 17 (40%) had T2DM and were taking metformin. All participants were cognitively healthy, as those with any history of neurological conditions would have been excluded from the trial. The participants reported good tolerance to carnosine, with none reporting any side effects.

Cognitive Performance Outcomes

For the Digit Symbol Substitution Test (DSST) (Table 2 and Supplementary Section S2), change values were not statistically different between groups (p = 0.46; Table 2). Multivariable regression analyses (Table 3) adjusting for baseline DSST scores, diabetic status, education and age also showed no significant effects (all $p \geq 0.20$; Table 3), and there were no interactions by sex (p = 0.96). Subgroup analyses also did not show significant differences between carnosine and placebo groups (all $p > 0.30$) (Tables S2.1, S2.2, S2.3 and S2.4).

Stroop Test results (Tables 2, 3 and S3 and Supplementary Section S2) showed no significant differences in change values for "Off Time" (p = 0.75), "Off Time + On Time" (p = 0.99), or interference state "On time–Off time" ($p \geq 0.68$) between groups. Multivariable regression models adjusted for baseline Stroop scores, diabetic status, education level and age did not alter results (all $p > 0.80$) (Tables 3, S3.1 and S3.2), and there were no interaction effects by sex ($p > 0.80$). Subgroup analyses (Table S3.3) comparing participants with prediabetes to those with T2DM (Tables S3.3.1, S3.3.2, S3.3.3 and S3.3.4) also showed no significant results (all $p \geq 0.40$).

For the Trail Making Test (TMT-A & B) (Table 2 and Supplementary Section S2), there were no significant differences in change values for TMT-A (p = 0.76), TMT-B (p = 0.42), or TMT-B:A ratio (p = 0.66) between carnosine and placebo groups. These results remained unchanged after adjustment for baseline scores, diabetic status, education and age (all $p \geq 0.20$) and in the interaction analyses ($p > 0.20$, as well as in subgroup analyses (all $p > 0.40$) (Tables S4.1, S4.2, S4.3 and S4.4).

In the CANTAB assessments (Tables 2, 3 and S5.1), no significant differences were found across any test domains. For the Delayed Match to Sample (DMS) test, key variables such as percentage correct, median latency and probability of error showed no group differences in change values ($p \geq 0.46$), including in adjusted analyses (Table 3) and interaction effects with sex ($p > 0.31$). Similarly, in the Paired Associates Learning test (Table 3), there were no significant differences in measures such as first-attempt memory score, total errors, mean errors to success or total attempts, including after adjustment for covariates ($p \geq 0.18$). There were no interactions by sex ($p > 0.36$), and multivariable subgroup analyses comparing prediabetes and T2DM groups also yielded no significant findings (all $p > 0.18$; Tables S5.2.1, S5.2.2, S5.2.3 and S5.2.4) were observed.

Changes in Pattern Recognition Memory (PRM), including percent correct latency or median correct latency, did not significantly differ between groups in either immediate or delayed measures (Table 2). This result remained consistent across univariable, multivariable, interaction and subgroup analyses ($p \geq 0.40$; Tables 2, 3, S5.2.1, S5.2.2, S5.2.3 and S5.2.4). Likewise, for the Reaction Time Index (RTI) and the Rapid Visual Processing (RVP) domains (Tables 2 and 3), the latter including key variables such as median response latency and probability of false alarms, there were no significant changes detected between groups in univariable, adjusted or subgroup analyses (all $p > 0.46$) or in interaction analyses by sex ($p > 0.53$).

Table 2. Cognitive test scores between carnosine supplementation and placebo.

Test Variable	Placebo			Carnosine			p *	p(adj)
	Baseline	Follow-Up	Δ	Baseline	Follow-Up	Δ		
Digit Symbol Test								
Score	71.37 ± 10.58	75.67 ± 10.71	3.67 ± 9.48	65.47 ± 17.85	76.00 ± 13.95	10.53 ± 12.90	0.08	0.46
Trail Making test								
Trail Making Test A (s)	17.05 ± 5.13	17.36 ± 5.00	0.31 ± 6.2	16.75 ± 4.90	15.67 ± 4.85	−1.09 ± 5.72	0.46	0.76
Trail Making Test B (seconds)	58.38 ± 31.07	61.71 ± 36.82	2.26 ± 26.0	63.18 ± 39.56	46.84 ± 10.95	−16.34 ± 42.35	0.1	0.42
B:A (s)	3.59 ± 1.6	3.66 ± 2.1	−0.01 ± 1.55	3.76 ± 1.90	3.13 ± 0.80	−0.63 ± 1.86	0.26	0.66
Stroop								
Off Time (s)	66.81 ± 7.90	64.22 ± 10.44	−2.45 ± 12.87	70.14 ± 13.62	72.24 ± 10.01	0.56 ± 7.84	0.05	0.75
On Time(s)	75.81 ± 8.74	81.99 ± 19.41	6.18 ± 17.81	83.38 ± 16.19	90.05 ± 22.06	6.66 ± 20.28	0.29	0.67
Off Time + On Time(s)	142.62 ± 15.48	166.19 ± 97.22	23.57 ± 97.17	153.52 ± 28.90	184.49 ± 79.96	30.97 ± 83.10	0.62	0.84
On time—Off time(s)	9.00 ± 6.19	13.79 ± 14.17	4.4 ± 14.34	13.25 ± 7.73	11.73 ± 4.52	−1.12 ± 7.53	0.28	0.68
Successful times x attempts (Off)	380.31 ± 74.61	361.14 ± 107.19	−12.33 ± 116.04	389.67 ± 97.76	399.54 ± 70.46	−3.81 ± 74.89	0.29	0.64
Successful times x attempts (On)	439.99 ± 112.74	458.21 ± 100.92	12.97 ± 117.89	470.05 ± 98.02	505.21 ± 128.93	28.65 ± 88.31	0.57	0.85
CANTAB								
DMS Percent Correct (All Delays)	84.7 ± 9.00	87 ± 10.76	2.60 ± 14.32	84.10 ± 13.70	85 ± 8.86	0.90 ± 17.81	0.74	0.70
DMS percent correct (Simultaneous)	88.25 ± 6.74	89.52 ± 8.05	1.75 ± 10.29	86.91 ± 11.67	87.38 ± 7.35	0.48 ± 15.08	0.70	0.85
DMS median correct latency	3569.20 ± 914.96	3459.86 ± 1235.52	−97.75 ± 1109.50	3427.29 ± 1747	3248.98 ± 1548.87	−178.31 ± 1467.79	0.84	0.88
DMS Probability of error given error	0.02 ± 0.90	0.09 ± 0.16	0.06 ± 0.20	0.07 ± 0.19	0.10 ± 0.15	0.03 ± 0.27	0.68	0.85
PALFAMS (Paired Associates Learning First attempt memory score)	12.20 ± 3.00	14.32 ± 3.92	2.11 ± 3.25	12.70 ± 4.05	12.40 ± 4.02	−0.37 ± 4.81	0.07	0.54

Table 2. *Cont.*

Test Variable	Placebo			Carnosine			p *	p(adj)
	Baseline	Follow-Up	Δ	Baseline	Follow-Up	Δ		
PALMETS (Paired Associates Learning Mean Errors to Success)	2.05 ± 1.43	1.24 ± 1.00	−1.00 ± 1.49	1.50 ± 1.54	2.35 ± 1.35	0.84 ± 1.34	<0.001	0.05
PALTA (Paired Associates Learning Total Attempts)	8.32 ± 1.77	6.86 ± 1.77	−1.53 ± 1.47	7.65 ± 1.90	7.65 ± 1.66	−0.05 ± 2.09	0.02	0.46
PALTA 4 (Paired Associates Learning Total Attempts 4 Patterns)	1.58 ± 0.61	1.24 ± 0.70	−0.32 ± 0.89	1.25 ± 0.72	1.45 ± 0.83	0.21 ± 0.71	0.05	0.59
PALTEA (Paired Associates Learning Total errors (adjusted))	15.40 ± 10.66	12.37 ± 14.40	−3.00 ± 9.21	17.95 ± 14.40	13.95 ± 12.60	−4.26 ± 12.94	0.73	0.86
PRMPCD (Pattern Recognition Memory Percent Correct Delayed)	94.91 ± 7.08	93.33 ± 7.66	−0.49 ± 9.07	87.084 ± 11.93	84.53 ± 13.77	−3.33 ± 17.19	0.53	0.84
PRMMDCLD (Pattern Recognition Memory Median correct latency)–Delayed	2065.92 ± 626.63	1814.38 ± 391.45	−255.94 ± 633.16	1900.22 ± 457.70	1968.23 ± 679.11	68.00 ± 766.33	0.17	0.65
PRMMDCLI (Pattern Recognition Memory median correct latency)–Immediate	1633.93 ± 386.86	1540.95 ± 280.27	−94.50 ± 312.68	1617.26 ± 326.25	1570.38 ± 328.71	−46.88 ± 211.89	0.57	0.87
PRMPCI (Pattern Recognition Memory Percent Correct Immediate)	93.34 ± 9.97	96.49 ± 6.40	3.51 ± 11.22	95.24 ± 6.26	94.05 ± 11.83	−1.19 ± 9.96	0.17	0.6
RTIFMMT (Reaction Time Index–mean five choice movement time)	292.09 ± 82.54	267.26 ± 63.07	−24.83 ± 81.86	255.14 ± 86.82	271.17 ± 103.42	16.03 ± 48.68	0.06	0.55
RTIFMDMT (RTI Median Five-Choice Movement Time)	290.38 ± 80.76	268.81 ± 64.88	−21.57 ± 82.07	253.57 ± 86.25	268.95 ± 102.64	15.38 ± 50.00	0.09	0.46
RTIFMDRT (RTI Median Five-Choice Reaction Time)	401.07 ± 46.76	407.50 ± 50.94	6.43 ± 34.95	402.67 ± 41.52	399.24 ± 46.23	−3.43 ± 32.34	0.35	0.64

Table 2. *Cont.*

Test Variable	Placebo			Carnosine			p *	p(adj)
	Baseline	Follow-Up	Δ	Baseline	Follow-Up	Δ		
RTIFMTSD (Reaction Time Index -five choice movement time (SD))	40.31 ± 17.22	38.19 ± 20.97	−2.12 ± 24.70	37.49 ± 14.09	36.86 ± 12.49	−0.63 ± 13.06	0.81	0.87
RTISES (Reaction time Index–Simple error Score)	1.91 ± 2.39	0.33 ± 0.56	−0.24 ± 3.21	2.48 ± 5.45	0.43 ± 1.12	0.29 ± 4.3491	0.66	0.84
RTIMSMT (Reaction Time Index–Mean simple movement time)	232.70 ± 75.09	237.12 ± 58.91	4.42 ± 56.76	207.12 ± 79.63	220.89 ± 75.64	13.77 ± 64.70	0.62	0.86
RTIMSRT (Reaction Time Index–Mean simple reaction time)	353.96 ± 38.80	373.28 ± 41.00	19.32 ± 31.79	350.28 ± 42.60	357.92 ± 40.72	7.64 ± 34.67	0.26	0.75
RTISMDRT (RTI Simple Median Reaction Time)	345.07 ± 36.25	360.90 ± 37.40	15.83 ± 26.95	342.10 ± 41.28	347.67 ± 36.55	5.57 ± 31.62	0.26	0.7
RTISMDMT (RTI Simple Median Movement Time)	228.67 ± 72.67	234.45 ± 57.43	5.79 ± 55.44	205.64 ± 78.83	216.71 ± 72.15	11.07 ± 61.23	0.77	0.84
RVPA (Rapid Visual Processing A prime)	0.88 ± 0.06	0.90 ± 0.39	0.02 ± 0.052	0.91 ± 0.04	0.92 ± 0.06	0.009 ± 0.044	0.35	0.62
RVPMDL (Rapid Visual Processing–median response latency)	493.88 ± 116.66	465.53 ± 88.86	−28.35 ± 69.75	481.91 ± 60.09	472.68 ± 61.38	−11.53 ± 62.04	0.43	0.73
RVPPFA (RVP Probability of False Alarm)	0.04 ± 0.117	0.012 ± 0.008	−0.03 ± 0.12	0.007 ± 0.011	0.01 ± 0.037	0.007 ± 0.028	0.19	0.62
SWMBE (Spatial Working Memory–between errors)	11.80 ± 9.80	12.35 ± 10.16	0.55 ± 9.59	12.33 ± 7.84	9.43 ± 8.16	−2.90 ± 8.32	0.22	0.67
SWMS (Spatial Working memory–Strategy 6–8 boxes)	6.70 ± 3.25	6.85 ± 3.31	0.15 ± 2.18	7.48 ± 2.68	6.76 ± 3.40	−0.71 ± 3.21	0.32	0.67

(Δ): follow-up—baseline values. All data are represented as mean ± standard deviation. * p-value for differences between groups estimated by independent samples t-test for change (Δ). p(adj): Adjusted p-value for false discovery rate using the Benjamini–Hochberg correction method.

Table 3. Multivariate regression analysis for the differences in change of cognitive test variables between carnosine and placebo supplementation adjusted for covariates.

	Cognitive Tests							
	Models	Change (Δ)						
		β	95% CI	SE	R2	p *	P2 (Pooled)	p(adj)
			Digit Symbol Test Variables					
Score	Model 1	3.99	−2.51, 10.49	3.2	0.38	0.22	0.19	0.34
	Model 2	3.93	−2.82, 10.69	3.32	0.38	0.24	0.21	0.34
	Model 3	3.71	−2.97, 10.40	3.28	0.42	0.27	0.25	0.34
	Model 4	4.03	−2.84, 10.89	3.36	0.42	0.24	0.25	0.34
	Model 5	−0.22	−8.2, −7.77	3.92	0.40	0.96	0.90	0.96
			Trail Making Test variables					
Trail Making Test A (s)	Model 1	−2.20	−4.98, 0.58	1.37	0.36	0.12	0.10	0.26
	Model 2	−1.83	−4.73, 1.06	1.43	0.38	0.21	0.17	0.30
	Model 3	−1.83	−4.78, 1.11	1.45	0.38	0.22	0.18	0.30
	Model 4	−2.11	−4.95, 0.73	1.40	0.45	0.14	0.12	0.26
	Model 5	−2.81	−5.75, 0.14	1.45	0.47	0.06	0.05	0.22
Trail Making Test B (s)	Model 1	−17.56	−33.58, −1.54	7.90	0.55	0.03	0.03	0.22
	Model 2	−14.53	−30.71, 1.66	7.97	0.58	0.08	0.07	0.22
	Model 3	−14.81	−31.31, 1.69	8.12	0.58	0.08	0.07	0.22
	Model 4	−15.68	−32.35, 0.99	8.19	0.59	0.06	0.06	0.22
	Model 5	−15.37	−33.10, 2.35	8.71	0.57	0.09	0.09	0.22
B:A (s)	Model 1	−0.59	−1.52, 0.33	0.46	0.37	0.20	0.21	0.30
	Model 2	−0.47	−1.42, 0.48	0.47	0.39	0.32	0.36	0.37
	Model 3	−0.48	−1.45, 0.49	0.48	0.39	0.32	0.36	0.37
	Model 4	−0.46	−1.45, 0.53	0.49	0.39	0.35	0.38	0.37
	Model 5	−0.26	−1.30, 0.79	0.51	0.38	0.62	0.69	0.62

Table 3. *Cont.*

Cognitive Tests								
	Models	Change (Δ)						
		β	95% CI	SE	R2	*p* *	P2 (Pooled)	*p*(adj)
Stroop test variables								
Off Time	Model 1	4.82	−2.27, 11.92	3.45	0.30	0.17	0.09	0.84
	Model 2	4.56	−2.85, 11.98	3.6	0.30	0.22	0.08	0.84
	Model 3	4.31	−3.29, 11.90	3.68	0.31	0.25	0.08	0.84
	Model 4	3.83	−4.11, 11.77	3.84	0.32	0.33	0.15	0.84
	Model 5	0.25	−8.57, 9.07	4.26	0.29	0.95	0.93	0.95
On Time	Model 1	1.77	−12.29, 15.83	6.87	0.03	0.8	0.8	0.89
	Model 2	2.95	−11.27, 17.17	6.94	0.07	0.67	0.67	0.84
	Model 3	2.91	−11.01, 16.83	6.78	0.15	0.67	0.67	0.84
	Model 4	0.82	−12.65, 14.29	6.55	0.25	0.90	0.90	0.93
	Model 5	−4.74	−19.65, 10.18	7.26	0.27	0.52	0.51	0.84
Off Time + On Time	Model 1	11.06	−55.00, 77.12	32.3	0.03	0.38	0.73	0.84
	Model 2	18.58	−47.12, 84.29	32.08	0.10	0.57	0.56	0.84
	Model 3	19.25	−43.94, 82.44	30.8	0.20	0.54	0.53	0.84
	Model 4	8.13	−53.51, 69.76	29.99	0.30	0.79	0.79	0.89
	Model 5	−13.58	−81.90, 54.74	33.24	0.30	0.69	0.68	0.84
On Time–Off Time	Model 1	−2.82	−11.40, 5.76	4.17	0.21	0.51	0.53	0.84
	Model 2	−2.97	−11.81, 5.86	4.29	0.21	0.49	0.54	0.84
	Model 3	−2.83	−11.94, 6.29	4.42	0.21	0.53	0.54	0.84
	Model 4	−4.55	−13.85, 4.75	4.50	0.28	0.32	0.33	0.84
	Model 5	−2.47	−12.35, 7.42	4.78	0.25	0.61	0.52	0.84
Successful times x attempts (Off)	Model 1	22.61	−43.72, 88.95	32.27	0.25	0.49	0.27	0.84
	Model 2	20.19	−48.72, 89.11	33.46	0.26	0.55	0.25	0.84
	Model 3	16.03	−54.28, 86.34	34.07	0.28	0.64	0.25	0.84
	Model 4	16.49	−57.67, 90.66	35.85	0.28	0.65	0.35	0.84
	Model 5	19.37	−60.32, 99.05	38.52	0.28	0.62	0.63	0.84

Table 3. *Cont.*

Cognitive Tests								
	Models	Change (Δ)						
		β	95% CI	SE	R2	p *	P2 (Pooled)	p(adj)
Successful times x attempts (On)	Model 1	27.76	−47.70, 103.23	36.71	0.16	0.46	0.4	0.84
	Model 2	21.87	−55.82, 99.56	37.72	0.18	0.57	0.4	0.84
	Model 3	14.23	−60.01, 88.46	35.97	0.29	0.7	0.42	0.84
	Model 4	−4.22	−75.03, 66.59	34.23	0.42	0.9	0.66	0.93
	Model 5	−19.89	−96.05, 56.27	36.82	0.43	0.59	0.69	0.84
CANTAB tests								
DMS Percent Correct (All Delays)	Model 1	−2.37	−8.55, 3.80	3.05	0.65	0.44	0.58	0.75
	Model 2	−4.59	−10.76, 1.58	3.05	0.69	0.14	0.31	0.51
	Model 3	−4.96	−10.772, 0.856	2.87	0.74	0.09	0.22	0.50
	Model 4	−5.01	−10.724, 0.698	2.81	0.75	0.08	0.16	0.50
	Model 5	−6.86	−12.60, −1.11	2.83	0.77	0.02	0.03	0.31
DMS percent correct (Simultaneous)	Model 1	−2.75	−7.63, 2.13	2.41	0.66	0.26	0.34	0.58
	Model 2	−4.39	−9.36, 0.59	2.46	0.69	0.11	0.21	0.50
	Model 3	−4.63	−9.40, 0.15	2.36	0.73	0.08	0.15	0.50
	Model 4	−4.67	−9.29, −0.052	2.28	0.75	0.06	0.10	0.50
	Model 5	−0.97	−6.57, 4.66	2.77	0.57	0.73	0.67	0.92
DMS Percent Correct (0 Second Delay)	Model 1	4.933	−5.30, 15.17	5.05	0.66	0.34	0.30	0.68
	Model 2	2.868	−7.82, 13.56	5.28	0.67	0.59	0.48	0.83
	Model 3	2.134	−8.21, 12.48	5.10	0.70	0.68	0.57	0.90
	Model 4	2.097	−8.25, 12.44	5.10	0.71	0.68	0.62	0.90
	Model 5	4.09	6.4, 14.57	5.16	0.72	0.43	0.40	0.74
DMS Percent Correct (4 Second Delay)	Model 1	−6.04	−16.41, 4.34	5.13	0.51	0.25	0.39	0.58
	Model 2	−8.81	−19.65, 2.04	5.35	0.54	0.11	0.27	0.50
	Model 3	−9.14	−20.09, 1.80	5.40	0.55	0.1	0.24	0.50
	Model 4	−9.03	−20.13, 2.07	5.47	0.55	0.11	0.25	0.50
	Model 5	−13.03	−24.37, −2.24	5.45	0.58	0.02	0.03	0.31

Table 3. *Cont.*

Cognitive Tests								
	Models	Change (Δ)						
		β	95% CI	SE	R2	p *	P2 (Pooled)	p(adj)
DMS Percent Correct (12 Second Delay)	Model 1	−5.98	−16.53, 4.57	5.21	0.60	0.26	0.27	0.58
	Model 2	−6.94	−17.89, 4.01	5.40	0.61	0.21	0.23	0.54
	Model 3	−7.74	−18.51, 3.04	5.31	0.63	0.15	0.16	0.51
	Model 4	−8.28	−18.61, 2.06	5.09	0.67	0.11	0.09	0.50
	Model 5	−9.92	−20.19, 0.35	5.06	0.68	0.06	0.05	0.50
DMS median correct latency	Model 1	−140.46	−886.88, 605.95	368.71	0.21	0.71	0.72	0.92
	Model 2	−120.18	−908.07, 667.70	388.85	0.21	0.76	0.77	0.92
	Model 3	−115.96	−916.68, 684.76	394.81	0.21	0.77	0.78	0.92
	Model 4	−126.76	−904.05, 650.54	382.88	0.28	0.74	0.67	0.92
	Model 5	−50.32	−844.91, 744.26	391.4	0.27	0.9	0.87	0.97
DMS Probability of error given error	Model 1	0.02	−0.09, 0.13	0.05	0.62	0.70	0.79	0.91
	Model 2	0	−0.12, 0.12	0.06	0.62	0.99	0.60	0.99
	Model 3	−0.01	−0.13, 0.12	0.06	0.63	0.9	0.56	0.97
	Model 4	0	−0.13, 0.12	0.06	0.65	0.94	0.58	0.97
	Model 5	−0.04	−0.15, 0.08	0.06	0.65	0.50	0.52	0.79
PALFAMS (Paired Associates Learning First)	Model 1	−2.19	−4.60, 0.23	1.19	0.3	0.07	0.06	0.50
	Model 2	−2.93	−5.49, −0.37	1.26	0.34	0.03	0.03	0.36
	Model 3	−2.95	−5.55, −0.34	1.28	0.34	0.03	0.03	0.36
	Model 4	−2.83	−5.46, −0.21	1.29	0.36	0.04	0.04	0.41
	Model 5	−3.22	−5.84, −0.61	1.28	0.36	0.02	0.006	0.31
PALMETS (Paired Associates Learning Mean Errors to Success)	Model 1	1.491	0.81, 2.17	0.34	0.65	0.001	0.001	0.15
	Model 2	1.72	1.01, 2.43	0.35	0.68	0.001	0.001	0.41
	Model 3	1.76	1.06, 2.47	0.35	0.7	0.001	0.001	0.31
	Model 4	1.70	1.00, 2.39	0.34	0.72	0.001	0.001	0.31
	Model 5	1.42	0.63, 2.22	0.39	0.65	0.001	0.001	0.50

Table 3. *Cont.*

Cognitive Tests								
	Models	Change (Δ)						
		β	95% CI	SE	R2	p *	P2 (Pooled)	p(adj)
PALTA (Paired Associates Learning Total Attempts)	Model 1	1.10	0.08, 2.13	0.50	0.41	0.04	0.03	0.73
	Model 2	1.47	0.42, 2.52	0.52	0.47	0.01	0.01	0.73
	Model 3	1.44	0.39, 2.48	0.51	0.49	0.01	0.01	0.74
	Model 4	1.30	0.31, 2.29	0.49	0.57	0.01	0.02	0.54
	Model 5	1.40	0.38, 2.41	0.50	0.57	0.008	0.01	0.97
PALTA 4 (Paired Associates Learning Total Attempts 4 patterns)	Model 1	0.46	−0.04, 0.96	0.25	0.24	0.07	0.06	0.90
	Model 2	0.25	−0.35, 0.85	0.29	0.29	0.40	0.19	0.90
	Model 3	0.25	−0.35, 0.85	0.30	0.30	0.40	0.19	0.91
	Model 4	0.24	−0.37, 0.85	0.30	0.31	0.42	0.21	0.58
	Model 5	0.36	−0.19, 0.91	0.27	0.30	0.20	0.09	0.36
PALTEA (Paired Associates Learning Total errors (adjusted))	Model 1	−0.33	−7.32, 6.66	3.45	0.14	0.92	0.89	0.31
	Model 2	1.517	−5.94, 8.97	3.67	0.19	0.68	0.88	0.31
	Model 3	1.53	−6.044, 9.10	3.72	0.19	0.68	0.87	0.31
	Model 4	1.459	−6.252, 9.17	3.79	0.19	0.70	0.86	0.31
	Model 5	4.42	−3.28, 12.12	3.78	0.22	0.25	0.23	0.67
PRMPCD (Pattern Recognition Memory Percent Correct Delayed)	Model 1	−9.21	−17.38, −1.05	4.02	0.37	0.03	0.05	0.54
	Model 2	−10.9	−19.47, −2.32	4.22	0.4	0.01	0.04	0.54
	Model 3	−10.72	−19.36, −2.08	4.24	0.41	0.02	0.05	0.54
	Model 4	−10.73	−19.52, −1.93	4.31	0.41	0.02	0.05	0.50
	Model 5	−11.27	−20.23,−2.31	4.39	0.42	0.02	0.04	0.82
PRMMDCLD (Pattern Recognition Memory Median correct latency)–Delayed	Model 1	188.12	−194.09, 570.33	188.07	0.42	0.32	0.26	0.92
	Model 2	263.75	−144.49, 671.99	200.66	0.44	0.20	0.15	0.92
	Model 3	261.01	−143.24, 665.25	198.46	0.47	0.20	0.17	0.94
	Model 4	257.24	−156.45, 670.93	202.84	0.47	0.21	0.20	0.92
	Model 5	358.25	−39.9, −756.41	195.22	0.49	0.08	0.09	0.62

Table 3. *Cont.*

	Cognitive Tests							
	Models	Change (Δ)						
		β	95% CI	SE	R2	*p* *	P2 (Pooled)	*p*(adj)
PRMMDCLI (Pattern Recognition Memory median correct latency)–Immediate	Model 1	40.2	−102.57, 182.97	70.46	0.32	0.57	0.43	0.58
	Model 2	20.18	−131.65, 172.02	74.87	0.33	0.79	0.53	0.58
	Model 3	22.45	−131.53, 176.43	75.85	0.33	0.77	0.51	0.58
	Model 4	15.91	−139.09, 170.92	76.27	0.35	0.84	0.61	0.53
	Model 5	24.53	−129.81, 178.87	75.95	0.35	0.75	0.64	0.51
PRMPCI (Pattern Recognition Memory Percent Correct)–Immediate	Model 1	−3.26	−9.28, 2.75	2.97	0.29	0.28	0.31	0.50
	Model 2	−3.62	−10.01, 2.76	3.15	0.29	0.26	0.32	0.50
	Model 3	−3.68	−10.17, 2.81	3.20	0.29	0.26	0.31	0.51
	Model 4	−3.77	−10.36, 2.81	3.24	0.29	0.25	0.29	0.56
	Model 5	−4.45	−10.98, 2.09	3.21	0.31	0.18	0.18	0.54
RTIFMMT (Reaction Time Index–mean five choice movement time)	Model 1	29.6	−10.70, 69.89	19.92	0.22	0.15	0.14	0.53
	Model 2	33.62	−8.32, 75.56	20.72	0.23	0.11	0.100	0.51
	Model 3	35.96	−4.07, 75.98	19.75	0.32	0.08	0.07	0.54
	Model 4	31.13	−8.99, 71.24	19.78	0.36	0.12	0.12	0.62
	Model 5	25.16	−15.72, 66.04	20.16	0.34	0.22	0.21	0.97
RTIFMDMT (RTI Median Five-Choice Movement Time)	Model 1	25.81	−15.07, 66.69	20.21	0.20	0.21	0.20	0.97
	Model 2	29.31	−13.24, 71.87	21.02	0.21	0.17	0.16	0.93
	Model 3	31.55	−9.22, 72.32	20.12	0.30	0.13	0.12	0.92
	Model 4	26.72	−14.20, 67.64	20.18	0.33	0.19	0.19	0.93
	Model 5	21.88	−19.71, 93.3	20.51	0.32	0.29	0.29	0.80
RTIFMTSD (Reaction Time Index -five choice movement time (SD))	Model 1	−0.45	−10.95, 10.06	5.19	0.3	0.93	0.93	0.83
	Model 2	0.50	−10.44, 11.43	5.40	0.31	0.93	0.93	0.80
	Model 3	1.29	−9.04, 11.63	5.10	0.40	0.80	0.80	0.81
	Model 4	1.43	−9.06, 11.92	5.17	0.40	0.78	0.78	0.92
	Model 5	1.27	−9.55, 12.1	5.34	0.40	0.81	0.81	0.97

Table 3. *Cont.*

Cognitive Tests								
	Models	Change (Δ)						
		β	95% CI	SE	R2	*p* *	P2 (Pooled)	*p*(adj)
RTISES (Reaction time Index–Simple error Score)	Model 1	0.29	−0.64, 1.22	0.46	0.09	0.53	0.52	0.92
	Model 2	0.26	−0.71, 1.23	0.48	0.09	0.59	0.58	0.92
	Model 3	0.30	−0.67, 1.27	0.48	0.12	0.54	0.53	0.97
	Model 4	0.29	−0.70, 1.28	0.49	0.12	0.55	0.55	0.79
	Model 5	−0.35	−2.88, 2.18	1.25	0.14	0.78	0.78	0.53
RTIMSMT (Reaction Time Index–Mean simple movement time)	Model 1	−1.54	−34.35, 31.28	16.22	0.30	0.92	0.92	0.53
	Model 2	4.38	−29.24, 38.01	16.61	0.33	0.79	0.79	0.51
	Model 3	5.39	−27.92, 38.69	16.44	0.36	0.74	0.74	0.53
	Model 4	2.12	−31.15, 35.39	16.4	0.40	0.90	0.90	0.85
	Model 5	−10.97	−44.42, 22.49	16.5	0.40	0.50	0.51	0.53
RTIMSRT (Reaction Time Index–Mean simple reaction time)	Model 1	−12.89	−32.14, 6.36	9.52	0.19	0.18	0.18	0.51
	Model 2	−13.81	−33.88, 6.26	9.91	0.19	0.17	0.16	0.51
	Model 3	−14.44	−34.56, 5.67	9.93	0.22	0.15	0.15	0.51
	Model 4	−13.66	−33.88, 6.55	9.97	0.24	0.18	0.17	0.50
	Model 5	−19.53	−39.99, 0.93	10.09	0.27	0.61	0.05	0.92
RTISMDRT (RTI Simple Median Reaction Time)	Model 1	−11.25	−27.94, 5.44	8.25	0.22	0.18	0.17	0.98
	Model 2	−12.52	−29.87, 4.83	8.57	0.23	0.15	0.14	0.97
	Model 3	−13.23	−30.47, 4.01	8.51	0.26	0.13	0.12	0.97
	Model 4	−12.34	−29.49, 4.82	8.46	0.29	0.15	0.14	0.74
	Model 5	−15.31	−32.87, 2.25	8.66	0.31	0.09	0.08	0.94
RTISMDMT (RTI Simple Median Movement Time)	Model 1	−4.54	−35.65, 26.57	15.38	0.31	0.77	0.77	0.94
	Model 2	0.62	−31.41, 32.65	15.82	0.34	0.97	0.97	0.94
	Model 3	1.55	−30.21, 33.32	15.68	0.37	0.92	0.92	0.94
	Model 4	−1.15	−33.04, 30.75	15.73	0.39	0.94	0.94	0.87
	Model 5	−12.68	−44.72, 19.37	15.8	0.40	0.43	0.42	0.75

Table 3. *Cont.*

Cognitive Tests								
	Models	Change (Δ)						
		β	95% CI	SE	R2	p *	P2 (Pooled)	p(adj)
RVPA (Rapid Visual Processing A prime)	Model 1	0	−0.03, 0.03	0.01	0.20	0.84	0.75	0.77
	Model 2	0	−0.03, 0.03	0.02	0.20	0.84	0.69	0.73
	Model 3	0	−0.04, 0.03	0.02	0.20	0.85	0.7	0.73
	Model 4	0	−0.04, 0.03	0.02	0.21	0.85	0.69	0.74
	Model 5	0.01	−0.02, 0.04	0.02	0.22	0.63	0.89	0.92
RVPMDL (Rapid Visual Processing–median response latency)	Model 1	12.81	−22.02, 47.65	17.19	0.35	0.46	0.30	0.97
	Model 2	12.92	−24.16, 50.01	18.29	0.35	0.48	0.28	0.97
	Model 3	15.91	−20.31, 52.13	17.84	0.41	0.38	0.20	0.98
	Model 4	15.58	−0.59, −0.15	17.95	0.42	0.39	0.25	0.68
	Model 5	15.03	−22.29, 52.36	18.36	0.42	0.42	0.33	0.75
RVPPFA (RVP Probability of False Alarm)	Model 1	0.002	−0.02, 0.02	0.01	0.90	0.79	0.78	0.80
	Model 2	0.001	−0.02, 0.02	0.01	0.90	0.95	0.92	0.80
	Model 3	0.001	−0.02, 0.02	0.01	0.90	0.95	0.92	0.77
	Model 4	0	−0.02, 0.02	0.01	0.91	0.97	0.90	0.80
	Model 5	−0.001	−0.03, 0.01	0.01	0.91	0.34	0.35	0.54
SWMS (Spatial Working memory–Strategy 6–8 boxes)	Model 1	−0.64	−2.33, 1.06	0.84	0.12	0.45	0.43	0.58
	Model 2	−0.54	−2.31, 1.24	0.88	0.13	0.54	0.51	0.53
	Model 3	−0.56	−2.36, 1.24	0.89	0.13	0.53	0.50	0.51
	Model 4	−0.61	−2.34, 1.11	0.85	0.22	0.48	0.39	0.62
	Model 5	0.57	−1.19, 2.33	0.87	0.22	0.52	0.55	0.67
SWMBE (Spatial Working Memory–between errors)	Model 1	−3.2	−8.28, 1.88	2.51	0.25	0.21	0.20	0.75
	Model 2	−3.2	−8.56, 2.17	2.65	0.25	0.24	0.22	0.73
	Model 3	−3.56	−8.62, 1.50	2.50	0.35	0.16	0.14	0.74
	Model 4	−3.68	−8.67, 1.32	2.46	0.39	0.14	0.11	0.84
	Model 5	−2.73	−7.9, 2.44	2.55	0.37	0.29	0.26	0.50

Table 3. *Cont.*

Cognitive Tests								
	Models	Change (Δ)						
		β	95% CI	SE	R2	*p* *	P2 (Pooled)	*p*(adj)
SWMBE4 (SWM Between Errors 4 Boxes)	Model 1	−0.34	−1.01, 0.34	0.33	0.33	0.32	0.37	0.51
	Model 2	−0.27	−0.96, −0.34	0.35	0.34	0.45	0.51	0.50
	Model 3	−0.30	−0.99, 0.40	0.34	0.37	0.40	0.45	0.50
	Model 4	−0.29	−1.00, 0.42	0.35	0.38	0.41	0.47	0.79
	Model 5	−0.19	−0.91, 0.53	0.36	0.37	0.60	0.63	0.82
SWMBE6 (Spatial Working Memory–between errors 6 boxes)	Model 1	−1.68	−3.40, 0.05	0.85	0.47	0.06	0.04	0.75
	Model 2	−1.38	−3.17, 0.40	0.88	0.49	0.12	0.08	0.70
	Model 3	−1.46	−3.21, 0.28	0.86	0.53	0.10	0.06	0.68
	Model 4	−1.49	−3.24, 0.26	0.86	0.54	0.09	0.06	0.70
	Model 5	−0.60	−2.46, 1.25	0.91	0.50	0.51	0.46	0.75
SWMBE8 (Spatial Working Memory–between errors 8 boxes)	Model 1	−1.1	−5.03, 2.83	1.94	0.27	0.57	0.56	0.51
	Model 2	−1.57	−5.69, 2.55	2.03	0.28	0.45	0.45	0.50
	Model 3	−1.81	−5.77, 2.15	1.95	0.36	0.36	0.35	0.50
	Model 4	−1.90	−5.81, 2.01	1.92	0.39	0.33	0.29	0.31
	Model 5	−1.83	−5.82, 2.17	1.97	0.39	0.36	0.33	0.58

Model 1: Adjusted for baseline value. Model 2: Adjusted for baseline value, diabetic status. Model 3: Adjusted for baseline value, diabetic status and level of education. Model 4: Adjusted for baseline value, diabetic status, level of education and age. Model 5: Interaction term (Group × Sex) and adjusted for baseline value, diabetic status, level of education and age. * *p*-values are estimated by Analysis of Covariance (ANCOVA). P2(Pooled): Pooled *p*-values estimated by ANCOVA after 5 imputations using predictive mean matching to replace missing data. *p*(adj): Adjusted *p*-value for false discovery rate using the Benjamini–Hochberg correction method. (β) Unstandardized beta-coefficient. (CI) confidence interval. (SE) standard error, and. (R2) R-square value.

Lastly, in the Spatial Working Memory (SWM) domain, measures such as between errors and strategy scores showed no significant differences between carnosine and placebo groups (Tables 2 and 3). Results were unchanged in multivariable regression models ($p \geq 0.31$), subgroup analyses (all $p \geq 0.83$) (Tables S5.2.2 and S5.2.4) and interaction analysis by sex ($p > 0.50$).

Carnosine was well tolerated, with no adverse effects linked to the supplementation. The sole reported concern was minor pain and bruise at the blood draw site experienced by one participant.

3. Discussion

To our knowledge, this is the first double-blind RCT investigating the effects of carnosine supplementation on cognitive function in individuals with prediabetes or T2DM. Our findings showed that short-term carnosine supplementation had no significant effect on cognitive function despite the use of comprehensive neuropsychological assessments, including the CANTAB series of computerised cognitive tests. These findings remained unchanged after controlling for key factors known to influence cognition, including diabetic status, age, sex and level of education, suggesting that carnosine supplementation may not provide cognitive benefits in this population.

No differences were observed between the carnosine and placebo groups across cognitive tests assessing executive function, attention, cognitive flexibility and processing speed. In particular, the Paired Associates Learning measures of the CANTAB series, which are highly sensitive to mild cognitive impairment (MCI) and early Alzheimer's pathology [28–30], were unchanged by carnosine supplementation, including after adjustment for covariates. One possible explanation for the lack of observed effects is that participants in this study had no known pre-existing cognitive impairment, potentially limiting the ability to detect measurable cognitive benefits. However, three previous studies in participants who were similarly healthy or had MCI have reported conflicting findings, showing that orally ingested carnosine improved cognitive performance after 12 weeks [31–33]. These trials involved older participants (mean age over 60 years) who were also more homogeneous (all recruited from the Tokyo metropolitan area), in contrast to the present RCT, which included a younger and more ethnically diverse cohort, including Caucasian, South American, Middle Eastern, South Asian and Southeast Asian participants. Additionally, although the average dose of carnosine used was lower than in the current study (ranging from 250 mg to 1 g daily compared with 2 g daily), two studies administered a combination of carnosine and anserine, making it difficult to isolate the specific effects of carnosine.

Importantly, previous RCTs investigating the effects of carnosine on cognition [31–36], including those noted above, have been constrained by limited numbers and types of neuropsychological testing, typically using assessments such as the Mini Mental State Examination (MMSE), Alzheimer's Disease Assessment Scale (ADAS), Clinical Dementia Rating (CDR), WMS (Wechsler Memory Scale), Short Test of Mental Status (STMS) or AVLT (Auditory Verbal Learning Test). While these tools are efficient in screening for specific cognitive deficits, none except the MMSE can derive a global assessment of cognitive functioning, and most lack the granularity to detect subtle changes in cognitive functioning. This contrasts with the domain-specific approach used in the current study, which is the first RCT to employ a comprehensive battery of objective cognitive assessments—including the gold-standard CANTAB, Stroop, DSST, and Trail Making Tests—to evaluate the cognitive effects of carnosine in prediabetes or T2DM. This specific test combination was chosen for its ability to assess diverse memory domains and complex cognitive functions, providing a more detailed analysis of cognitive performance. The use of computerised tests such as the CANTAB also minimises ceiling effects, enabling greater sensitivity in detecting subtle cognitive changes. Moreover, the more detailed statistical analysis used in this study suggests that many of the effects of carnosine on cognition reported previously may be confounded by variables known to affect cognition and/or potentially erroneous data due to multiple tests.

Despite the absence of an effect in this study, a potential effect of carnosine on neurocognitive function remains plausible from a mechanistic perspective. Recent findings from the NEAT trail [37] indicated cognitive benefits in younger healthy adults (23–35 years), suggesting age-dependent effects. The NEAT trial [37] included a larger and healthy cohort, whereas the participants from our trial had metabolic conditions, such as impaired glucose metabolism, that could influence cognitive outcomes, particularly in those with prediabetes and T2DM. Increased levels of fasting plasma glucose, 2 h postprandial glucose, HbA1c and fasting plasma insulin are important determinants in the development of cognitive impairment [38], especially in carriers of the APOE4 gene [39]. A meta-analysis of 122 studies reported a significant increase in the risk of developing cognitive disorders and all-cause dementia, Alzheimer's disease and vascular dementia in those with T2DM and prediabetes [38]. Carnosine has the ability to improve glucose metabolism in those with prediabetes and T2DM, as shown by our group previously [40,41]. Further, carnosine, along with anserine, has the ability to cross the blood–brain barrier (BBB) and induce the expression of neurotrophic genes in human neuronal cells and in glial cells, which produce brain-derived neurotrophic factor (BDNF) and neuronal growth factor (NGF) in the brain [42]. However, there is limited evidence of carnosine's penetrance of the BBB into neural tissues in vivo in humans. Carnosine is rapidly hydrolysed by the enzyme carnosinase to its constituents in the gut, limiting its ability to saturate distal tissue sites, and this may explain in part the lack of significant differences in this study. Future research aiming to elucidate the true pharmacodynamics of carnosine in human neural tissues should utilise phosphate MR-spectroscopy to image changes in metabolite concentrations and fractional volumes of brain grey and white matter post-supplementation [43,44].

The primary limitation of this study is its small sample size, as it is a secondary analysis of an RCT originally designed to examine the effects of carnosine on glycaemic parameters rather than on cognitive performance. This study was, therefore, likely underpowered to detect the smaller effect sizes typically seen in cognitive research. A post hoc power analysis suggests that future trials would require much larger sample sizes, with approximately 350 participants per group, to achieve 90% power to detect the small effect sizes commonly seen in cognitive outcome studies. Additionally, our study population did not include participants with cognitive dysfunction, limiting the generalisability of our results to these populations. Participants had relatively well-controlled diabetes (HbA1c < 8%) and typically shorter durations since diagnosis of T2DM (2 months to 6 years). Evidence suggests that cognitive impairment in prediabetes and T2DM is minor in those with shorter duration of diabetes compared with those with long-standing chronic diabetes (>13 years) [45], suggesting that supplementation-induced changes may be more detectable in populations with longer disease durations and concomitant cognitive impairment. The dosage (2 g) and duration (14 weeks) of carnosine supplementation used in this trial may also have been insufficient to affect cognitive measures to an extent detectable within the constraints of the sample size and statistical power. Given that longer durations (at least 24 months) have been recommended for interventional studies of cognitive function in Alzheimer's disease and MCI [46], future studies should consider extended follow-up periods to assess cumulative cognitive effects. Finally, the average age of participants was 54 years, and it is possible that carnosine is more effective in older populations with early indications of cognitive decline. This is supported by a previous meta-analysis [47] by our group, which found that carnosine supplementation improved delayed recall in older groups (>65 years) but not in younger cohorts.

Notwithstanding these limitations, this is the first RCT examining carnosine supplementation for cognitive function in prediabetes and T2DM. We utilised comprehensive neuropsychological testing in a well-characterised cohort, albeit with a likely smaller sample size than required to detect significant differences. While the cognitive benefits of carnosine could not be demonstrated in the present study, potential effects cannot be ruled out, and our data generate important insights to advance this area of study. Future trials should aim to recruit larger sample sizes with diverse baseline risk profiles, age groups and ethnicities. Key factors such as physical activity levels, pre-existing cognitive impairment, T2DM durations and diagnosis of T2DM using American Diabetes Association (ADA) guidelines, which incorporate HbA1c [48], should be carefully considered to ensure a more representative study population. Trials should also incorporate domain-specific neuropsychological testing to improve internal and external validity and clarify the effects of carnosine, if any, on cognitive performance in high-risk populations.

4. Materials and Methods

4.1. Study Design and Participants

This is a secondary analysis of a double-blind placebo-controlled RCT investigating the effects of 14 weeks of carnosine supplementation on glycaemic control in individuals with prediabetes or T2DM, the primary results of which are published elsewhere [41]. Detailed methodology is provided in our published protocol [49]. Briefly, we included participants aged 18–70 years with prediabetes or T2DM diagnosed using oral glucose tolerance test (OGTT) (as per World Health Organization [WHO] guidelines [50,51]) and who were diet controlled and not taking any medications except metformin, which participants continued taking during the trial. Participants did not undergo cognitive testing prior to recruitment and were assumed to be cognitively healthy based on the history they provided. Those with haemoglobin A1c (HbA1c) higher than 8% at the time of screening were excluded. Furthermore, participants with a body mass index (BMI) > 40 kg/m^2; fluctuating body weight (>5 kg weight change in the prior 12 months); smoking, or alcohol consumption [52] (standard drinks > 10 per week or >4/day); concomitant central nervous system, cardiovascular, respiratory, haematological or gastrointestinal diseases; and women who were pregnant or lactating were also excluded. Participants were instructed not to alter their diet or physical activity during the trial.

4.2. Recruitment

Primary advertising for the trial was conducted via newspapers, radio and posters. Volunteers were screened via a telephone-based questionnaire and, if eligible, were invited to the Clinical Trials Centre of the Monash Health Translational Research Precinct for an in-person screening visit. At the screening visit, prospective participants underwent a 75 g OGTT to confirm prediabetes/T2DM status using WHO (2006) criteria [50] and blood tests to exclude other underlying conditions. All participants were assessed against the inclusion and exclusion criteria noted above prior to formal inclusion and randomisation. Participants were free to withdraw at any time they desired and were encouraged to speak to the study physician. They were informed that all personal data would be deidentified, with only clinical data retained.

4.3. Ethics

All participants provided written informed consent before attending the baseline screening investigations. The trial was registered on clinicaltrials.gov (NCT02917928,

28/09/16) and conducted as per the published protocol [49] in line with the Standardised Protocol Interventions: Recommendations for Interventional Trials [53], with reporting conforming to the CONSORT guidelines [54]. The Monash Health Human Research Ethics Committee provided ethics approval for the trial (Ref: 16061A), and all trial processes complied with the Declaration of Helsinki [55].

4.4. Intervention and Randomisation

Computer-generated randomisation codes were provided by the study statistician using block sizes of four by sex, which were then forwarded to the clinical trials pharmacist. Participants were randomised to 2 g of oral carnosine (1 g twice daily, CarnoPure™ Flamma S.p.A, Chignolo d'Isola (BG), Italy), including on the clinical testing days, or an equivalent placebo group receiving 2 g of oral methylcellulose (1 g twice daily; Pharmaceutical Packaging Pty Ltd., Melbourne, Australia). Both groups were instructed to take the assigned intervention for 14 weeks. The sample size, intervention dosages and duration utilised were decided based on a pilot study and previous meta-analysis conducted by our group [40,56]. To ensure double-blinding of participants and researchers, both carnosine and placebo were provided in identical capsules within indistinguishable 60-capsule containers. All participants and trial personnel, including study physicians, nurses and research assistants, remained blinded to the intervention allocation assigned by the trial pharmacists until after trial closure and primary analyses were complete. The carnosine and the placebo powder were assessed for quality and crystallinity by an independent chemical laboratory and deemed to be free of impurities. Carnosine supplementation at these dosages has been used safely in previous studies with no reported side effects or toxicity. During informed consent, participants were advised that should any side effects arise, such as light-headedness, nausea or transient sensations of feeling hot, they should immediately inform the study physician. Treatment compliance was self-reported by participants to the study physicians. Compliance was assessed using the return of containers and counting of remaining capsules at the last follow-up visit.

4.5. Outcome Measures

The primary outcome of the RCT was a change in 2 h glucose levels after 14 weeks of carnosine supplementation, with results reported elsewhere showing beneficial effects [28]. This study examined secondary cognitive outcomes assessed in English through four tests in written and digital formats, detailed in Supplementary S1 and includes the following: (1) The Digit Symbol Substitution Test, performed in a paper format using a pre-printed questionnaire. The instruction set displayed at the top of the questionnaire had a row of numbers from '1 to 9' with corresponding non-language symbols to assess cognitive flexibility, attention and executive function; (2) The Stroop test was administered via the Encephalapp (www.encephalapp.com) application [57] and is intended to measure cognitive flexibility and processing speed; (3) The Trail Making Tests (A&B) were administered using the "Trail Making Test UK/XIF5/1014/0071" application (Norgine Pharmaceuticals Ltd., Harefield, UK) available during the trial, and assess executive functioning; and (4) The Cambridge Neuropsychological Automated Battery (CANTAB) tests were conducted on a digital tablet (iPad iOS v.10) to collect several metrics of cognitive function through different tasks.

For the CANTAB, we tested six domains as follows: (i) delayed match to sample to test the cognitive domains of attention and short-term visual recognition memory [58]; (ii) paired associates learning to test visual episodic memory [58] via a multi-stage process of remembering patterns and locations of patterns; (iii) pattern recognition memory to assess visual recognition memory [58], where participants select a previously seen pattern after being shown a series of visually complex patterns in a continuous sequence (iv); reaction time index to examine the domains of processing and psychomotor speed [58]; (v) rapid visual processing to test sustained attention, administered as a random sequence of numbers ticking in a white box in the centre of the screen, and participants press a button when the target sequence appears; and (vi) spatial working memory which assesses working memory and strategy [58] by measuring the ability to process and store spatial memory and apply it in answering the test questions.

All participants were tested at baseline (prior to randomisation) and after 14 weeks of supplementation (follow-up). Participants were contacted at week 4 and week 10 via phone to enquire about treatment side effects and compliance. Testing was conducted in the same location but not at the same time of day, and participants received a brief explanation of the method for each test before commencing their attempt. Participants were not fasting during testing and were seated in a relaxed, bright and controlled setting to limit external stimuli (noise, distractions), with only the participant and researcher present in the room.

4.6. Statistical Analysis

For this analysis, data were analysed using JASP (v0.18.3, University of Amsterdam) and SPSS (v29, IBM Corp, Armonk, NY, USA). Initially, a complete-case analysis was considered, but Little's MCAR (missing completely at random) test indicated that some data were missing at random (MAR), with no variable exceeding 10% missing data. Consequently, a modified intention-to-treat (mITT) approach was applied, including all randomised participants who completed at least one follow-up cognitive assessment after initiating treatment. Participants lost to follow-up before contributing cognitive follow-up data were excluded, while those who withdrew post-randomisation but had follow-up data were retained. Additionally, participants with incorrectly collected cognitive data were excluded.

Baseline characteristics (Table 1) were compared using independent-sample t-tests. A power analysis confirmed 80% power to detect effect sizes between 0.91 and 1.17, whereas no cognitive variable exceeded an effect size of 0.61. Missing data were imputed using predictive mean matching with five imputations. Sensitivity analysis compared mITT and imputed datasets by assessing pooled estimates from multiple imputations using Rubin's rules to evaluate whether imputation significantly altered results.

Cognitive variables were assessed for normality using histograms and the Shapiro–Wilk test. Descriptive statistics were reported as means with standard deviations (SDs) or medians with interquartile ranges (IQRs) for non-normal data. Change (delta) values were calculated by subtracting follow-up from baseline values, with between-group differences analysed via independent samples t-tests. Effect sizes were estimated using Cohen's δ.

A general linear model (GLM) was fitted to both original and imputed datasets, yielding pooled mean estimates for each variable while controlling for baseline values, intervention group (placebo; carnosine), diabetes status (prediabetes; T2DM), education level (primary; secondary; tertiary and above) and age. Exploratory analyses included an interaction term between sex and intervention group and subgroup analyses for participants with prediabetes or T2DM.

Following univariable analysis, delta values were included in multivariable linear regression models. The first model adjusted for baseline cognitive values, while subsequent models incorporated adjustments for diabetes status (Model 2), education (Model 3), age (Model 4), and sex-by-intervention interaction (Model 5). For the CANTAB test, key outcome variables were selected based on CANTAB guidelines [34], presented in Tables 2 and 3, with additional variables in the Supplementary Materials. To correct for multiple comparisons, p-values were adjusted using the Benjamini–Hochberg procedure [59,60].

Adjusted p-values were used to determine statistical significance at a two-tailed threshold of $p < 0.05$.

5. Conclusions

In this double-blind, placebo-controlled RCT, carnosine supplementation did not improve cognitive function in individuals with prediabetes or well-controlled T2DM compared with placebo. While this study was unable to detect potentially subtle cognitive effects, it highlights key considerations for future research, namely the need for larger, longer-duration trials with comprehensive neuropsychological testing. Such data will help establish more definitively whether carnosine can mitigate the cognitive impairment commonly seen in metabolic disorders such as T2DM.

Supplementary Materials: The following supporting information can be downloaded at https://www.mdpi.com/article/10.3390/ph18050630/s1.

Author Contributions: Conceptualisation, B.d.C.; methodology, R.H., A.M. (Aya Mousa), M.S. and B.d.C.; software, R.H. and J.F.; validation, R.H., A.M. (Aya Mousa), J.F. and B.d.C.; formal analysis, R.H., A.M. (Aya Mousa), J.F. and S.M.B.; investigation, R.H., A.M. (Aya Mousa), and B.d.C.; resources, B.d.C.; data curation, R.H.; writing—original draft preparation, R.H.; writing—review and editing, R.H., A.M. (Aya Mousa), K.M., J.F., B.U., J.U., M.S., A.M. (Arshad Majid), G.A., M.d.C., J.C., S.M.B. and B.d.C.; supervision, A.M. (Aya Mousa), J.F., S.M.B. and B.d.C.; project administration, R.H., K.M.; funding acquisition, B.d.C. All authors have read and agreed to the published version of the manuscript.

Funding: R.H. is supported by an Australian Government Research Training Program (RTP) Scholarship. A.M. (Aya Mousa) is supported by a fellowship from the National Health and Medical Research Council (NHMRC) of Australia. S.M.B. is supported by an Academy of Medical Sciences Starter Grants for Clinical Lecturers Scheme (Ref: SGL028\1097) and funding from the NIHR Sheffield Biomedical Research Centre award (NIHR 203321). This is a summary of independent research carried out in conjunction with the NIHR Sheffield Biomedical Research Centre (Translational Neuroscience). The views expressed are those of the author(s) and not necessarily those of the NHS, the NIHR or the Department of Health and Social Care (DHSC). Activities of J.U., B.U. and M.S. related to this work were supported by Slovak Research and Development Agency grant APVV20-0466, grant VEGA2/0076/22, VEGA-2/0161/24 and Austrian Science Fund FWF-KLI-1122.

Institutional Review Board Statement: The trial was registered on clinicaltrials.gov (NCT02917928, 28/09/16) and conducted as per the published protocol [49] in line with the Standardised Protocol Interventions: Recommendations for Interventional Trials, with reporting conforming to the CONSORT guidelines. The Monash Health Human Research Ethics Committee provided ethics approval for the trial (Ref: 16061A, 14 April 2016), and all trial processes complied with the Declaration of Helsinki.

Informed Consent Statement: Written informed consent was obtained from all subjects involved in the study.

Data Availability Statement: The data presented in this study can be made available upon reasonable request to the corresponding author. The data are not publicly available due to participant confidentiality agreements, per the conditions of the ethics approval for the trial.

Acknowledgments: We acknowledge all the participants of this trial for their time and efforts in participation. We acknowledge funding agencies including CASS (Contributing to Australian Scholarship and Science) and Royal Australasian College of Physicians foundations. We acknowledge Flamma Group for supplying carnosine for the trial.

Conflicts of Interest: The authors declare no conflicts of interest.

References

1. Whiting, D.R.; Guariguata, L.; Weil, C.; Shaw, J. IDF Diabetes Atlas: Global estimates of the prevalence of diabetes for 2011 and 2030. *Diabetes Res. Clin. Pract.* **2011**, *94*, 311–321. [CrossRef] [PubMed]
2. Sun, H.; Saeedi, P.; Karuranga, S.; Pinkepank, M.; Ogurtsova, K.; Duncan, B.B.; Stein, C.; Basit, A.; Chan, J.C.N.; Mbanya, J.C.; et al. IDF Diabetes Atlas: Global, regional and country-level diabetes prevalence estimates for 2021 and projections for 2045. *Diabetes Res. Clin. Pr.* **2022**, *183*, 109119. [CrossRef]
3. Klein, S.; Gastaldelli, A.; Yki-Järvinen, H.; Scherer, P.E. Why does obesity cause diabetes? *Cell Metab.* **2022**, *34*, 11–20. [CrossRef]
4. Drewnowski, A.; Darmon, N. The economics of obesity: Dietary energy density and energy cost. *Am. J. Clin. Nutr.* **2005**, *82*, 265S–273S. [CrossRef] [PubMed]
5. World Health Organization. *Obesity and Overweight*; World Health Organization: Geneva, Switzerland, 2024.
6. Athanasaki, A.; Melanis, K.; Tsantzali, I.; Stefanou, M.I.; Ntymenou, S.; Paraskevas, S.G.; Kalamatianos, T.; Boutati, E.; Lambadiari, V.; Voumvourakis, K.I.; et al. Type 2 Diabetes Mellitus as a Risk Factor for Alzheimer's Disease: Review and Meta-Analysis. *Biomedicines* **2022**, *10*, 778. [CrossRef]
7. Chohan, H.; Senkevich, K.; Patel, R.K.; Bestwick, J.P.; Jacobs, B.M.; Bandres Ciga, S.; Gan-Or, Z.; Noyce, A.J. Type 2 Diabetes as a Determinant of Parkinson's Disease Risk and Progression. *Mov. Disord.* **2021**, *36*, 1420–1429. [CrossRef]
8. Goldstein, B.J. Insulin resistance as the core defect in type 2 diabetes mellitus. *Am. J. Cardiol.* **2002**, *90*, 3–10. [CrossRef] [PubMed]
9. Geroldi, C.; Frisoni, G.B.; Paolisso, G.; Bandinelli, S.; Lamponi, M.; Abbatecola, A.M.; Zanetti, O.; Guralnik, J.M.; Ferrucci, L. Insulin Resistance in Cognitive Impairment: The InCHIANTI Study. *Arch. Neurol.* **2005**, *62*, 1067–1072. [CrossRef]
10. Kim, B.; Feldman, E.L. Insulin resistance as a key link for the increased risk of cognitive impairment in the metabolic syndrome. *Exp. Mol. Med.* **2015**, *47*, e149. [CrossRef]
11. Park, H.L.; O'Connell, J.E.; Thomson, R.G. A systematic review of cognitive decline in the general elderly population. *Int. J. Geriatr. Psychiatry* **2003**, *18*, 1121–1134. [CrossRef]
12. Khan, M.A.B.; Hashim, M.J.; King, J.K.; Govender, R.D.; Mustafa, H.; Al Kaabi, J. Epidemiology of Type 2 Diabetes—Global Burden of Disease and Forecasted Trends. *J. Epidemiol. Glob. Health* **2020**, *10*, 107–111. [CrossRef] [PubMed]
13. Biessels, G.J.; Despa, F. Cognitive decline and dementia in diabetes mellitus: Mechanisms and clinical implications. *Nat. Rev. Endocrinol.* **2018**, *14*, 591–604. [CrossRef] [PubMed]
14. Biessels, G.J.; Staekenborg, S.; Brunner, E.; Brayne, C.; Scheltens, P. Risk of dementia in diabetes mellitus: A systematic review. *Lancet Neurol.* **2006**, *5*, 64–74. [CrossRef]
15. Boldyrev, A.A.; Aldini, G.; Derave, W. Physiology and Pathophysiology of Carnosine. *Physiol. Rev.* **2013**, *93*, 1803–1845. [CrossRef] [PubMed]
16. Caruso, G.; Godos, J.; Castellano, S.; Micek, A.; Murabito, P.; Ferri, R.; Grosso, G.; Caraci, F. The Therapeutic Potential of Carnosine/Anserine Supplementation Against Cognitive Decline: A Systematic Review With Meta-Analysis. *Biomedicines* **2021**, *9*, 253. [CrossRef]
17. Mahomoodally, M.F.; Dilmar, A.S.; Khadaroo, S.K. Chapter 4.2—Carnosine. In *Antioxidants Effects in Health*; Nabavi, S.M., Silva, A.S., Eds.; Elsevier: Amsterdam, The Netherlands, 2022; pp. 251–268.
18. Cesak, O.; Vostalova, J.; Vidlar, A.; Bastlova, P.; Student, V., Jr. Carnosine and Beta-Alanine Supplementation in Human Medicine: Narrative Review and Critical Assessment. *Nutrients* **2023**, *15*, 1770. [CrossRef]
19. Sweeney, K.M.; Wright, G.A.; Brice, A.G.; Doberstein, S.T. The effect of β-alanine supplementation on power performance during repeated sprint activity. *J. Strength. Cond. Res.* **2010**, *24*, 79–87. [CrossRef]
20. Baierle, M.; Nascimento, S.N.; Moro, A.M.; Brucker, N.; Freitas, F.; Gauer, B.; Durgante, J.; Bordignon, S.; Zibetti, M.; Trentini, C.M.; et al. Relationship between inflammation and oxidative stress and cognitive decline in the institutionalized elderly. *Oxid. Med. Cell Longev.* **2015**, *2015*, 804198. [CrossRef]
21. Chatterjee, K.; Pal, A.; Padhy, D.S.; Saha, R.; Chatterjee, A.; Bharadwaj, M.; Sarkar, B.; Mazumder, P.M.; Banerjee, S. Vitamin K2 Ameliorates Diabetes-Associated Cognitive Decline by Reducing Oxidative Stress and Neuroinflammation. *J. Neuroimmune Pharmacol.* **2024**, *19*, 56. [CrossRef]
22. Papadopoulou, P.; Polissidis, A.; Kythreoti, G.; Sagnou, M.; Stefanatou, A.; Theoharides, T.C. Anti-Inflammatory and Neuroprotective Polyphenols Derived from the European Olive Tree, Olea europaea L., in Long COVID and Other Conditions Involving Cognitive Impairment. *Int. J. Mol. Sci.* **2024**, *25*, 11040. [CrossRef]
23. Yang, Y.; Xu, L.; Yao, X.; Wang, Y.; Fang, M.; Zhou, D.; Li, N.; Hou, Y. Isoamericanin A ameliorates neuronal damage and alleviates vascular cognitive impairments by inhibiting oxidative stress through activation of the Nrf2 pathway. *Int. Immunopharmacol.* **2024**, *143*, 113366. [CrossRef] [PubMed]
24. Chen, P.; Zhang, Z.; Lei, J.; Zhu, J.; Liu, G. Ellagitannin Component Punicalin Ameliorates Cognitive Dysfunction, Oxidative Stress, and Neuroinflammation via the Inhibition of cGAS-STING Signaling in the Brain of an Aging Mouse Model. *Phytother. Res.* **2024**, *38*, 5690–5712. [CrossRef] [PubMed]

25. Schön, M.; Mousa, A.; Berk, M.; Chia, W.L.; Ukropec, J.; Majid, A.; Ukropcová, B.; de Courten, B. The Potential of Carnosine in Brain-Related Disorders: A Comprehensive Review of Current Evidence. *Nutrients* **2019**, *11*, 1196. [CrossRef]
26. Bell, S.M.; Hariharan, R.; Laud, P.J.; Majid, A.; de Courten, B. Histidine-Containing Dipeptide Supplementation Improves Delayed Recall: A Systematic Review and Meta-Analysis. *Nutr. Rev.* **2023**, *82*, 1372–1385. [CrossRef] [PubMed]
27. Kinattingal, N.; Mehdi, S.; Undela, K.; Wani, S.U.D.; Almuqbil, M.; Alshehri, S.; Shakeel, F.; Imam, M.T.; Manjula, S.N. Prevalence of Cognitive Decline in Type 2 Diabetes Mellitus Patients: A Real-World Cross-Sectional Study in Mysuru, India. *J. Pers. Med.* **2023**, *13*, 524. [CrossRef]
28. Blackwell, A.D.; Sahakian, B.J.; Vesey, R.; Semple, J.M.; Robbins, T.W.; Hodges, J.R. Detecting Dementia: Novel Neuropsychological Markers of Preclinical Alzheimer's Disease. *Dement. Geriatr. Cogn. Disord.* **2003**, *17*, 42–48. [CrossRef]
29. De Jager, C.; Blackwell, A.D.; Budge, M.M.; Sahakian, B.J. Predicting Cognitive Decline in Healthy Older Adults. *Am. J. Geriatr. Psychiatry* **2005**, *13*, 735–740. [CrossRef]
30. O'Connell, H.; Coen, R.; Kidd, N.; Warsi, M.; Chin, A.-V.; Lawlor, B.A. Early detection of Alzheimer's disease (AD) using the CANTAB paired Associates Learning Test. *Int. J. Geriatr. Psychiatry* **2004**, *19*, 1207–1208. [CrossRef]
31. Rokicki, J.; Li, L.M.; Imabayashi, E.; Kaneko, J.; Hisatsune, T.; Matsuda, H. Daily Carnosine and Anserine Supplementation Alters Verbal Episodic Memory and Resting State Network Connectivity in Healthy Elderly Adults. *Front. Aging Neurosci.* **2015**, *7*. [CrossRef]
32. Masuoka, N.; Yoshimine, C.; Hori, M.; Tanaka, M.; Asada, T.; Abe, K.; Hisatsune, T. Effects of Anserine/Carnosine Supplementation on Mild Cognitive Impairment With APOE4. *Nutrients* **2019**, *11*, 1626. [CrossRef]
33. Hisatsune, T.; Kaneko, J.; Kurashige, H.; Cao, Y.; Satsu, H.; Totsuka, M.; Katakura, Y.; Imabayashi, E.; Matsuda, H. Effect of anserine/carnosine supplementation on verbal episodic memory in elderly people. *J. Alzheimer's Dis.* **2016**, *50*, 149–159. [CrossRef] [PubMed]
34. Cornelli, U. Treatment of Alzheimer's disease with a cholinesterase inhibitor combined with antioxidants. *Neurodegener. Dis.* **2010**, *7*, 193–202. [CrossRef]
35. Szcześniak, D.; Budzeń, S.; Kopeć, W.; Rymaszewska, J. Anserine and carnosine supplementation in the elderly: Effects on cognitive functioning and physical capacity. *Arch. Gerontol. Geriatr.* **2014**, *59*, 485–490. [CrossRef] [PubMed]
36. Baraniuk, J.N.; El-Amin, S.; Corey, R.; Rayhan, R.U.; Timbol, C.R. Carnosine treatment for gulf war illness: A randomized controlled trial. *Glob. J. Health Sci.* **2013**, *5*, 69. [CrossRef] [PubMed]
37. O'Toole, T.E.; Amraotkar, A.R.; Gao, H.; Sears, C.G.; Rai, S.N.; Basner, M.; Bhatnagar, A. Carnosine supplementation improves cognitive outcomes in younger participants of the NEAT trial. *Neurotherapeutics* **2025**, *22*, e00541. [CrossRef]
38. Xue, M.; Xu, W.; Ou, Y.-N.; Cao, X.-P.; Tan, M.-S.; Tan, L.; Yu, J.-T. Diabetes mellitus and risks of cognitive impairment and dementia: A systematic review and meta-analysis of 144 prospective studies. *Ageing Res. Rev.* **2019**, *55*, 100944. [CrossRef]
39. Dash, S.K. Cognitive impairment and diabetes. *Recent. Pat. Endocr. Metab. Immune Drug Discov.* **2013**, *7*, 155–165. [CrossRef]
40. De Courten, B.; Jakubova, M.; De Courten, M.P.; Kukurova, I.J.; Vallova, S.; Krumpolec, P.; Valkovic, L.; Kurdiova, T.; Garzon, D.; Barbaresi, S. Effects of carnosine supplementation on glucose metabolism: Pilot clinical trial. *Obesity* **2016**, *24*, 1027–1034. [CrossRef]
41. Hariharan, R.; Cameron, J.; Menon, K.; Mesinovic, J.; Jansons, P.; Scott, D.; Lu, Z.X.; de Courten, M.; Feehan, J.; de Courten, B. Carnosine supplementation improves glucose control in adults with pre-diabetes and type 2 diabetes: A randomised controlled trial. *Nutr. Metab. Cardiovasc. Dis.* **2024**, *34*, 485–496. [CrossRef]
42. Yamashita, S.; Sato, M.; Mutoh, T.; Kadooka, K.; Hasegawa, T.; Fujimura, T.; Katakura, Y. Mechanisms of Carnosine-Induced Activation of Neuronal Cells. *Biosci. Biotechnol. Biochem.* **2018**, *82*, 683–688. [CrossRef]
43. Zhu, H.; Barker, P.B. MR Spectroscopy and Spectroscopic Imaging of the Brain. In *Magnetic Resonance Neuroimaging: Methods and Protocols*; Modo, M., Bulte, J.W.M., Eds.; Humana Press: Totowa, NJ, USA, 2011; pp. 203–226.
44. Dobrota, D.; Tkáè, I.; Mlynárik, V.; Liptaj, T.; Boldyrev, A.A.; Stvolinsky, S.L. Carnosine Protective Effect on Ischemic Brain in Vivo Study Using Proton Magnetic Resonance Spectroscopy. In *Neurochemistry: Cellular, Molecular, and Clinical Aspects*; Teelken, A., Korf, J., Eds.; Springer: Boston, MA, USA, 1997; pp. 177–182.
45. Dybjer, E.; Nilsson, P.M.; Engström, G.; Helmer, C.; Nägga, K. Pre-diabetes and diabetes are independently associated with adverse cognitive test results: A cross-sectional, population-based study. *BMC Endocr. Disord.* **2018**, *18*, 91. [CrossRef] [PubMed]
46. Macready, A.L.; Butler, L.T.; Kennedy, O.B.; Ellis, J.A.; Williams, C.M.; Spencer, J.P.E. Cognitive tests used in chronic adult human randomised controlled trial micronutrient and phytochemical intervention studies. *Nutr. Res. Rev.* **2010**, *23*, 200–229. [CrossRef]
47. Bell, S.M.; Hariharan, R.; Laud, P.; Majid, A.; Courten, B. Carnosine Supplementation Improves Delayed Recall: A Systematic Review and Meta-Analysis. *Alzheimer's Dement.* **2023**, *19*, e071004. [CrossRef]
48. American Diabetes Association Professional Practice Committee. 2. Diagnosis and Classification of Diabetes: Standards of Care in Diabetes—2024. *Diabetes Care* **2023**, *47*, S20–S42. [CrossRef]

49. Baye, E.; Menon, K.; de Courten, M.P.; Earnest, A.; Cameron, J.; de Courten, B. Does supplementation with carnosine improve cardiometabolic health and cognitive function in patients with pre-diabetes and type 2 diabetes? study protocol for a randomised, double-blind, placebo-controlled trial. *BMJ Open* **2017**, *7*, e017691. [CrossRef]
50. World Health Organization. *Definition and Diagnosis of Diabetes Mellitus and Intermediate Hyperglycaemia: Report of a WHO/IDF Consultation*; World Health Organization: Geneva, Switzerland, 2006.
51. Alberti, K.G.; Mayer, M.; Zimmet, P.Z. Definition, Diagnosis and Classification of Diabetes Mellitus and Its Complications. Part 1: Diagnosis and Classification of Diabetes Mellitus. Provisional Report of a Who Consultation. *Diabet. Med.* **1998**, *15*, 539–553. [CrossRef]
52. Australian Guidelines to Reduce Health Risks from Drinking Alcohol. National Health and Medical Research Council. Available online: https://www.nhmrc.gov.au/about-us/publications/australian-guidelines-reduce-health-risks-drinking-alcohol (accessed on 17 April 2025).
53. Chan, A.W.; Tetzlaff, J.M.; Gotzsche, P.C.; Altman, D.G.; Mann, H.; Berlin, J.A.; Dickersin, K.; Hrobjartsson, A.; Schulz, K.F.; Parulekar, W.R.; et al. SPIRIT 2013 explanation and elaboration: Guidance for protocols of clinical trials. *BMJ* **2013**, *346*, e7586. [CrossRef]
54. Schulz, K.F.; Altman, D.G.; Moher, D.; Group, C. CONSORT 2010 statement: Updated guidelines for reporting parallel group randomized trials. *Ann. Intern. Med.* **2010**, *152*, 726–732. [CrossRef]
55. World Medical Association Declaration of Helsinki: Ethical principles for medical research involving human subjects. *JAMA* **2013**, *310*, 2191–2194. [CrossRef]
56. Menon, K.; Marquina, C.; Liew, D.; Mousa, A.; de Courten, B. Histidine-containing dipeptides reduce central obesity and improve glycaemic outcomes: A systematic review and meta-analysis of randomized controlled trials. *Obes. Rev.* **2020**, *21*, e12975. [CrossRef]
57. Bajaj, J.S.; Heuman, D.M.; Sterling, R.K.; Sanyal, A.J.; Siddiqui, M.; Matherly, S.; Luketic, V.; Stravitz, R.T.; Fuchs, M.; Thacker, L.R.; et al. Validation of EncephalApp, Smartphone-Based Stroop Test, for the Diagnosis of Covert Hepatic Encephalopathy. *Clin. Gastroenterol. Hepatol.* **2015**, *13*, 1828–1835.e1821. [CrossRef] [PubMed]
58. Cantab Connect Research: Admin Application User Guide. 2021. Available online: https://gbiomed.kuleuven.be/english/research/50000737/research/pash/pasoca/documenten/CANTAB-Connect-Research-Admin-Application-User-Guide.pdf (accessed on 17 April 2025).
59. Benjamini, Y.; Hochberg, Y. Controlling the false discovery rate: A practical and powerful approach to multiple testing. *J. R. Stat. Soc. Ser. B* **1995**, *57*, 289–300. [CrossRef]
60. Yekutieli, D.; Benjamini, Y. Resampling-based false discovery rate controlling multiple test procedures for correlated test statistics. *J. Stat. Plan. Inference* **1999**, *82*, 171–196. [CrossRef]

pharmaceuticals

MDPI

Article

Effects of Ganjianglingzhu Decoction on Lean Non-Alcoholic Fatty Liver Disease in Mice Based on Untargeted Metabolomics

Nan Tang [1], Lei Ji [2], Xinyu Shi [1], Yalan Xiong [1], Xinying Xiong [1], Hanhua Zhao [3], Hualing Song [1], Jianying Wang [1], Lei Zhang [1], Shengfu You [4], Guang Ji [1,4,5], Baocheng Liu [1,5,*] and Na Wu [1,5,*]

[1] School of Public Health, Shanghai Innovation Center of Traditional Chinese Medicine Health Service, Shanghai University of Traditional Chinese Medicine, Shanghai 201203, China; tangnan@shutcm.edu.cn (N.T.); 22022547@shutcm.edu.cn (X.S.); yalanxiongg@shutcm.edu.cn (Y.X.); 0022023573@shutcm.edu.cn (X.X.); 99shl@163.com (H.S.); wjy8310@163.com (J.W.); zhanglei37@sina.com (L.Z.); jg@shutcm.edu.cn (G.J.)

[2] Bio-X Institutes, Key Laboratory for the Genetics of Developmental and Neuropsychiatric Disorders, Shanghai Jiao Tong University, Shanghai 200030, China; amber_jl@sjtu.edu.cn

[3] Department of Sport Science, College of Education, Zhejiang University, Hangzhou 310058, China; 12003024@zju.edu.cn

[4] Institute of Digestive Diseases, Longhua Hospital, Shanghai University of Traditional Chinese Medicine, Shanghai 200032, China; yoosf@sina.com

[5] State Key Laboratory of Integration and Innovation of Classic Formula and Modern Chinese Medicine, Shanghai University of Traditional Chinese Medicine, Shanghai 201203, China

* Correspondence: baochliu_lab@163.com (B.L.); wuna0308@163.com (N.W.); Tel.: +86-021-51322155 (N.W.)

Abstract: Non-alcoholic fatty liver disease (NAFLD) is usually associated with obesity. However, it is crucial to recognize that NAFLD can also occur in lean individuals, which is frequently overlooked. Without an approved pharmacological therapy for lean NAFLD, we aimed to investigate whether the Ganjianglingzhu (GJLZ) decoction, a representative traditional Chinese medicine (TCM), protects against lean NAFLD and explore the potential mechanism underlying these protective effects. The mouse model of lean NAFLD was established with a methionine-choline-deficient (MCD) diet in male C57BL/6 mice to be compared with the control group fed the methionine-choline-sufficient (MCS) diet. After four weeks, physiological saline, a low dose of GJLZ decoction (GL), or a high dose of GJLZ decoction (GH) was administered daily by gavage to the MCD group; the MCS group was given physiological saline by gavage. Untargeted metabolomics techniques were used to explore further the potential mechanism of the effects of GJLZ on lean NAFLD. Different doses of GJLZ decoction were able to ameliorate steatosis, inflammation, fibrosis, and oxidative stress in the liver; GL performed a better effect on lean NAFLD. In addition, 78 candidate differential metabolites were screened and identified. Combined with metabolite pathway enrichment analysis, GL was capable of regulating the glucose and lipid metabolite pathway in lean NAFLD and regulating the glycerophospholipid metabolism by altering the levels of sn-3-O-(geranylgeranyl)glycerol 1-phosphate and lysoPC(P-18:0/0:0). GJLZ may protect against the development of lean NAFLD by regulating glucose and lipid metabolism, inhibiting the levels of sn-3-O-(geranylgeranyl)glycerol 1-phosphate and lysoPC(P-18:0/0:0) in glycerophospholipid metabolism.

Keywords: Ganjianglingzhu decoction; lean NAFLD; glycerophospholipid metabolism

1. Introduction

As the most prevalent chronic liver disease, the overall morbidity of non-alcoholic fatty liver disease (NAFLD) worldwide has significantly increased, from 25.5% to 37.8% in the last 20 years [1]. NAFLD covers a series of illnesses, including liver steatosis and non-alcoholic steatohepatitis (NASH), and leads to liver fibrosis and hepatocellular carcinoma [2]. Increasing evidence has demonstrated NAFLD is closely related to metabolic syndrome, covering type 2 diabetes mellitus, dyslipidemia, obesity, and hypertension [3].

Of note, NAFLD is not exclusive to overweight or obese individuals; it is also discovered in lean people. NAFLD in lean individuals is far from uncommon, with prevalence rates around 14.5%, but it is easier to ignore than NAFLD in overweight or obese individuals, which leads to severe consequences [4].

Lean NAFLD represents a proportion of NAFLD cases that have a normal body mass index (BMI); an estimated 13.11% of individuals with NAFLD have lean body habitus [5,6]. The World Health Organization's standard defines normal weight as a BMI between 18.5 and 24.9 kg/m^2 [7]. Otherwise, visceral fat accumulation is detrimental to lean NAFLD patients, making waist circumference a supplementary indicator of BMI [8]. Some reports show that lean NAFLD patients exhibit a higher fibrosis-4 index and mortality than obese NAFLD patients [9–11]. At present, the pathophysiology of lean NAFLD remains obscure.

The current treatment for lean NAFLD is to lose 3–5% of weight through lifestyle intervention, including exercise and dietary changes [12]. Nevertheless, the majority of patients have difficulty maintaining a lifestyle intervention in practice. Moreover, the lack of effective therapeutic medicine for lean NAFLD remains a serious problem. The current medicines for NAFLD are vitamin E, metformin, glucagon-like peptide-1 agonists (liraglutide), and pioglitazone. Still, their therapeutic role in lean NAFLD needs to be further explored [5,12]. Therefore, there is an urgent need to conduct research into lean NAFLD's pathogenesis and undertake drug development.

The active ingredients in a large number of traditional Chinese medicines (TCMs) significantly affect NAFLD [13,14]. Due to the lack of pharmaceutical options in lean NAFLD, we intended to discover a kind of TCM that is effective for lean NAFLD. The Ganjianglingzhu (GJLZ) decoction is a representative formula that successfully alleviates hepatic steatosis and inflammation in NAFLD rats [15,16]. Whether it is also effective against lean NAFLD is unclear.

Therefore, we utilized the methionine-choline-deficient (MCD) diet to imitate the progression of NAFLD, as first proposed by Shinozuka. In this model, steatohepatitis develops rapidly, with apparent steatohepatitis lesions at about three weeks, liver fibrosis at eight weeks, and significant weight loss [17]. The pathological lesions caused by MCD diet are similar to those of human NAFLD. In addition, we investigated the effects of the GJLZ decoction on lean NAFLD through untargeted metabolomics. The potential metabolic biomarkers related to lean NAFLD were identified, and the underlying mechanism was explored. Our findings might also guide the optimization of TCM treatment for lean NAFLD.

2. Results

2.1. The Analysis of GJLZ Compositions

A total of 37 compounds of GJLZ were identified by UPLC-Q-TOF/MS. The chromatograms are exhibited in Figure 1, and the detailed information about the compounds is summarized in Table S3.

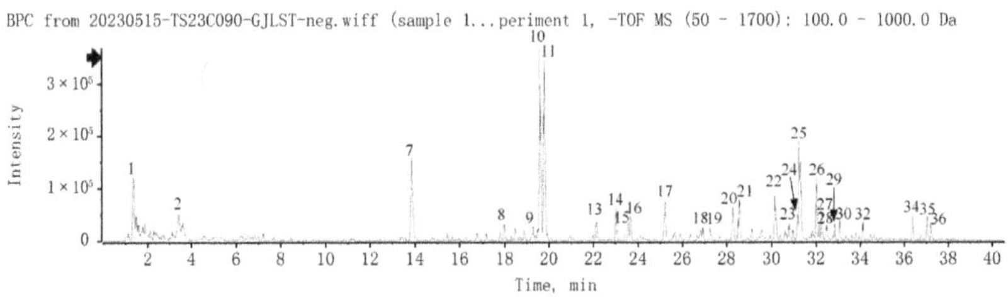

(a)

Figure 1. *Cont.*

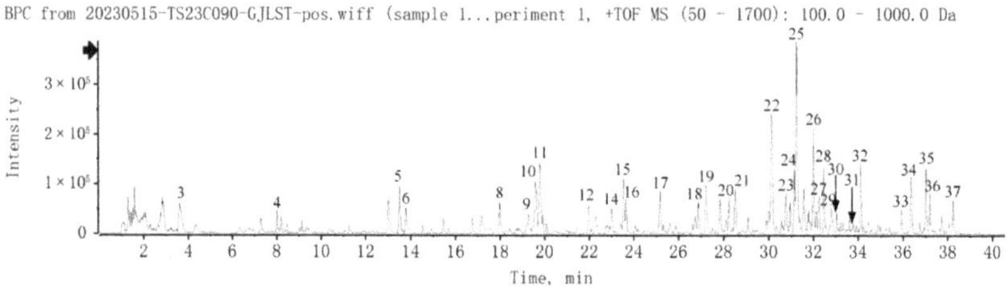

(b)

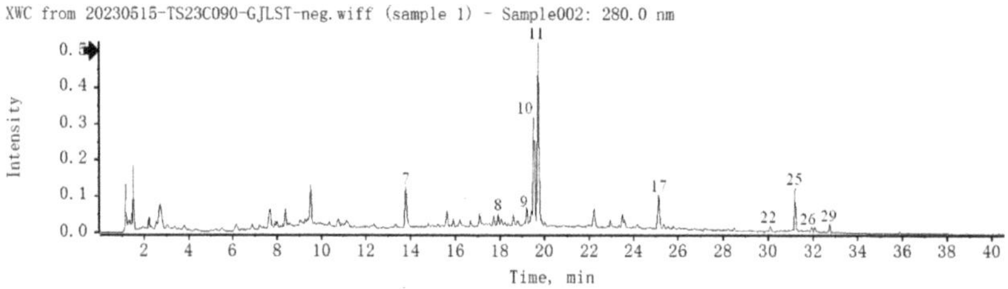

(c)

Figure 1. UPLC-Q-TOF/MS analysis of GJLZ decoction. (**a**) The base peak chromatogram of GJLZ decoction via UPLC-HRMS in negative ion mode. (**b**) The base peak chromatogram of GJLZ decoction via UPLC-HRMS in positive ion mode. (**c**) The UV chromatogram of GJLZ decoction at 280 nm. Each number of the peak was identified as the ingredient of GJLZ, the detail information is summarized in Table S3. GJLZ, Ganjianglingzhu.

2.2. *Evaluation of the Lean NAFLD Mode*

2.2.1. Body Weight of Mice

After one week of adaptive feeding, no significant difference was observed in body weight between the MCS and the MCD groups. From the first week to the fourth week, the body weight significantly reduced in the MCD group compared with the MCS group, as shown in Figure 2a.

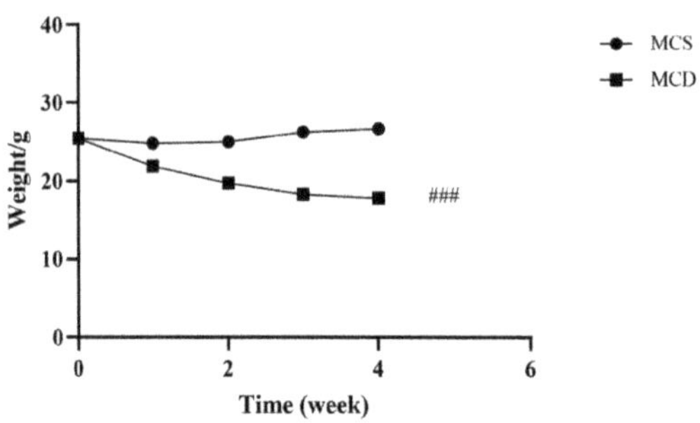

(a)

Figure 2. *Cont.*

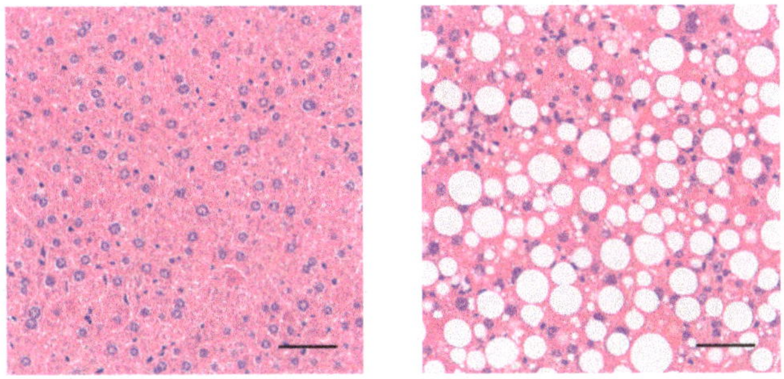

MCS **MCD**

(**b**)

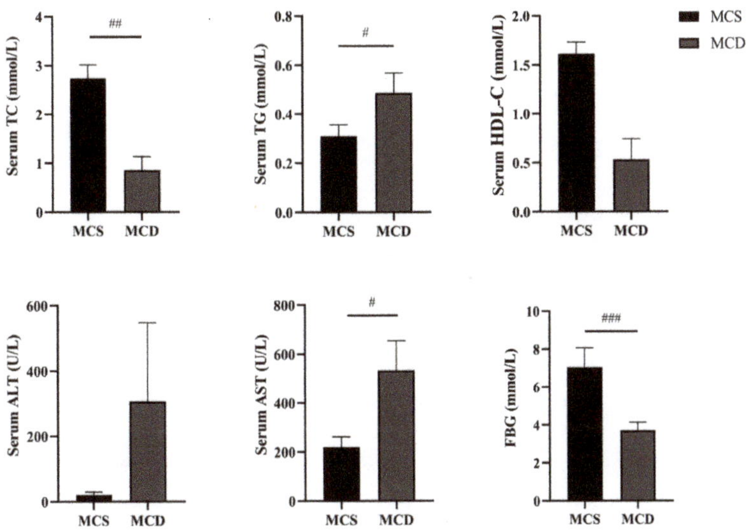

(**c**)

Figure 2. Evaluation of the lean NAFLD model in the fourth week. (**a**) Weight changes in the fourth week. (**b**) H&E staining of hepatic tissue (magnification 200×, the scale bar refers to 50 μm). (**c**) The levels of serum TC, TG, HDL-C, ALT, AST, and FBG. ALT, alanine transaminase; AST, aspartate transaminase; FBG, fasting blood glucose; HDL-C, high-density lipoprotein cholesterol; MCD, methionine-choline-deficient; MCS, methionine-choline-sufficient; NAFLD, non-alcoholic fatty liver disease; TC, total cholesterol; TG, triglyceride. # $p < 0.050$, ## $p < 0.010$ and ### $p < 0.001$: MCD group compared with the MCS group.

2.2.2. Liver Histology

Morphologic evaluations provided visual evidence of injury from MCD diet-induced NAFLD (Figure 2b). The H&E results showed typical hepatocytes with well-preserved cytoplasm, obvious nucleus and nucleolus, liver lobules, and no steatosis in the MCS group. In the MCD group, we observed the hepatocyte's steatosis and inflammatory cell infiltration.

2.2.3. Changes in Serum Index of Mice

Compared with the MCS group, serum TG and AST ($p < 0.05$) were significantly increased, and serum TC ($p < 0.01$) and FBG ($p < 0.001$) were significantly decreased, in the MCD group. Serum HDL-C was decreased and serum ALT was increased mainly in the MCD group, although no significant difference was exhibited (Figure 2c). Our results demonstrated that the MCD diet could increase levels of serum liver enzymes, contributing to dyslipidemia and impairing both liver function and lipid metabolism. Based on the abovementioned results, the lean NAFLD model succeeded after four weeks.

2.3. Effects of GJLZ on Body Weight

After eight weeks of the experiment, compared with the MCS group, the body weight ($p < 0.001$) was significantly reduced in the MCD group. Nevertheless, there was no significant difference among MCD, GL, and GH groups. During the treatment, MCD, GL, and GH groups all displayed the trend of weight loss, as shown in Figure 3a.

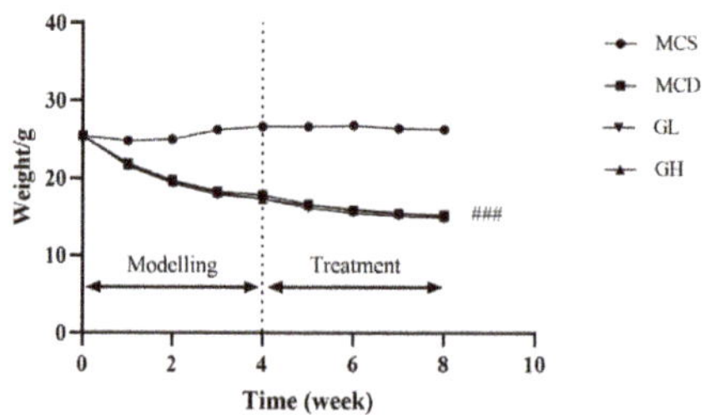

(**a**)

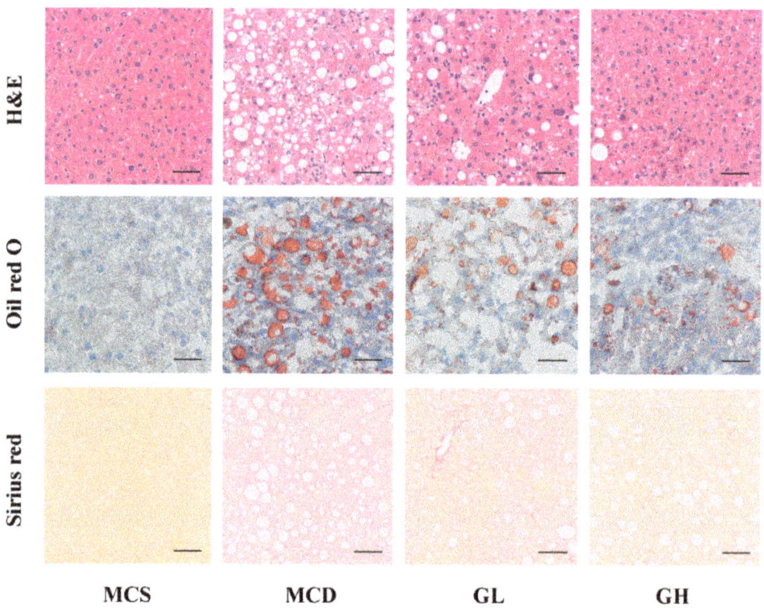

(**b**)

Figure 3. *Cont.*

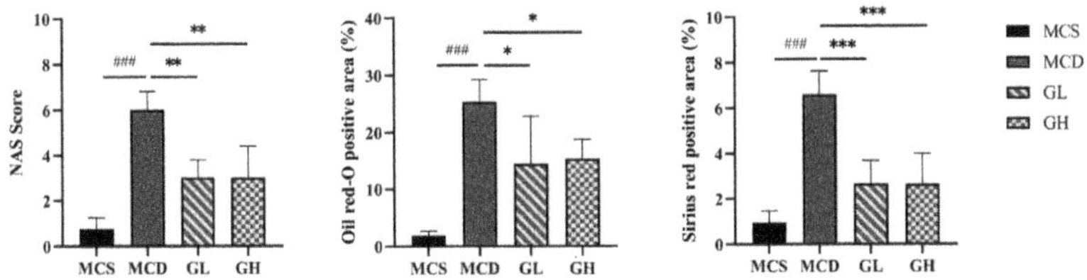

(c)

Figure 3. GJLZ ameliorated lean NAFLD induced by the MCD diet. (**a**) Weight changes in the four groups. (**b**) Representative images of hepatic H&E staining, Oil Red O staining, and Sirius Red staining (magnification 200×, the scale bar refers to 50 μm). (**c**) NAS score of liver and histomorphometric analysis of the positive area with Oil Red O staining and Sirius Red staining. GH, high dose of GJLZ; GJLZ, Ganjianglingzhu; GL, low dose of GJLZ; MCD, methionine-choline-deficient; MCS, methionine-choline-sufficient; NAFLD, non-alcoholic fatty liver disease; NAS, NAFLD activity score. ### $p < 0.001$: MCD group compared with the MCS group; * $p < 0.050$, ** $p < 0.010$ and *** $p < 0.001$: GL group and GH group compared with the MCD group.

2.4. Effects of GJLZ on Liver Morphology

The liver morphological results revealed severe structural destruction of liver tissue in the MCD group, heavy fat infiltration, hepatomegaly, and inflammatory cell infiltration and fibrosis (Figure 3b). The liver morphology and structure were relatively complete; hepatocellular ballooning was ameliorated, with less inflammatory cell infiltration and fibrosis in the GL and GH groups compared with the MCD group (Figure 3b,c). According to the hepatic histological changes, GL and GH could also significantly decrease NAFLD activity score (NAS) (Figure 3c).

2.5. Effects of GJLZ on Serum Index

Compared with the MCS group, serum TG ($p < 0.05$), ALT, AST ($p < 0.001$), and TBIL ($p < 0.05$) were significantly increased, and serum TC, HDL-C ($p < 0.01$), and FBG ($p < 0.001$) were significantly decreased, in the MCD group. Serum TG ($p < 0.01$), ALT, AST, and TBIL ($p < 0.05$) were significantly decreased, and serum HDL-C ($p < 0.05$) was significantly increased, in the GL group; serum TG, ALT, and TBIL ($p < 0.05$) were significantly decreased, and serum HDL-C ($p < 0.05$) was increased, in the GH group, compared with the MCD group (Figure 4a).

2.6. Antioxidative Effects of GJLZ

Previous studies have shown that oxidative stress is of great importance in lean NAFLD. The liver SOD ($p < 0.001$) and T-AOC ($p < 0.05$) were significantly decreased, and the liver MDA ($p < 0.001$) was significantly increased in the MCD group, compared with the MCS group (Figure 4b). The liver SOD and T-AOC were higher, while the liver MDA was lower, in the GL and GH groups than those in the MCD group (SOD, $p < 0.01$; T-AOC, $p < 0.05$; MDA, $p < 0.01$ in the GL group; SOD, $p < 0.05$; MDA, $p < 0.001$ in the GH group, Figure 4b). Overall, the results manifested that GJLZ had the effect of anti-oxidation and alleviating lean NAFLD symptoms.

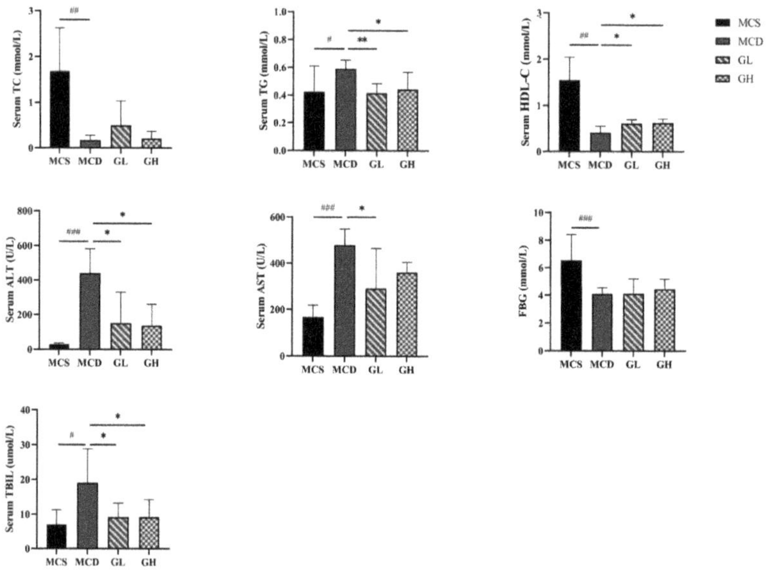

(a)

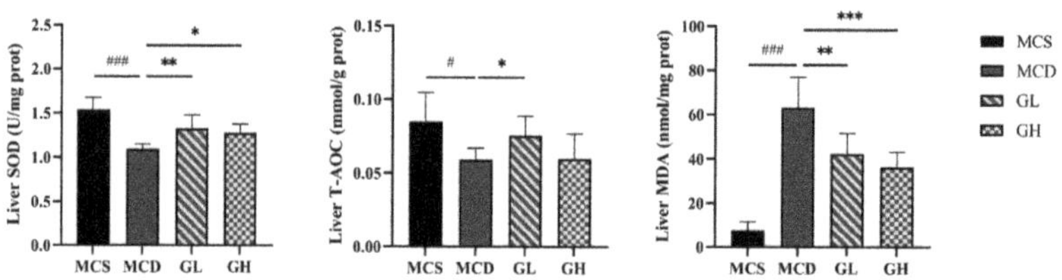

(b)

Figure 4. Serum index and liver oxidative stress index among the four groups. (**a**) The levels of serum TC, TG, HDL-C, ALT, AST, FBG, and TBIL. (**b**) The levels of liver SOD, T-AOC, and MDA. ALT, alanine transaminase; AST, aspartate transaminase; FBG, fasting blood glucose; GH, high dose of GJLZ; GJLZ, Ganjianglingzhu; GL, low dose of GJLZ; HDL-C, high-density lipoprotein cholesterol; MCD, methionine-choline-deficient; MCS, methionine-choline-sufficient; MDA, malondialdehyde; SOD, superoxide dismutase; TBIL, total bilirubin; TC, total cholesterol; TG, triglyceride; T-AOC, total antioxidant capacity. # $p < 0.050$, ## $p < 0.010$ and ### $p < 0.001$: MCD group compared with the MCS group; * $p < 0.050$, ** $p < 0.010$ and *** $p < 0.001$: GL group and GH group compared with the MCD group.

2.7. Untargeted Metabolomics Analysis

2.7.1. Quality Control

PCA plots demonstrated a significant separation of liver metabolites between the MCS and MCD groups, as well as a significant separation between the MCD and GL groups (Figure 5a–c). Based on the established OPLS-DA model, the predictive index of the model (Q2) was assessed using seven-fold cross-validation and 200 RPT. Significant segregation of liver metabolites was observed between the MCS group and the MCD group (Figure 5d), as well as between the MCD group and the GL group (Figure 5f), in OPLS-DA models. All samples were within the 95% confidence interval. In the OPLS-DA model, the R2 and Q2 values were (0.0, 0.911) and (0.0, −0.737) between the MCS group and MCD group

(Figure 5e), while the R2 and Q2 values were (0.0, 0.894) and (0.0, −0.629) between the MCD group and GL group (Figure 5g).

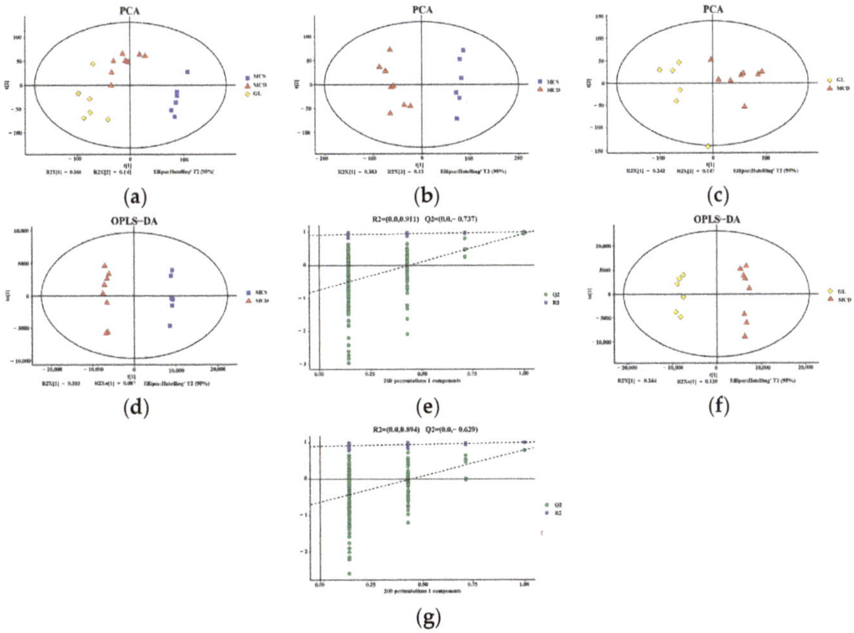

Figure 5. Quality control of the metabolomics data. (**a**) PCA score plot among the three groups. PCA showed a clear group separation between the three groups. (**b**) PCA score plot shows the metabolic state difference between the MCS group and the MCD group. (**c**) PCA score plot showing the difference in the metabolic state between the GL group and MCD group. (**d**,**e**) Score plots of OPLS-DA between the MCS group and the MCD model group and the corresponding coefficient of loading plots. The OPLS-DA models indicated significant metabolic variations between the MCS group and the MCD group. (**f**,**g**) Score plots of OPLS-DA between the GL group and the MCD group and the corresponding coefficient of loading plots. The OPLS-DA models indicated significant metabolic variations between the GL group and the MCD group. GJLZ, Ganjianglingzhu; GL, low dose of GJLZ; MCD, methionine-choline-deficient; MCS, methionine-choline-sufficient; OPLS-DA, orthogonal partial least-squares-discriminant analysis; PCA, principal component analysis.

2.7.2. Cluster Analysis

Differential metabolite analysis was performed between the MCS and the MCD groups (VIP > 1 and $p < 0.05$), and a total of 553 liver differential metabolites were identified (Figure 6a); a total of 351 liver differential metabolites were detected between the MCD and the GL groups (VIP > 1 and $p < 0.05$) (Figure 6b). Figure 6c shows that fatty acyls, glycerophospholipids, prenol lipids, steroids, and steroid derivatives were the differential metabolites between MCS and MCD groups, indicating the successful NAFLD modeling. The cluster analysis of the metabolites between MCD and GL groups showed that 44.73% of metabolites were related to fatty acyls, glycerolipids, glycerophospholipids, prenol lipids, steroids, and steroid derivatives (Figure 6d). To more intuitively represent the differences in metabolites, cluster analysis heatmaps were used to classify the top 50 liver differential metabolites between MCS and MCD groups, as well as the principal 50 liver differential metabolites between MCD and GL groups (Figure 6e,f). We selected 78 metabolites that kept the same trends between the MCS and GL groups after comparing them with the MCD group (Tables 1 and S4).

Table 1. List of the top 10 identified metabolites of the intersection statistics between MCS vs. MCD and MCD vs. GL in positive and negative ion modes based on UHPLC-Q-TOF/MS.

m/z	Retention Time (min)	Ion Mode	Formula	Metabolites	VIP	*p*-Value	FC	
							MCS vs. MCD	MCD vs. GL
453.2860415	7.848233333	neg	C24H40O5	alpha-Muricholic acid	16.06769146	0.001366585	0.226549791	4.844474413
854.5920444	11.47483333	neg	C46H84NO8P	PE(22:4(7Z,10Z,13Z,16Z)/19:0)	11.85212432	0.000161857	1.861265702	0.653574112
373.2735342	8.718383333	pos	C24H36O3	3alpha-Hydroxy-5beta-chola-7,9(11)-dien-24-oic Acid	10.53291874	0.001324031	0.254796555	4.932638804
469.2808627	6.996783333	neg	C24H40O6	3alpha,6alpha,7beta,12alpha-Tetrahydroxy-5beta-cholan-24-oic Acid	9.722835203	0.00032875	0.108749729	5.89703359
786.6001094	12.6016	pos	C44H86NO9P	PS(O-20:0/18:1(9Z))	9.283616715	0.016021262	1.313988022	0.796299615
526.2928203	10.2723	pos	C27H44NO7P	LysoPE(0:0/22:6(4Z,7Z,10Z,13Z,16Z,19Z))	9.248142084	0.002656101	0.589762419	1.94542687
475.2678339	7.848233333	neg	C26H38O5	15-keto Latanoprost	7.181839741	0.001131022	0.312034456	3.641811108
837.5497715	7.848233333	neg	C43H83O13P	PI(18:0/16:0)	5.834670211	0.002426321	0.074756485	17.15141474
113.0713445	14.8042	pos	C5H5NO	2-Hydroxypyridine	5.509739735	7.52517×10^{-6}	1.075065689	0.845072861
165.113551	14.23996667	pos	C8H14N4O	Carcinine	5.38750534	0.000454935	1.071885203	0.879479787

FC, fold change; GJLZ, Ganjianglingzhu; GL, low dose of GJLZ; MCD, methionine-choline-deficient; MCS, methionine-choline-sufficient; VIP, variable importance of projection.

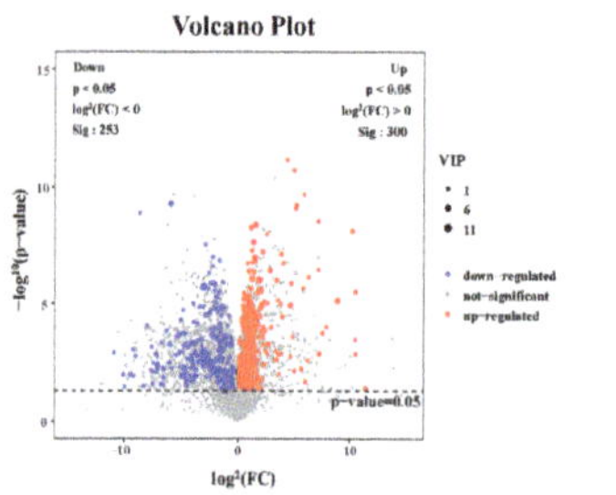

(a)

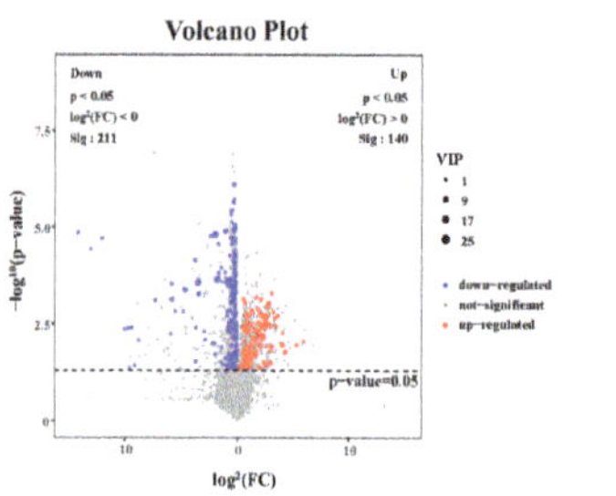

(b)

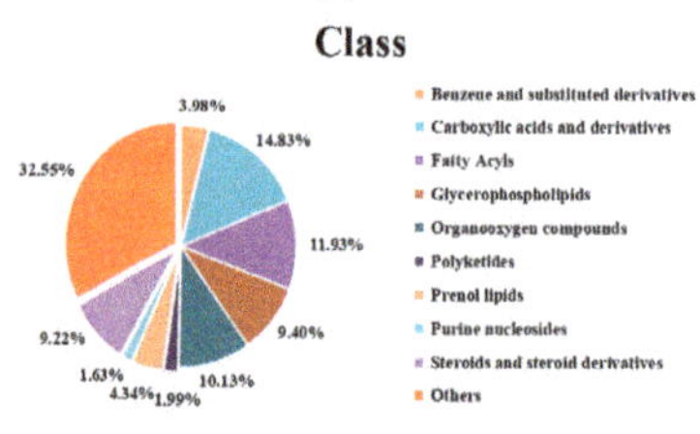

(c)

Figure 6. *Cont.*

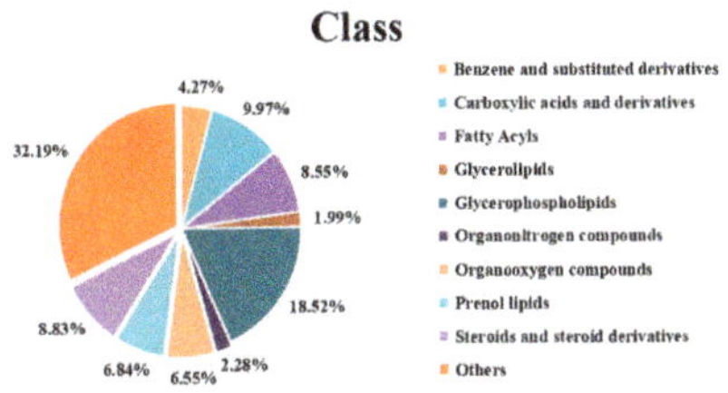

(**d**)

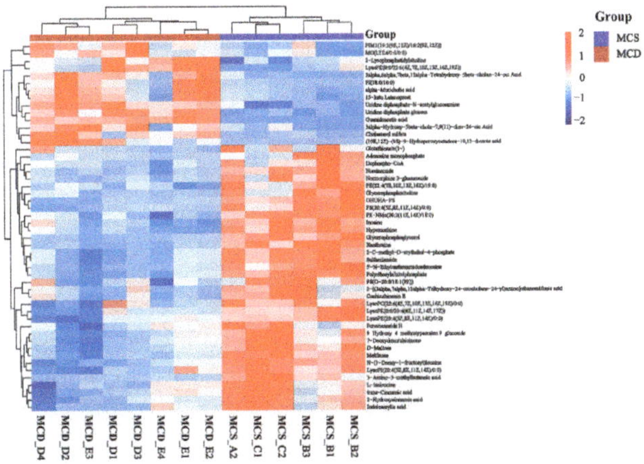

(**e**)

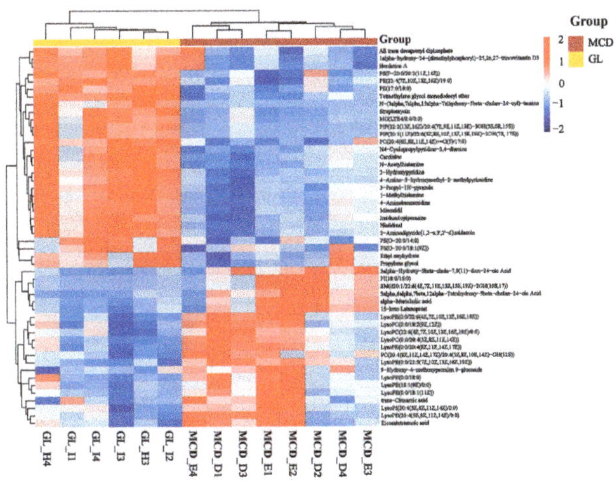

(**f**)

Figure 6. Analysis of different metabolites among three groups. (**a**) Volcano plot for differential metabolites in MCS vs. MCD. (**b**) Volcano plot for differential metabolites in GL vs. MCD. (**c**) Classification of differential metabolites between MCS and MCD groups. (**d**) Classification of differential metabolites between MCD and GL groups. (**e**) Hierarchical cluster analysis heat map of top 50 liver content metabolites in MCS vs. MCD. (**f**) Hierarchical cluster analysis heat map of top 50 liver content metabolites in GL vs. MCD. GJLZ, Ganjianglingzhu; GL, low dose of GJLZ; MCD, methionine-choline-deficient; MCS, methionine-choline-sufficient; VIP, variable importance of projection.

2.7.3. Metabolite Pathway Enrichment Analysis

The KEGG database was applied to explore the relevant metabolic pathway of differential metabolites between the MCS and the MCD groups and between the MCD and the GL groups. The analysis of differential metabolic pathways showed significantly affected pathways ($p < 0.05$) and the number of metabolites. When lean NAFLD mice were fed a MCD diet, the perturbed metabolites were primarily concerned with ABC transporters, purine metabolism, pantothenate and CoA biosynthesis, choline metabolism in cancer, pyrimidine metabolism, protein digestion and absorption, beta-alanine metabolism, aminoacyl-tRNA biosynthesis, glycerophospholipid metabolism, arachidonic acid metabolism, central carbon metabolism in cancer, amino sugar and nucleotide sugar metabolism, galactose metabolism, cGMP-PKG signaling pathway, carbohydrate digestion and absorption, linoleic acid metabolism, mineral absorption, morphine addiction, ascorbate and aldarate metabolism, regulation of lipolysis in adipocytes, sphingolipid signaling pathway, vascular smooth muscle contraction, and glutathione metabolism (Figure 7a). After treatment with GL (Figure 7b), the metabolites were related to histidine metabolism, ABC transporters, choline metabolism in cancer, primary bile acid biosynthesis, glycerophospholipid metabolism, citrate cycle (tricarboxylic acid cycle, TCA cycle), bile secretion, glucagon signaling pathway, carbohydrate digestion and absorption, alanine, aspartate and glutamate metabolism, pyruvate metabolism, sulfur metabolism, taste transduction, central carbon metabolism in cancer, and glycerolipid metabolism. We found that citric acid and succinic acid, belonging to the TCA cycle, glucagon signaling pathway, alanine, aspartate, and glutamate metabolism, were significantly increased in the GL group; D-Lactic acid was also elevated in the GL group, which belongs to pyruvate metabolism (Figure 7c). In the glycerophospholipid metabolism pathway, sn-3-O-(geranylgeranyl)glycerol 1-phosphate and lysoPC(P-18:0/0:0) were all higher in the MCD group than in the MCS and GL groups (Figure 7d). Therefore, we focused on the change in sn-3-O-(geranylgeranyl)glycerol 1-phosphate and lysoPC(P-18:0/0:0) in three groups.

2.8. Spearman Correlation Analysis of Serum Biochemical Indicators, Liver Antioxidant Indicators, and Differential Metabolites

The Spearman correlation analysis was conducted between serum biochemical indicators, liver antioxidant indicators, and the 78 metabolites selected above (Table S5). Through this analysis, we discovered that two metabolites belonging to the glycerophospholipid metabolism pathway were closely associated with these indicators. Sn-3-O-(geranylgeranyl)glycerol 1-phosphate was positively correlated with serum TG, AST, and liver MDA, while it was negatively correlated with liver SOD; lysoPC(P-18:0/0:0) was positively correlated with serum ALT, AST, and liver MDA, while it was also negatively correlated with serum HDL-C, liver SOD, and T-AOC (Table 2).

Table 2. The correlation between biochemical indicators and the metabolites.

	TG	HDL-C	ALT	AST	TBIL	SOD	T-AOC	MDA
sn-3-O-(geranylgeranyl)glycerol 1-phosphate	0.560 *	−0.443	0.475	0.569 *	0.29	−0.624 **	−0.354	0.649 **
LysoPC(P-18:0/0:0)	0.362	−0.896 **	0.741 **	0.800 **	0.293	−0.706 **	−0.737 **	0.738 **

ALT, alanine transaminase; AST, aspartate transaminase; HDL-C, high-density lipoprotein cholesterol; MDA, malondialdehyde; SOD, superoxide dismutase; TBIL, total bilirubin; TG, triglyceride; T-AOC, total antioxidant capacity. * Correlation is significant at the 0.05 level (2-tailed); ** correlation is significant at the 0.01 level (2-tailed).

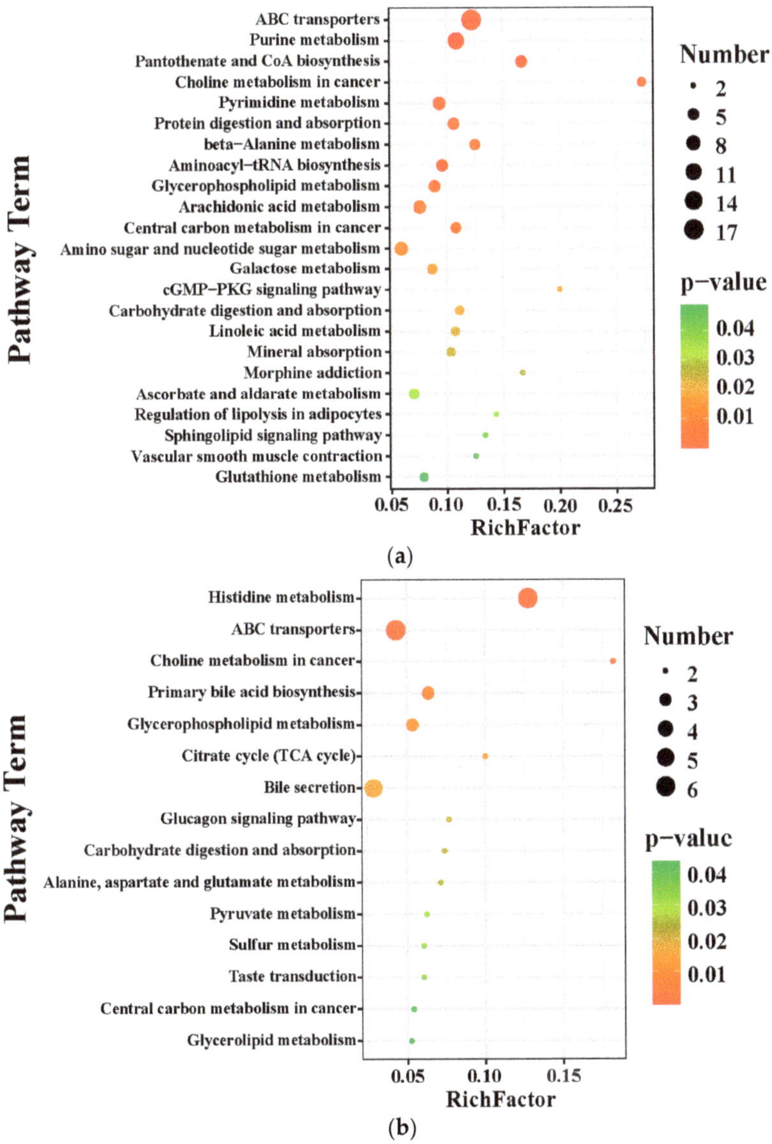

Figure 7. *Cont.*

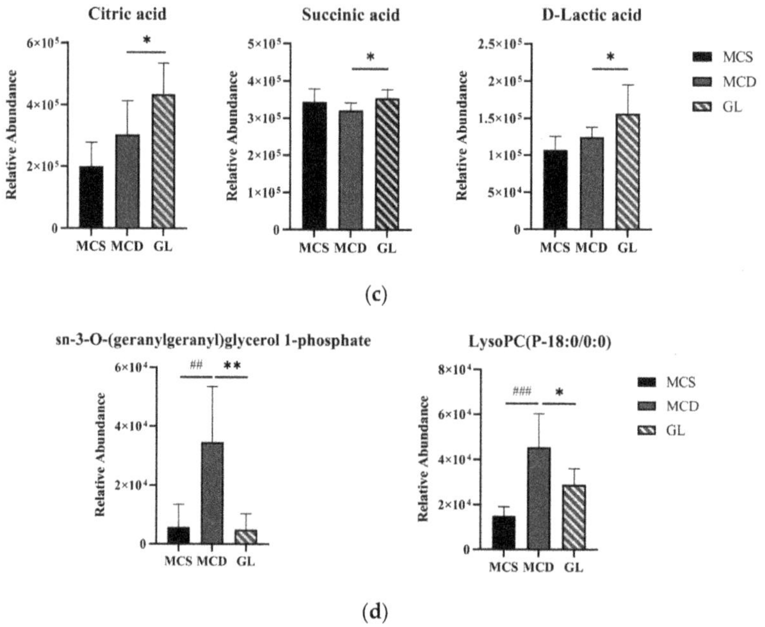

Figure 7. Metabolite pathway enrichment analysis. (**a**) KEGG pathway enrichment analysis between the MCS group and the MCD group. (**b**) KEGG pathway enrichment analysis between the GL group and the MCD group. (**c**) After treatment with GL, the specific differential metabolites in the tricarboxylic acid cycle, glucagon signaling pathway, alanine, aspartate and glutamate metabolism, and pyruvate metabolism. (**d**) In the glycerophospholipid metabolism pathway, sn-3-O-(geranylgeranyl)glycerol 1-phosphate and LysoPC(P-18:0/0:0) were all higher in the MCD group than in the MCS and GL groups. GJLZ, Ganjianglingzhu; GL, low dose of GJLZ; MCD, methionine-choline-deficient; MCS, methionine-choline-sufficient. ## $p < 0.010$ and ### $p < 0.001$: MCD group compared with the MCS group; * $p < 0.050$, and ** $p < 0.01$: GL group compared with the MCD group.

3. Discussion

Lean NAFLD patients exhibit a normal BMI but have insulin resistance, excessive visceral adiposity, and metabolic dysfunction, which are typically observed in obese individuals [18]. At present, there is an increasing consensus that lean NAFLD may be associated with genetic and environmental factors [19–21]. At the same time, there is no proven medical treatment for lean NAFLD [22]. Therefore, we designed an experiment to verify whether GJLZ is effective in treating lean NAFLD. The results showed the following: (1) GJLZ can alleviate the degree of steatosis, inflammation, fibrosis, and oxidative stress injury in the liver and antagonize the accumulation of lipids in serum. (2) GJLZ improves glucose and lipid metabolism in lean NAFLD. (3) GJLZ can regulate glycerophospholipid metabolism, and the two metabolites from the glycerophospholipid metabolism pathway: sn-3-O-(geranylgeranyl)glycerol 1-phosphate and lysoPC(P-18:0/0:0) might become novel targets for lean NAFLD.

In this research, we measured body weight and serum biochemical parameters and evaluated liver morphology to trial the effect of the MCD diet in modeling lean NAFLD and the effectiveness of GJLZ in treating lean NAFLD. The MCD diet was able to reduce weight, FBG, serum TC, and HDL-C; elevate serum TG, ALT, AST, and TBIL; and cause steatosis, inflammation lobular, hepatocellular ballooning, and fibrosis in the liver, which was consistent with the results of previous research [23]. After treatment with GJLZ, we found different doses of GJLZ ameliorate steatosis, inflammation, and fibrosis in the liver, lessen serum lipid accumulation, and reduce liver damage. This is consistent with the research of Dang et al., which showed that GJLZ decoction improved liver steatosis and inflammation, alleviated the liver injury, and considerably reduced serum AST and ALT contents in NAFLD [15].

Oxidative stress in the liver is important in the progression of lean NAFLD. SOD, T-AOC, and MDA are the leading indices that measure the antioxidant capacity. Liver MDA is the lipid peroxidation product that was elevated in the MCD group when compared with the MCS, GL, and GH groups; SOD, which is an antioxidant enzyme that makes significant contributions to diminish oxidative stress, was lower in the MCD group when compared with MCS, GL, and GH groups [24,25]. The liver T-AOC level was lower in the MCD group than in the MCS and GL groups. The MCD diet increased liver oxidative stress and decreased the antioxidant capacity, exacerbating lean NAFLD. GL and GH reduced the MDA level and improved the liver SOD level; GL also raised liver T-AOC. Those findings illustrate that different doses of GJLZ improved liver oxidative stress by enhancing the content of SOD and suppressing the production of MDA; GJLZ could be a prophylactic medicine in lean NAFLD. The same results for Poria cocos polysaccharides in improving liver T-AOC and reducing liver MDA levels, one of the components in Poria from GJLZ, support our research [26].

To further explore the therapeutic mechanism of GJLZ in lean NAFLD, we chose GL as a better dosage for treating lean NAFLD according to the careful consideration of serum biochemicals, hepatic oxidative stress level, and histological analysis. Based on metabolomics analysis, we discovered an abundance of differential metabolic pathways between MCS and MCD groups; glycerophospholipid metabolism, arachidonic acid metabolism, galactose metabolism, carbohydrate digestion and absorption, linoleic acid metabolism, regulation of lipolysis in adipocytes, and sphingolipid signaling pathway were related to glucose and lipid metabolism, indicating that MCD diets not only cause liver lipid accumulation, but also induce glucose and lipid metabolism disorder. This is in accordance with the research of Ye et al. on metabolic disorders in lean NAFLD, which showed that metabolic diseases such as hypercholesterolemia, diabetes, and elevated blood pressure, or both elevated blood pressure and hypercholesterolemia, should be the screening criteria for lean NAFLD, besides BMI [27]. After GL treatment, the pathways related to glucose and lipid metabolism: glycerophospholipid metabolism, glucagon signaling pathway, carbohydrate digestion and absorption, and glycerolipid metabolism were altered. Glucagon can stimulate lipolysis in adipocytes. The activation of the glucagon signaling pathway may illustrate that GL can enhance the lipolysis of the adipocytes in the liver to alleviate lean NAFLD [28,29]. The accumulation of hepatocyte lipids in NAFLD triggers the production of reactive oxygen species and the rise in oxidative stress [30]. These processes ultimately lead to mitochondrial dysfunction, which may cause the abnormal process of the TCA cycle. Research shows that decreased glycolytic/TCA cycle metabolites are associated with cirrhosis; we can infer that the down-regulation of glycolytic/TCA cycle metabolites may be linked to liver injury [29]. In the fasted state, lactate and amino acids fail to produce glucose via gluconeogenesis. TCA cycle intermediates accumulate in hepatocytes, leading to hepatic steatosis [31]. The up-regulation of the TCA cycle and pyruvate metabolism pathway and their metabolites suggests that GL may improve glucose and lipid metabolism in lean NAFLD.

Lipids are a group of complex and diverse molecules; lipid alterations are a common cause and consequence of NAFLD, alcoholic hepatitis, and steatohepatitis [32]. Glycerophospholipids are involved in cellular signal transduction, the major component of cellular membranes. The phospholipid family is classified into phosphatidic acid (PA), phosphatidylcholine (PC), phosphatidylethanolamine (PE), phosphatidylinositol (PI), phosphatidylserine (PS), cardiolipin (CL), etc. [33]. Glycerophospholipid metabolism involves diseases like type 2 diabetes mellitus and atherosclerosis, psoriasis, and tuberculosis comorbidity [34–36]. When analyzing the 78 common metabolites in three groups, we focused on two metabolites in glycerophospholipid metabolism: sn-3-O-(geranylgeranyl)glycerol 1-phosphate and lysoPC(P-18:0/0:0), which decreased in the MCS and GL groups and increased in the MCD group. LysoPC has diverse roles in cellular processes, including regulating inflammation, cell differentiation, immune responses, and signaling pathways in various cell types [37–39]. The elevated lysoPC(15:0) content was causally related to the risk of high uric acid, high insulin, high homeostasis model assessment of insulin resistance (HOMA-IR), dyslipidemia, and overweight/obesity, which shows that abnormal lysoPC metabolism may be connected to the metabolic risk [33,40]. Likewise, the dynamic changes in sn-3-O-(geranylgeranyl)glycerol 1-phosphate and lysoPC(P-18:0/0:0) may reflect the injury and recovery of the liver. This suggests that the GL treatment is effective in lean NAFLD, probably by regulating the glycerophospholipid metabolism. Moreover, sn-3-O-(geranylgeranyl)glycerol 1-phosphate and lysoPC(P-18:0/0:0) may serve as biomarkers for lean NAFLD and have a negative effect on lean NAFLD.

To provide more evidence that the level of sn-3-O-(geranylgeranyl)glycerol 1-phosphate and lysoPC(P-18:0/0:0) may be associated with the severity of lean NAFLD, we conducted a correlation analysis of serum biochemical indicators and liver antioxidant indicators, sn-3-O-(geranylgeranyl)glycerol 1-phosphate and lysoPC(P-18:0/0:0). They were positively correlated with serum ALT and AST, indicating sn-3-O-(geranylgeranyl)glycerol 1-phosphate and lysoPC(P-18:0/0:0) may be involved in liver damage. They were positively correlated with serum TG, while being negatively correlated with serum HDL-C; this shows that sn-3-O-(geranylgeranyl)glycerol 1-phosphate and lysoPC(P-18:0/0:0) could lead to dyslipidemia in lean NAFLD. This is consistent with the outcomes of Han et al., which showed that patients with coexisting HBV infection, NAFLD, and T2DM exhibit higher levels of sn-3-o-(geranylgeranyl) glyceroll-phosphate and serum TG, which may infer that the increase in sn-3-o-(geranylgeranyl) glyceroll-phosphat indicates the excessive lipogenesis [41]. Sn-3-O-(geranylgeranyl)glycerol, 1-phosphate, and lysoPC(P-18:0/0:0) were positively associated with MDA and inversely associated with T-AOC and SOD, suggesting that sn-3-O-(geranylgeranyl)glycerol, 1-phosphate, and lysoPC(P-18:0/0:0) may exacerbate oxidative stress in the liver. Our discovery is in accordance with the study of Pang et al., which showed that the HFD diet induced NAFLD with higher HDL, LDL, TC, TG, FBG, ALT, and AST levels that were positively correlated with the PC and PE levels [42]. Furthermore, Zhou et al. reported that metabolism of glycerophospholipid was highly associated with the hepatic injury triggered by Concanavalin A (Con A), which showed that the glycerophospholipid metabolism pathway was of great importance in Con A-induced hepatic injury [43]. The correlation analysis of serum biochemical indicators, liver antioxidant indicators, sn-3-O-(geranylgeranyl)glycerol 1-phosphate, and lysoPC(P-18:0/0:0) demonstrated that GL may regulate glycerophospholipid metabolism by reducing sn-3-O-(geranylgeranyl)glycerol 1-phosphate and lysoPC(P-18:0/0:0) levels, thereby ameliorating glucose and lipid metabolism disorder and oxidative stress in liver, as well as hepatic injury. In summary, treating GJLZ could enhance the antioxidant capacity of liver cells, recover the TCA cycle function, and improve pyruvate and glycerophospholipid metabolism. Restoration of glycerophospholipid metabolism leads to the downregulation of sn-3-O-(geranylgeranyl)glycerol 1-phosphate and lysoPC(P-18:0/0:0) levels. It is associated with the elevation of serum HDL-C, hepatic T-AOC, and SOD, and the reduction in serum TG and hepatic MDA, thereby restoring glucose and lipid metabolism (Figure 8).

We made several discoveries in this study. Firstly, we found that GJLZ, an effective medication from TCM, may treat lean NAFLD. Secondly, according to untargeted metabolomics analysis, we found that GL ameliorated lean NAFLD by regulating glucose and lipid metabolism, and sn-3-O-(geranylgeranyl)glycerol 1-phosphate and lysoPC(P-18:0/0:0) were screened from the glycerophospholipid metabolism pathway. However, this research has some limitations. First, the number of mice was six to eight in each group; therefore, a larger sample size is required to verify the accuracy of our experimental outcomes. Second, there are no general methods to model lean NAFLD in mice. Thus, the MCD diet mouse model was constructed to model lean NAFLD, which significantly impacted the mouse's longevity and failed to demonstrate metabolic features, including the usual insulin resistance and visceral fat accumulation, in lean NAFLD patients. Still, it is of interest to study the pathogenesis of lean NAFLD. Third, lipidomics must be applied in subsequent research after we revealed the importance of lipid metabolism in the treatment of lean NAFLD using GJLZ. Fourth, in our research we did not explore the beneficial effects of GJLZ supplementation on lean NAFLD due to direct effects on the liver or due to indirect effects via other tissues; thus, more experiments are needed to further investigate the beneficial effects of GJLZ on lean NAFLD. Finally, genomics, transcriptomics, and proteomics should be utilized in the continuing exploration to systematically search for the mechanism.

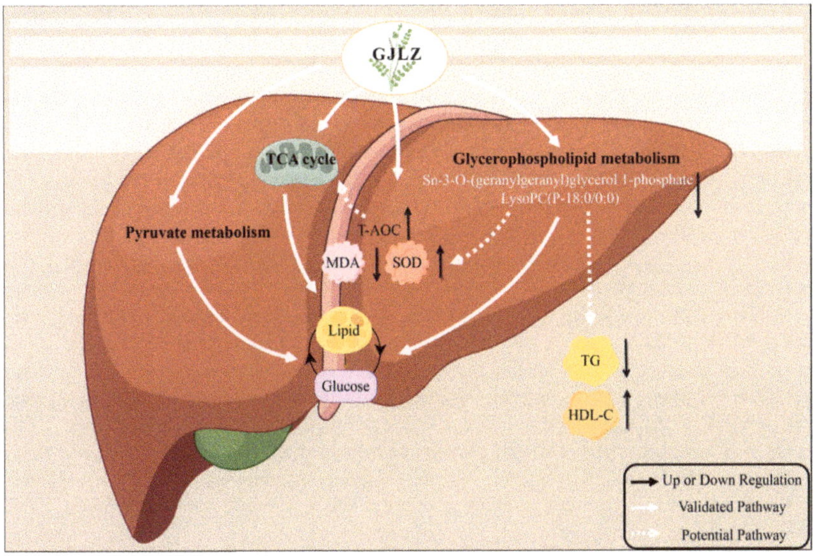

Figure 8. The mechanisms underlying the therapeutic effects of GJLZ in treating lean NAFLD. GJLZ, Ganjianglingzhu; HDL-C, high-density lipoprotein cholesterol; MDA, malondialdehyde; NALFD, non-alcoholic fatty liver disease; SOD, superoxide dismutase; TCA cycle, tricarboxylic acid cycle; TG, triglyceride; T-AOC, total antioxidant capacity. The cartoon components originated from www.figdraw.com for model drawing (accessed on 28 November 2023).

4. Materials and Methods

4.1. Preparation of GJLZ Decoction

The original prescription of the GJLZ decoction comprised Glycyrrhizae Radix et Rhizoma (6 g), Zingiberis Rhizoma (12 g), Poria (12 g), and Macrocephalae Rhizoma (6 g), which was set as the low-dose group of the GJLZ decoction (GL group). The dosage of the high-dose group of the GJLZ decoction (GH group) was 1.5 times that of the GL group. We purchased granules from Sichuan Neo-Green Pharmaceutical Technology Development Co., Ltd. (Chengdu, China). A quantity of 1g of Glycyrrhizae Radix et Rhizoma, Zingiberis Rhizoma, Poria, and Macrocephalae Rhizoma granules was equivalent to 7 g, 21 g, 17 g, and 7 g of herbs, respectively. The granules were mixed according to the proportion of the GJLZ decoction. The dose of intragastric administration in mice was calculated as 12.33 times the clinical adult dose; the low dose (614.70 $g \cdot kg^{-1} \cdot d^{-1}$) and high dose (922.05 $g \cdot kg^{-1} \cdot d^{-1}$) of the GJLZ decoction were administered to mice in the experiment.

4.2. Component Analysis of GJLZ Decoction

The composition of the GJLZ decoction was analyzed by UPLC-Q-TOF/MS. The ultra-high-performance liquid chromatography (UPLC) system was Waters H-Class UPLC system (Waters Corporation, Milford, MA, USA), the chromatographic column was a Waters ACQUITY UPLC® HSS T3 (2.1 × 150 mm, 1.8 μm, Waters Corporation, Milford,

MA, USA), and the column temperature was 30 °C. The sample injection volume was 2 μL. The mobile phase was an aqueous solution of acetonitrile (A) and 0.1% formic acid (B); the DAD wavelength ranged from 190 to 400 nm. The flow rate was 0.3 mL/min. The gradient elution program is exhibited in Table S1.

The AB Sciex Triple TOF® 4600 system (AB SCIEX LLC, Framingham, MA, USA) with an ESI ion source was used to perform MS analysis. Samples were analyzed in negative and positive ion modes; the parameter set is shown in Table S2.

4.3. *Mouse Preparation and Sampling*

Male C57BL/6 mice (9-week-old; n = 38) were immediately kept in a specific pathogen-free room after being purchased from the Vital River (Beijing, China). After being adaptively fed for one week and weighed, they were randomly divided into a lean NAFLD model group (provided with the MCD diet, #519580, Dyets, Wuxi, China), having 27 mice, and a control group (provided with the methionine-choline-sufficient (MCS) diet, #519581, Dyets, Wuxi, China), having 11 mice. After feeding of the MCD and MCS diets for four weeks, three mice from the MCD diet model and MCS diet control groups were sacrificed. To estimate the model, serum total cholesterol (TC), triglyceride (TG), high-density lipoprotein cholesterol (HDL-C), alanine transaminase (ALT), aspartate transaminase (AST), and fasting blood glucose (FBG) were determined, and the liver tissues of mice were stained with hematoxylin, eosin (H&E).

Subsequently, the lean NAFLD model group was randomly divided into three groups: model group (MCD group, n = 8), GL group (n = 8, 614.70 $g\cdot kg^{-1}\cdot d^{-1}$), and GH group (n = 8, 922.05 $g\cdot kg^{-1}\cdot d^{-1}$). The GL group and GH group received intragastric administration of varying concentrations of the GJLZ decoction; the control group (MCS group, n = 8) and MCD group were given 7.5 $mL\cdot kg^{-1}\cdot d^{-1}$ physiological saline by gavage. In the eighth week, the mice from each group were sacrificed, and arterial blood and liver tissue were taken and immediately stored at −80 °C. The animal experiments were approved by the Animal Ethics Committee of the Shanghai Model Organisms Center (IACUC NO. 2022-0034-1).

4.4. *Histological Analysis of Liver Tissue*

The liver tissues of mice fixed with paraformaldehyde were made into paraffin sections and stained with H&E and Sirius Red. Frozen sections were utilized for Oil Red O staining. The staining area was calculated by ImageJ-win64.

4.5. *Serum Biochemical and Liver Oxidative Stress Indicator Analysis*

An automatic biochemical analyzer detected the serum TC, TG, HDL-C, ALT, AST, and total bilirubin (TBIL) (Chemray 240, Rayto, Shenzhen, China). The liver malondialdehyde (MDA), superoxide dismutase (SOD), and total antioxidant capacity (T-AOC) were measured using the assay kits from Nanjing Jiancheng Bioengineering Institute according to the instructions (Nanjing, China).

4.6. *Untargeted Metabolomics Analysis*

L-2-chlorophenylalanine was purchased from Shanghai Heng Chuang Bio-technology Co., Ltd. (Shanghai, China). Acetonitrile, formic acid, methanol, and water were acquired from Thermo Fisher Scientific (Thermo Fisher Scientific, Waltham, MA, USA). All reagents were appropriate for the high-performance liquid chromatography analysis.

4.6.1. Metabolite Extraction

The liver sample was weighed (30 mg) and then transferred to a 1.5 mL tube with two small steel balls. A mixture of 400 μL of methanol and water (4/1, *v/v*) and 4 μg/mL of L-2-chlorophenylalanine (internal standard) were added to each sample. A quantity of 300 μL of the supernatant was taken after grinding the samples and centrifugation. A further 300 μL of methanol and water (1/4, *v/v*) was added to each sample and the supernatant (150 μL) was then collected in each tube. Aliquots of all samples were pooled to make quality control (QC) samples.

4.6.2. UPLC–MS/MS Analysis

The metabolic profiling was analyzed using the VION IMS QTOF mass spectrometer (Waters Corporation, Milford, MA USA) and ACQUITY UPLC I-Class system (Waters Corporation, Milford, MA, USA). The chromatographic column was an ACQUITY UPLC HSS® T3 (2.1 × 100 mm, 1.8 μm), and the column temperature was 45 °C. The sample injection volume was 3 μL. The mobile phase was composed of an aqueous solution of A (water) and B (acetonitrile/methanol 2/3 (*v*/*v* 0.1%) plus 0.1% formic acid; the flow rate was 0.4 mL/min. The data were collected using a combination of full scan mode (m/z ranging from 50 to 1000) and MSE mode, alternating two independent scans during operation with different collision energies. The QCs were utilized to provide the data that could be evaluated for reproducibility by periodically injecting them throughout the analysis.

4.6.3. Bioinformatics Analysis

The raw LC-MS data were processed by the Proggenesis QI V2.3 software (Nonlinear, Dynamics, Newcastle, UK) for baseline filtering, peak identification, peak extraction, peak alignment, and normalization. Compounds were identified by secondary fragmentation, mass-to-charge ratio, and isotopic distribution. The qualitative analysis was based on the Human Metabolome Database (HMDB), Lipidmaps (V2.3), EMDB, PMDB, METLIN, and self-built databases. The data matrix consisted of a combination of positive and negative ion data.

Principal component analysis (PCA) was utilized for estimating the analysis process's stability and the samples' distribution through R. Differential metabolites between groups were identified by orthogonal partial least-squares-discriminant analysis (OPLS-DA). Seven-fold cross-validation and 200 response permutation testing (RPT) were used to prevent model overfitting. The two-tailed Student's *t*-test and the variable importance of projection (VIP) values in the OPLS-DA model were used to screen out differential metabolites (VIP > 1.0 and $p < 0.05$). The KEGG database (http://www.kegg.jp) was used to identify the differential biological pathways of metabolite data, which was accessed on 14 September 2023.

4.7. Statistical Analysis

SPSS 26.0 software was used for statistical analyses. The two-tailed Student's *t*-test (between two groups) and one-way analysis of variance (ANOVA) (between multiple groups) were used for the data that had a normal distribution, and the nonparametric test was utilized for non-normal distributions. Data are presented as the mean ± SD in this study.

5. Conclusions

The efficacy and mechanism of GJLZ in treating lean NAFLD were studied for the first time, and the low dose (i.e., the original prescription dose) was found to have a better therapeutic effect on lean NAFLD. The analysis of untargeted metabolomics exhibited that GL may regulate glucose and lipid metabolism to alleviate lean NAFLD. Glycerophospholipid metabolism plays a crucial role in the treatment of lean NAFLD using GL. Furthermore, sn-3-O-(geranylgeranyl)glycerol 1-phosphate and lysoPC(P-18:0/0:0) are likely to be involved in aggravating lean NAFLD and may serve as diagnostic and therapeutic biomarkers for lean NAFLD in the future.

Supplementary Materials: The following supporting information can be downloaded at: https://www.mdpi.com/article/10.3390/ph17040502/s1, Table S1: Elution gradient; Table S2: Mass parameters (Sciex Triple TOF 4600 LC-MS); Figure S1: Food intake of mice; Table S3: Main component identification of GJLZ decoction [44–48]; Table S4: List of the identified metabolites of the intersection statistics between MCS vs. MCD and MCD vs. GL in positive and negative ion mode based on UHPLC-Q-TOF/MS; Table S5: The correlation between biochemical indicators and the metabolites.

Author Contributions: Conceptualization, N.W., B.L., G.J. and S.Y.; methodology, N.W., B.L. and N.T.; validation, N.W., B.L. and N.T.; formal analysis, N.T., X.S. and Y.X.; investigation, N.T., X.S., Y.X., X.X., H.Z., H.S., J.W. and L.Z.; resources, N.W., B.L. and L.Z.; data curation, N.T.; writing—original draft preparation, N.T.; writing—review and editing, N.W., L.J. and B.L.; visualization, N.T.; supervision, N.W. and B.L.; project administration, N.W. and B.L.; funding acquisition, N.W., B.L. and L.Z. All authors have read and agreed to the published version of the manuscript.

Funding: This research was funded by Three-year action plan for Shanghai (project number: ZY (2021-2023)-0211); National Natural Science Foundation of China (81973730); Local Colleges Faculty Constitution of Shanghai MSTC 2022 (22010504300); Shanghai Collaborative Innovation Center for Chronic Disease Prevention and Health Services (2021 Science and Technology 02-37); Shanghai Health Commission for Traditional Chinese Medicine Research (2022QN014); China Postdoctoral Science Foundation, No. 72 General Fund, 2022 (2022M722164); Shanghai 2023 "Science and Technology Innovation Action Plan" Qi Ming Xing Cultivation (Yang Fan Project, 23YF1447700); Subject Connotation Construction Project in School of Public Health, Shanghai University of Traditional Chinese Medicine, 2023 (GJ202303).

Institutional Review Board Statement: The study was approved by the Experimental Animal Ethics Committee in the Shanghai Model Organisms Center (IACUC NO. 2022-0034-1).

Informed Consent Statement: Not applicable.

Data Availability Statement: The data presented in this study are available on request from the corresponding author.

Conflicts of Interest: The authors declare no conflicts of interest.

Abbreviations

ALT: alanine transaminase; ANOVA: analysis of variance; AST: aspartate transaminase; BMI: body mass index; CL: cardiolipin; Con A: Concanavalin A; FBG: fasting blood glucose; FC: fold change; GH: high dose of GJLZ; GJLZ: Ganjianglingzhu; GL: low dose of GJLZ; HDL-C: high-density lipoprotein cholesterol; HMDB: human metabolome database; HOMA-IR: homeostasis model assessment of insulin resistance; H&E: hematoxylin, eosin; MCD: methionine-choline-deficient; MCS: methionine-choline-sufficient; MDA: malondialdehyde; NAFLD: non-alcoholic fatty liver disease; NAS: non-alcoholic fatty liver disease activity score; NASH: non-alcoholic steatohepatitis; OPLS-DA: orthogonal partial least-squares-discriminant analysis; PA: phosphatidic acid; PC: phosphatidylcholine; PCA: principal component analysis; PE: phosphatidylethanolamine; PI: phosphatidylinositol; PS: phosphatidylserine; QC: quality control; RPT: response permutation testing; SOD: superoxide dismutase; TBIL: total bilirubin; TC: total cholesterol; TCA cycle: tricarboxylic acid cycle; TCM: traditional Chinese medicine; TG: triglyceride; T-AOC: total antioxidant capacity; UPLC: ultra-high-performance liquid chromatography; VIP: variable importance of projection.

References

1. Riazi, K.; Azhari, H.; Charette, J.H.; Underwood, F.E.; King, J.A.; Afshar, E.E.; Swain, M.G.; Congly, S.E.; Kaplan, G.G.; Shaheen, A.-A. The prevalence and incidence of NAFLD worldwide: A systematic review and meta-analysis. *Lancet Gastroenterol. Hepatol.* **2022**, *7*, 851–861. [CrossRef]
2. Friedman, S.L.; Neuschwander-Tetri, B.A.; Rinella, M.; Sanyal, A.J. Mechanisms of NAFLD development and therapeutic strategies. *Nat. Med.* **2018**, *24*, 908–922. [CrossRef]
3. Chalasani, N.; Younossi, Z.; Lavine, J.E.; Charlton, M.; Cusi, K.; Rinella, M.; Harrison, S.A.; Brunt, E.M.; Sanyal, A.J. The diagnosis and management of nonalcoholic fatty liver disease: Practice guidance from the American Association for the Study of Liver Diseases. *Hepatology* **2017**, *67*, 328–357. [CrossRef]

4. Zou, Z.Y.; Wong, V.W.S.; Fan, J.G. Epidemiology of nonalcoholic fatty liver disease in non-obese populations: Meta-analytic assessment of its prevalence, genetic, metabolic, and histological profiles. *J. Dig. Dis.* **2020**, *21*, 372–384. [CrossRef]
5. Ahadi, M.; Molooghi, K.; Masoudifar, N.; Namdar, A.B.; Vossoughinia, H.; Farzanehfar, M. A review of non-alcoholic fatty liver disease in non-obese and lean individuals. *J. Gastroenterol. Hepatol.* **2020**, *36*, 1497–1507. [CrossRef]
6. Tang, A.; Ng, C.H.; Phang, P.H.; Chan, K.E.; Chin, Y.H.; Fu, C.E.; Zeng, R.W.; Xiao, J.; Tan, D.J.H.; Quek, J.; et al. Comparative Burden of Metabolic Dysfunction in Lean NAFLD vs. Non-lean NAFLD—A Systematic Review and Meta-analysis. *Clin. Gastroenterol. Hepatol.* **2023**, *21*, 1750–1760.e1712. [CrossRef]
7. Maier, S.; Wieland, A.; Cree-Green, M.; Nadeau, K.; Sullivan, S.; Lanaspa, M.A.; Johnson, R.J.; Jensen, T. Lean NAFLD: An underrecognized and challenging disorder in medicine. *Rev. Endocr. Metab. Disord.* **2021**, *22*, 351–366. [CrossRef]
8. Feng, R.-N.; Du, S.-S.; Wang, C.; Li, Y.-C.; Liu, L.-Y.; Guo, F.-C.; Sun, C.-H. Lean-non-alcoholic fatty liver disease increases risk for metabolic disorders in a normal weight Chinese population. *World J. Gastroenterol.* **2014**, *20*, 17932–17940. [CrossRef]
9. Chang, Y.; Cho, Y.K.; Cho, J.; Jung, H.-S.; Yun, K.E.; Ahn, J.; Sohn, C.I.; Shin, H.; Ryu, S. Alcoholic and Nonalcoholic Fatty Liver Disease and Liver-Related Mortality: A Cohort Study. *Am. J. Gastroenterol.* **2019**, *114*, 620–629. [CrossRef] [PubMed]
10. Golabi, P.; Paik, J.; Fukui, N.; Locklear, C.T.; de Avilla, L.; Younossi, Z.M. Patients with Lean Nonalcoholic Fatty Liver Disease Are Metabolically Abnormal and Have a Higher Risk for Mortality. *Clin. Diabetes* **2019**, *37*, 65–72. [CrossRef] [PubMed]
11. Zou, B.; Yeo, Y.H.; Nguyen, V.H.; Cheung, R.; Ingelsson, E.; Nguyen, M.H. Prevalence, characteristics and mortality outcomes of obese, nonobese and lean NAFLD in the United States, 1999–2016. *J. Intern. Med.* **2020**, *288*, 139–151. [CrossRef] [PubMed]
12. Long, M.T.; Noureddin, M.; Lim, J.K. AGA Clinical Practice Update: Diagnosis and Management of Nonalcoholic Fatty Liver Disease in Lean Individuals: Expert Review. *Gastroenterology* **2022**, *163*, 764–774.e761. [CrossRef] [PubMed]
13. Wang, R.-R.; Zhang, L.-F.; Chen, L.-P.; Wang, J.-Y.; Zhang, L.; Xu, Y.-S.; Yang, P.-L.; Ji, G.; Liu, B.-C.; Dominguez Perles, R. Structural and Functional Modulation of Gut Microbiota by Jiangzhi Granules during the Amelioration of Nonalcoholic Fatty Liver Disease. *Oxidative Med. Cell. Longev.* **2021**, *2021*, 2234695. [CrossRef]
14. Yue, S.-R.; Tan, Y.-Y.; Zhang, L.; Zhang, B.-J.; Jiang, F.-Y.; Ji, G.; Liu, B.-C.; Wang, R.-R. Gynostemma pentaphyllum polysaccharides ameliorate non-alcoholic steatohepatitis in mice associated with gut microbiota and the TLR2/NLRP3 pathway. *Front. Endocrinol.* **2022**, *13*, 885039. [CrossRef] [PubMed]
15. Dang, Y.; Xu, J.; Zhu, M.; Zhou, W.; Zhang, L.; Ji, G. Gan-Jiang-Ling-Zhu decoction alleviates hepatic steatosis in rats by the miR-138-5p/CPT1B axis. *Biomed. Pharmacother.* **2020**, *127*, 110127. [CrossRef] [PubMed]
16. Xu, Y.; Zhang, L.; Zhang, Y.; Gao, S.; Zhuo, Y. Effect of Modified Ganjiang Lingzhu Decoction on Nonalcoholic Fatty Liver in Mice and Its Mechanism Based on Network Pharmacology and Experiments. *World J. Integr. Tradit. West. Med.* **2023**, *18*, 74–84. [CrossRef]
17. Shinozuka, H.; Lombardi, B.; Sell, S.; Iammarino, R.M. Early histological and functional alterations of ethionine liver carcinogenesis in rats fed a choline-deficient diet. *Cancer Res.* **1978**, *38*, 1092–1098. [PubMed]
18. Chen, F.; Esmaili, S.; Rogers, G.B.; Bugianesi, E.; Petta, S.; Marchesini, G.; Bayoumi, A.; Metwally, M.; Azardaryany, M.K.; Coulter, S.; et al. Lean NAFLD: A Distinct Entity Shaped by Differential Metabolic Adaptation. *Hepatology* **2020**, *71*, 1213–1227. [CrossRef] [PubMed]
19. Wu, N.; Zhai, X.; Yuan, F.; Li, J.; Yu, N.; Zhang, F.; Li, D.; Wang, J.; Zhang, L.; Shi, Y.; et al. Fasting glucose mediates the influence of genetic variants of SOD2 gene on lean non-alcoholic fatty liver disease. *Front. Genet.* **2022**, *13*, 970854. [CrossRef]
20. Wu, N.; Zhai, X.; Yuan, F.; Li, J.; Li, D.; Wang, J.; Zhang, L.; Shi, Y.; Ji, G.; He, G.; et al. Genetic variation in TBC1 domain family member 1 gene associates with the risk of lean NAFLD via high-density lipoprotein. *Front. Genet.* **2023**, *13*, 1026725. [CrossRef]
21. Wu, N.; Li, J.; Zhang, J.; Yuan, F.; Yu, N.; Zhang, F.; Li, D.; Wang, J.; Zhang, L.; Shi, Y.; et al. Waist circumference mediates the association between rs1260326 in GCKR gene and the odds of lean NAFLD. *Sci. Rep.* **2023**, *13*, 6488. [CrossRef]
22. Kim, D.; Kim, W.R. Nonobese Fatty Liver Disease. *Clin. Gastroenterol. Hepatol.* **2017**, *15*, 474–485. [CrossRef] [PubMed]
23. Alshawsh, M.A.; Alsalahi, A.; Alshehade, S.A.; Saghir, S.A.M.; Ahmeda, A.F.; Al Zarzour, R.H.; Mahmoud, A.M. A Comparison of the Gene Expression Profiles of Non-Alcoholic Fatty Liver Disease between Animal Models of a High-Fat Diet and Methionine-Choline-Deficient Diet. *Molecules* **2022**, *27*, 858. [CrossRef] [PubMed]
24. Carillon, J.; Rouanet, J.-M.; Cristol, J.-P.; Brion, R. Superoxide Dismutase Administration, A Potential Therapy Against Oxidative Stress Related Diseases: Several Routes of Supplementation and Proposal of an Original Mechanism of Action. *Pharm. Res.* **2013**, *30*, 2718–2728. [CrossRef] [PubMed]
25. Ayala, A.; Muñoz, M.F.; Argüelles, S. Lipid Peroxidation: Production, Metabolism, and Signaling Mechanisms of Malondialdehyde and 4-Hydroxy-2-Nonenal. *Oxidative Med. Cell. Longev.* **2014**, *2014*, 360438. [CrossRef]
26. Tan, Y.-Y.; Yue, S.-R.; Lu, A.-P.; Zhang, L.; Ji, G.; Liu, B.-C.; Wang, R.-R. The improvement of nonalcoholic steatohepatitis by Poria cocos polysaccharides associated with gut microbiota and NF-κB/CCL3/CCR1 axis. *Phytomedicine* **2022**, *103*, 154208. [CrossRef] [PubMed]
27. Ye, Q.; Zou, B.; Yeo, Y.H.; Li, J.; Huang, D.Q.; Wu, Y.; Yang, H.; Liu, C.; Kam, L.Y.; Tan, X.X.E.; et al. Global prevalence, incidence, and outcomes of non-obese or lean non-alcoholic fatty liver disease: A systematic review and meta-analysis. *Lancet Gastroenterol. Hepatol.* **2020**, *5*, 739–752. [CrossRef] [PubMed]
28. Schade, D.S.; Woodside, W.; Eaton, R.P. The role of glucagon in the regulation of plasma lipids. *Metabolism* **1979**, *28*, 874–886. [CrossRef] [PubMed]

29. Gorden, D.L.; Myers, D.S.; Ivanova, P.T.; Fahy, E.; Maurya, M.R.; Gupta, S.; Min, J.; Spann, N.J.; McDonald, J.G.; Kelly, S.L.; et al. Biomarkers of NAFLD progression: A lipidomics approach to an epidemic. *J. Lipid Res.* **2015**, *56*, 722–736. [CrossRef]
30. Kartsoli, S.; Kostara, C.E.; Tsimihodimos, V.; Bairaktari, E.T.; Christodoulou, D.K. Lipidomics in non-alcoholic fatty liver disease. *World J. Hepatol.* **2020**, *12*, 436–450. [CrossRef]
31. Burgess, S.C.; Hausler, N.; Merritt, M.; Jeffrey, F.M.H.; Storey, C.; Milde, A.; Koshy, S.; Lindner, J.; Magnuson, M.A.; Malloy, C.R.; et al. Impaired Tricarboxylic Acid Cycle Activity in Mouse Livers Lacking Cytosolic Phosphoenolpyruvate Carboxykinase. *J. Biol. Chem.* **2004**, *279*, 48941–48949. [CrossRef]
32. Paul, B.; Lewinska, M.; Andersen, J.B. Lipid alterations in chronic liver disease and liver cancer. *JHEP Rep.* **2022**, *4*, 100479. [CrossRef] [PubMed]
33. Wang, R.; Li, B.; Lam, S.M.; Shui, G. Integration of lipidomics and metabolomics for in-depth understanding of cellular mechanism and disease progression. *J. Genet. Genom.* **2020**, *47*, 69–83. [CrossRef] [PubMed]
34. López-Hernández, Y.; Lara-Ramírez, E.E.; Salgado-Bustamante, M.; López, J.A.; Oropeza-Valdez, J.J.; Jaime-Sánchez, E.; Castañeda-Delgado, J.E.; Magaña-Aquino, M.; Murgu, M.; Enciso-Moreno, J.A. Glycerophospholipid Metabolism Alterations in Patients with Type 2 Diabetes Mellitus and Tuberculosis Comorbidity. *Arch. Med. Res.* **2019**, *50*, 71–78. [CrossRef] [PubMed]
35. Zeng, C.; Wen, B.; Hou, G.; Lei, L.; Mei, Z.; Jia, X.; Chen, X.; Zhu, W.; Li, J.; Kuang, Y.; et al. Lipidomics profiling reveals the role of glycerophospholipid metabolism in psoriasis. *GigaScience* **2017**, *6*, 1–11. [CrossRef]
36. Akerele, O.A.; Cheema, S.K. Fatty acyl composition of lysophosphatidylcholine is important in atherosclerosis. *Med. Hypotheses* **2015**, *85*, 754–760. [CrossRef]
37. Kelher, M.R.; McLaughlin, N.J.; Banerjee, A.; Elzi, D.J.; Gamboni, F.; Khan, S.Y.; Meng, X.; Mitra, S.; Silliman, C.C. LysoPCs induce Hck- and PKCδ-mediated activation of PKCγ causing p47phox phosphorylation and membrane translocation in neutrophils. *J. Leukoc. Biol.* **2017**, *101*, 261–273. [CrossRef]
38. Rikitake, Y.; Kawashima, S.; Yamashita, T.; Ueyama, T.; Ishido, S.; Hotta, H.; Hirata, K.; Yokoyama, M. Lysophosphatidylcholine inhibits endothelial cell migration and proliferation via inhibition of the extracellular signal-regulated kinase pathway. *Arter. Thromb. Vasc. Biol.* **2000**, *20*, 1006–1012. [CrossRef]
39. Sugiyama, S.; Kugiyama, K.; Ogata, N.; Doi, H.; Ota, Y.; Ohgushi, M.; Matsumura, T.; Oka, H.; Yasue, H. Biphasic regulation of transcription factor nuclear factor-kappaB activity in human endothelial cells by lysophosphatidylcholine through protein kinase C-mediated pathway. *Arter. Thromb. Vasc. Biol.* **1998**, *18*, 568–576. [CrossRef]
40. Wu, Q.; Li, J.; Sun, X.; He, D.; Cheng, Z.; Li, J.; Zhang, X.; Xie, Y.; Zhu, Y.; Lai, M. Multi-stage metabolomics and genetic analyses identified metabolite biomarkers of metabolic syndrome and their genetic determinants. *eBioMedicine* **2021**, *74*, 103707. [CrossRef]
41. Han, W.; Huang, C.; Ji, Y.; Zhou, L.; Chen, J.; Hou, J. Alterations in the Gut Microbiota and Hepatitis-B-Virus Infection in Southern Chinese Patients with Coexisting Non-Alcoholic Fatty Liver Disease and Type-2 Diabetes Mellitus. *Front. Med.* **2021**, *8*, 805029. [CrossRef]
42. Pang, Y.; Zheng, Y.; Yang, N.; Zan, M.; Zhang, L.; Ding, W. Potential novel biomarkers in small intestine for obesity/obesity resistance revealed by multi-omics analysis. *Lipids Health Dis.* **2022**, *21*, 98. [CrossRef]
43. Zhou, C.; Jia, H.-M.; Liu, Y.-T.; Yu, M.; Chang, X.; Ba, Y.-M.; Zou, Z.-M. Metabolism of glycerophospholipid, bile acid and retinol is correlated with the early outcomes of autoimmune hepatitis. *Mol. BioSystems* **2016**, *12*, 1574–1585. [CrossRef]
44. Li, G.; Nikolic, D.; van Breemen, R.B. Identification and Chemical Standardization of Licorice Raw Materials and Dietary Supplements Using UHPLC-MS/MS. *J. Agric. Food Chem.* **2016**, *64*, 8062–8070. [CrossRef]
45. Xue, G.; Su, S.; Yan, P.; Shang, J.; Wang, J.; Yan, C.; Li, J.; Wang, Q.; Xiong, X.; Xu, H. Integrative analyses of widely targeted metabolomic profiling and derivatization-based LC-MS/MS reveals metabolic changes of Zingiberis Rhizoma and its processed products. *Food Chem.* **2022**, *389*, 133068. [CrossRef]
46. Song, L.; Xie, X.-Y.; Sun, J.; Huang, S.-H.; Li, X.-L.; Peng, G.-P.; Gao, X.-L.; Zheng, Y.-F. Structural identification and comprehensive comparison of saponin-related impurities present in the three different compound glycyrrhizin tablets. *J. Pharm. Biomed. Anal.* **2023**, *229*, 115287. [CrossRef]
47. Sun, L.; Zhao, M.; Zhao, Y.; Jiang, X.; Wang, M.; Zhang, Y.; Zhao, C. Rapid characterization of chemical constituents of Shaoyao Gancao decoction using UHPLC coupled with Fourier transform ion cyclotron resonance mass spectrometry. *RSC Adv.* **2020**, *10*, 29528–29535. [CrossRef] [PubMed]
48. Wong, Y.F.; Cacciola, F.; Fermas, S.; Riga, S.; James, D.; Manzin, V.; Bonnet, B.; Marriott, P.J.; Dugo, P.; Mondello, L. Untargeted profiling of Glycyrrhiza glabra extract with comprehensive two-dimensional liquid chromatography-mass spectrometry using multi-segmented shift gradients in the second dimension: Expanding the metabolic coverage. *Electrophoresis* **2018**, *39*, 1993–2000. [CrossRef] [PubMed]

pharmaceuticals

MDPI

Article

Therapeutic Potential of Qilianxiaopi Formula: Targeting ADAM17-Mediated Chronic Inflammation in Atrophic Gastritis

Sijing Du [1,2,†], Tianxiang Wang [1,†], Zhiqiang Li [1,†], Ting Li [1], Zelong Miao [1], Yuling Chen [1], Songbiao Zhu [3], Wei Wei [2,*] and Haiteng Deng [1,*]

1 MOE Key Laboratory of Bioinformatics, Center for Synthetic and Systematic Biology, School of Life Sciences, Tsinghua University, Beijing 100084, China; ddusijing@163.com (S.D.)
2 Wangjing Hospital, China Academy of Chinese Medical Sciences, Beijing 100102, China
3 Chinese Institutes for Medical Research (CIMR), Beijing 100069, China
* Correspondence: sxxtyy@sina.com (W.W.); dht@mail.tsinghua.edu.cn (H.D.); Tel./Fax: +86-010-8473-9761 (W.W.); +86-010-6279-7838 (H.D.)
† These authors contributed equally to this work.

Abstract: Background: Gastric cancer (GC) is a leading cause of mortality worldwide, particularly in China. Chronic atrophic gastritis (CAG) and intestinal metaplasia (IM) are recognized as precancerous conditions contributing to GC development. Qilianxiaopi formula (QLXP), a traditional Chinese medicine (TCM), has demonstrated significant therapeutic effects on CAG and IM; however, its underlying mechanisms remain poorly understood. **Methods**: This study utilized chromatography-mass spectrometry to identify the major compounds in QLXP. Network pharmacology was used to predict the associated targets of these components. Thermal proteome profiling (TPP) pinpointed the potential binding proteins of QLXP, which were validated by bioinformatic analyses. Bio-layer interferometry (BLI) was used to analyze the interactions between QLXP and its key target proteins, thereby determining their binding components. Molecular docking predicted the binding modes between the components and proteins. **Results**: ADAM17 was identified as a key binding protein for QLXP. Further investigation revealed that QLXP inhibits the enzymatic activity of ADAM17, thereby reducing the secretion of the pro-inflammatory cytokine TNF-α, contributing to the anti-inflammatory properties of QLXP. BLI confirmed direct and reversible binding interactions between QLXP and ADAM17. Narirutin, isolated from the ADAM17 binding fraction, displayed the highest affinity for QLXP. **Conclusions**: This study highlights ADAM17 as a key molecular target of QLXP and narirutin as its principal binding component. The integrated approach combining chromatography-mass spectrometry, network pharmacology, TPP, BLI, and molecular docking provides a robust framework for elucidating the mechanisms of action of TCM.

Keywords: chronic atrophic gastritis; Qilianxiaopi formula; network pharmacology; thermal proteome profiling; bio-layer interferometry; ADAM17

1. Introduction

Gastric cancer (GC) is one of the biggest contributors to the global cancer burden. Despite an overall drop in age-adjusted incidence, GC remains the fifth leading cause of cancer-related mortality worldwide [1]. High-income Asian Pacific and East Asian areas had the highest age-standardized incidence rates in 2017, with almost half of the worldwide cases appearing in China [2]. Chronic atrophic gastritis (CAG) and intestinal metaplasia (IM) are precancerous conditions that independently increase the risk of GC [3]. Studies have reported cumulative GC incidences of 2.4% at 10 years and 2% at 20 years in patients with IM [4] and higher incidences in those with extensive endoscopic atrophy or IM in Japan (5.3–9.8% at 5 years) [5]. Even after endoscopic resection, IM in the corpus can significantly increase the risk of metachronous gastric lesions [6].

Helicobacter pylori (*H. pylori*) is the most common risk factor for developing GC, due to inducing a chronic inflammatory environment. ADAM17 acts as a molecular switch, regulating inflammation and tissue regeneration, thereby participating in the inflammation–cancer transition [7]. In addition to the eradication of *H. pylori*, endoscopic surveillance is considered the primary approach for patients with CAG or IM, especially in the advanced stages of atrophic gastritis [3]. Traditional Chinese medicine (TCM) has also shown clinical advantages in treating CAG and IM, it alleviates clinical symptoms as well as gastric mucosal lesions [8–10]. Banxia Xiexin Decoction is a traditional prescription used to treat epigastric distension by employing the "Xinkai Kujiang" approach, which involves the regulation of gastrointestinal functions with pungent and bitter medicinal herbs [10]. Given that chronic atrophic gastritis (CAG) is characterized by glandular atrophy and microvascular circulation impairment [11], we have modified the original formula by adding herbs that nourish qi and promote blood circulation to develop the Qilianxiaopi (QLXP) formula, thereby aligning more closely with the pathological changes of CAG. In clinical terms, our randomized controlled trial (RCT) showed that QLXP mitigates gastric mucosal atrophy and IM. Mechanistically, preliminary in vitro studies revealed that QLXP effectively inhibits the epithelial–mesenchymal transition (EMT) process.

Traditional Chinese herbal formulae often contain complex mixtures of bioactive compounds that simultaneously target multiple cellular pathways, contributing to holistic therapeutic effects [12]. However, the complexity of herbal formulae makes it challenging to identify their specific targets and mechanisms of action. This study therefore aimed to identify target proteins and interactive components of QLXP, aligning with the characteristics of TCM.

Network pharmacology is an emerging field that applies the principles of complex system biology to investigate the therapeutic mechanisms underlying TCM. It focuses on the intricate interactions between drugs and biological systems, especially at the molecular level, to predict potential targets and identify key nodes in drug-target-pathway networks [13,14]. To experimentally verify these predictions, thermal proteome profiling (TPP) offers a proteome-wide screening strategy. Based on the principle that ligand-bound proteins exhibit enhanced thermal stability, TPP subjects cell lysates to a temperature gradient and quantifies protein denaturation via mass spectrometry [15]. This technique has proven effective in identifying targets for diverse molecules, from cofactors to clinical drug candidates [16]. The integration of TPP with the cellular thermal shift assay (CETSA), which evaluates protein solubility in response to temperature changes, allows for a more rigorous validation of the temperature-dependent stabilization of target proteins [17,18]. Bio-layer interferometry (BLI) offers a sensitive and label-free approach for real-time biomolecular interaction analysis. By immobilizing target proteins, BLI enables the identification of binding partners through a process known as "affinity fishing" [19]. Molecular docking, a computational technique, simulates the binding modes and affinities of small molecules (ligands) with biological macromolecules (targets), facilitating the identification of the most promising drug candidates based on their predicted interactions [20]. The synergistic application of network pharmacology, TPP, BLI, and molecular docking provides a comprehensive framework for investigating the target proteins of QLXP. This integrated approach promises to yield insights into the molecular underpinnings of QLXP's therapeutic efficacy, thereby advancing our understanding of its mechanisms of action.

2. Results

2.1. Prediction of the QLXP Potential Targets Using Network Pharmacological Analysis

Utilizing UPLC-Orbitrap MS, we characterized the phytochemical composition of QLXP's aqueous extract. To pinpoint the primary constituents driving its therapeutic benefits, we applied two selection criteria: (1) We employed the "mzVault Best Match" over 80 to ensure reliable identification and reduce false positives. (2) We calculated the "Sample/Control Ratio" to assess the differential abundance in QLXP relative to placebo, focusing on compounds with a ratio exceeding 20. After data filtering, we identified 32 components in negative ion mode (Table 1) and 30 in positive ion mode (Table 2.), resulting in a consolidated list of 54 unique compounds after deduplication.

Table 1. Main components of QLXP in negative ion mode.

No.	Name	Formula	*m/z*	RT [min]	mzVault Best Match	Sample/ Control Ratio
1	*N*-Acetylglutamic acid	$C_7H_{11}NO_5$	188.05663	1.403	88.6	29.27
2	Forsythoside E	$C_{20}H_{30}O_{12}$	461.16685	5.795	88.3	43.39
3	Hastatoside	$C_{17}H_{24}O_{11}$	449.13039	5.972	84.3	40.19
4	Atractyloside A	$C_{21}H_{36}O_{10}$	493.22952	6.266	90.5	40.27
5	Purpureaside C	$C_{35}H_{46}O_{20}$	785.25233	7.471	90.2	50.63
6	Vicenin II	$C_{27}H_{30}O_{15}$	593.15181	7.583	89.5	33.36
7	Dihydromorin	$C_{15}H_{12}O_7$	303.05097	7.886	92	104.08
8	Isoforsythiaside	$C_{29}H_{36}O_{15}$	623.19852	8.252	91.1	109.93
9	Magnoloside A	$C_{29}H_{36}O_{15}$	623.19843	9.288	89.2	83.28
10	Apigenin 5-*O*-glucoside	$C_{21}H_{20}O_{10}$	431.09853	9.289	89.2	29.35
11	Narirutin	$C_{27}H_{32}O_{14}$	579.17223	9.721	90.9	43.45
12	Isoacteoside	$C_{29}H_{36}O_{15}$	623.19834	9.724	88.6	109.99
13	Rosmarinic acid	$C_{18}H_{16}O_8$	359.07738	10.035	82.8	97.41
14	Salvianolic acid A	$C_{26}H_{22}O_{10}$	493.11453	10.062	89.3	31.69
15	Puerarin	$C_{21}H_{20}O_9$	415.10377	10.097	84.2	85.09
16	Hesperetin	$C_{16}H_{14}O_6$	301.07183	10.225	92.8	40.93
17	Scutellarin	$C_{21}H_{18}O_{12}$	461.07282	10.605	84.9	32.96
18	Baicalein	$C_{15}H_{10}O_5$	269.04536	10.82	91	20.02
19	Oroxin A	$C_{21}H_{20}O_{10}$	431.09846	11.188	88.1	35.62
20	Dalbergioidin	$C_{15}H_{12}O_6$	287.05634	11.239	84.8	150.86
21	Baicalin	$C_{21}H_{18}O_{11}$	445.07751	11.446	87.1	33.50
22	Luteolin	$C_{15}H_{10}O_6$	285.04062	11.773	87.2	23.75
23	Oroxylin A	$C_{16}H_{12}O_5$	283.06125	11.788	90.4	24.75
24	Didymin	$C_{28}H_{34}O_{14}$	593.18798	12.009	90.1	33.26
25	Wogonoside	$C_{22}H_{20}O_{11}$	459.093	12.188	91.5	24.93
26	Hexahydrocurcumin	$C_{21}H_{26}O_6$	373.1659	12.613	85.4	30.01
27	Hispidulin	$C_{16}H_{12}O_6$	299.0562	12.707	89.2	36.79
28	Randaiol	$C_{15}H_{14}O_3$	241.08724	13.291	80.8	152.77
29	Formononetin	$C_{16}H_{12}O_4$	267.06628	13.61	88.7	49.00
30	Magnaldehyde D	$C_{16}H_{14}O_3$	253.0871	14.129	84.2	81.10
31	Wogonin	$C_{16}H_{12}O_5$	283.0611	14.291	89.9	23.53
32	Casticin	$C_{19}H_{18}O_8$	373.0929	14.435	80.1	109.01

Table 2. Main components of QLXP in positive ion mode.

No.	Name	Formula	*m/z*	RT [min]	mzVault Best Match	Sample/ Control Ratio
1	Hordenine	$C_{10}H_{15}NO$	166.1224	2.271	86.3	31.83
2	Indoleacrylic acid	$C_{11}H_9NO_2$	188.0704	5.299	84.4	35.78
3	Vicenin II	$C_{27}H_{30}O_{15}$	595.16551	7.568	86	45.71
4	*N*-Methylcoclaurine	$C_{18}H_{21}NO_3$	300.15912	7.754	89.6	21.01
5	Scutellarein	$C_{15}H_{10}O_6$	287.05462	8.886	81.2	26.26
6	Calycosin-7-*O*-β-D-glucoside	$C_{22}H_{22}O_{10}$	447.12807	8.968	82.9	25.81
7	Naringenin	$C_{15}H_{12}O_5$	273.07539	9.718	89.1	38.50
8	Narirutin	$C_{27}H_{32}O_{14}$	581.18599	9.718	89.8	35.54
9	Hesperetin	$C_{16}H_{14}O_6$	303.08563	10.229	89.8	42.68
10	Hesperidin	$C_{28}H_{34}O_{15}$	611.19639	10.231	89.4	34.81
11	Baicalein	$C_{15}H_{10}O_5$	271.05936	10.828	83.4	23.90
12	Baicalin	$C_{21}H_{18}O_{11}$	447.09099	10.829	80.5	24.28
13	Atractylenolide I	$C_{15}H_{18}O_2$	231.1376	11.217	83.9	31.00
14	Formononetin	$C_{16}H_{12}O_4$	269.08048	11.229	84.7	21.53
15	Jatrorrhizine	$C_{20}H_{19}NO_4$	338.13782	11.237	90.1	22.20
16	Oroxylin A	$C_{16}H_{12}O_5$	285.07512	11.791	83.1	27.36
17	Calycosin	$C_{16}H_{12}O_5$	285.07516	11.931	92.5	22.71
18	Wogonin	$C_{16}H_{12}O_5$	285.07495	12.195	82	24.61
19	Heterophyllin B	$C_{40}H_{58}N_8O_8$	779.44451	13.048	90.1	35.10
20	Isosinensetin	$C_{20}H_{20}O_7$	373.12749	13.374	93.1	46.46
21	5-*O*-Demethylnobiletin	$C_{20}H_{20}O_8$	389.12254	13.532	87.7	55.67
22	Sinensetin	$C_{20}H_{20}O_7$	373.12687	13.853	90	48.41
23	6-Demethoxytangeretin	$C_{19}H_{18}O_6$	343.11711	13.93	85.5	38.92
24	Nobiletin	$C_{21}H_{22}O_8$	403.13754	14.363	92.8	30.35
25	Tangeretin	$C_{20}H_{20}O_7$	373.1272	14.909	90.9	49.55
26	Curcumenol	$C_{15}H_{22}O_2$	235.16861	14.924	91.1	31.01
27	Zederone	$C_{15}H_{18}O_3$	247.13265	15.203	84.3	31.31
28	Dihydrotanshinone I	$C_{18}H_{14}O_3$	279.10093	15.657	87	48.06
29	Cryptotanshinone	$C_{19}H_{20}O_3$	297.1477	16.609	87.7	104.72
30	Tanshinone IIA	$C_{19}H_{18}O_3$	295.13229	17.508	93	33.04

In the Swiss Target Prediction database (http://swisstargetprediction.ch/, accessed on 12 May 2023), the targets for the 54 unique compounds were predicted and filtered based on a probability value threshold of ≥ 0.3, resulting in 86 targets corresponding to 38 components. These association data were then imported into Cytoscape 3.8.0 (https://cytoscape.org/, accessed on 15 May 2023) to generate a component-target network comprising 124 nodes and 225 edges (Figure 1A). The results of the GO enrichment analysis showed that the mechanisms of action of QLXP were mainly related to the regulation of the tube, blood vessel diameter maintenance, integral components of the postsynaptic membrane, and hydrolyase activity, whereas the results of the KEGG pathway analysis indicated that QLXP is involved in neuroactive ligand–receptor interactions, the serotonergic synapse, and nitrogen metabolism pathways (Figure 1B).

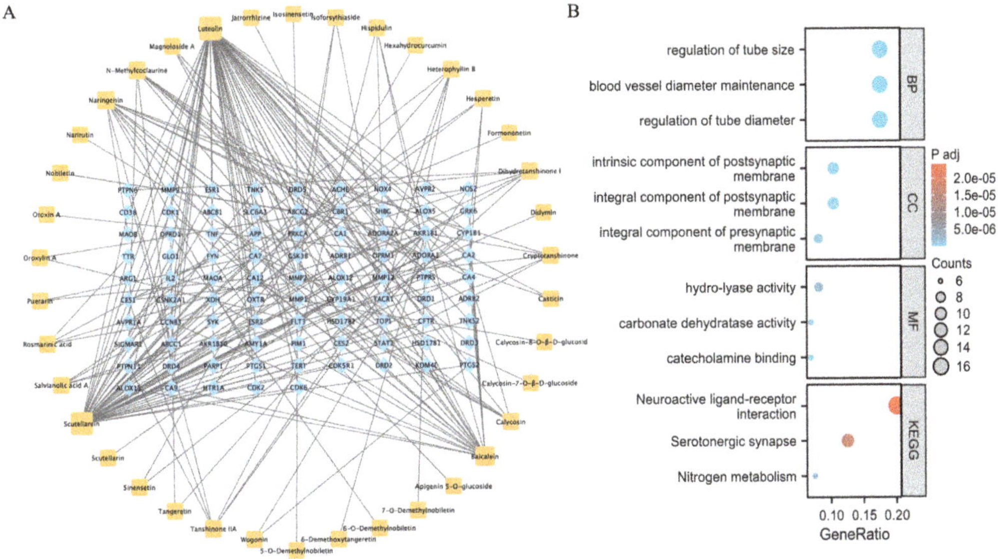

Figure 1. Network pharmacology analysis of QLXP. (**A**) The network of main components and predicted targets. Orange round rectangles represent components and blue diamond nodes represent relevant targets. (**B**) GO enrichment analysis and KEGG pathway enrichment analysis of predicted targets.

2.2. Identification of QLXP Targets Using Thermal Proteome Profiling

The TPP analysis revealed 5463 proteins across biological duplicates, of which 2374 were successfully quantified. After using a filtering criterion, 2338 proteins produced valid sigmoidal melting curves (Figure 2A), permitting the determination of melting temperature (Tm), which is the point at which half of the protein is denatured. After evaluating the reproducibility of our TPP-based QLXP assessment, we observed a robust Pearson's correlation coefficient between 0.83 and 0.93 for Tm values across biological replicates, indicating high consistency. Overall, the protein abundance decreased as the temperature increased (Figure 2B). The distribution of the Tm in the human proteome ranged from 45–70 °C (Figure 2C). To investigate the impact of QLXP on protein stability, we calculated the ΔTm (TmQLXP-TmCtrl) for each protein (Figure 2D). Using NPARC analysis to minimize false negatives, we pinpointed 263 potential interactors with statistical significance ($p < 0.05$), including 115 proteins that exhibited a marked QLXP-mediated shift ($p < 0.01$) in thermal stability. After applying a more rigorous threshold of adjusted $p < 0.1$, we identified 10 proteins as prime QLXP targets (Figure 3A). The gene set enrichment analysis (GSEA) revealed that ADAM17 and NF-κB1 are closely associated with cellular responses to tumor necrosis factor and *H. pylori* infection (Figure 3B). The melting curves of 10 prime targets with adjusted p values < 0.1 are shown in Figure 4.

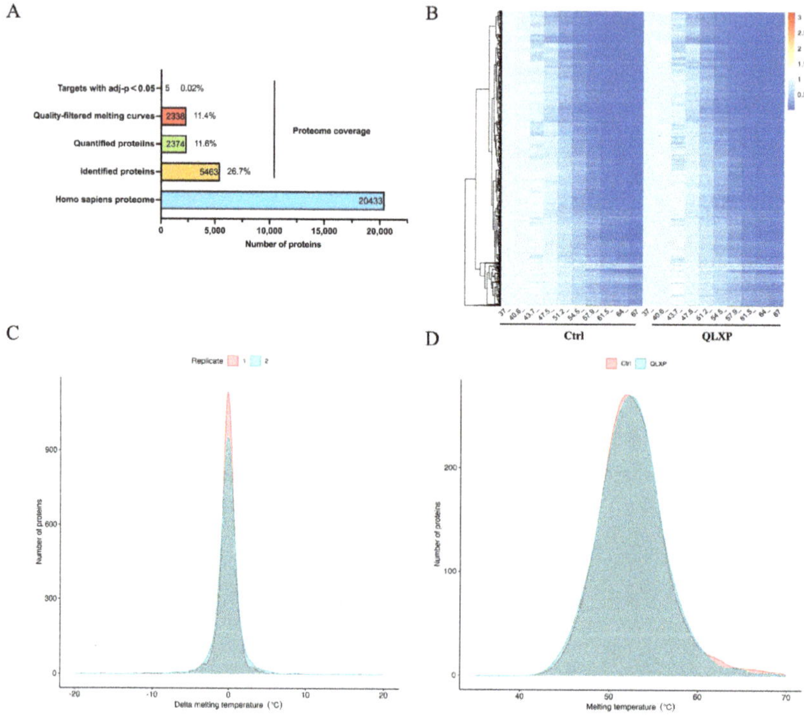

Figure 2. Comprehensive analysis of the thermal proteome profiling experiment for QLXP in GES-1 cell lysates. (**A**) Statistical numbers of TPP data compared to the proteome of *Homo sapiens*. (**B**) The representative heatmap of the non-denatured fraction under different temperatures of all proteins, which reflected the global precipitation behavior of proteins after heat treatment in control or QLXP-treated lysates. The colors suggest protein abundance levels of the non-denatured protein fractions after heat treatment at one of ten temperatures. Relative abundances were normalized to the abundance at 37 °C. (**C**) Tm differences (ΔTm) of proteins in two biological replicates are reproducible. (**D**) TPP experiments captured a large dynamic range of proteins and depicted the distribution of melting temperatures (Tm) in GES-1 cells.

A

ID	Protein Name	Symbol	*p*Val	*p*-Adj
P50225	Sulfotransferase 1A1	*SULT1A1*	1.84×10^{-6}	0.001447
Q15047	Histone-lysine N-methyltransferase SETDB1	*SETDB1*	4.98×10^{-5}	0.015057
Q9BPX3	Condensin complex subunit 3	*NCAPG*	8.4×10^{-5}	0.018018
P78536	Disintegrin and metalloproteinase domain-containing protein 17	*ADAM17*	0.000229	0.032359
Q9Y3D8	Adenylate kinase isoenzyme 6	*AK6*	0.000401	0.047257
Q5SWX8	Protein odr-4 homolog	*ODR4*	0.00046	0.050217
Q86YP4	Transcriptional repressor p66-alpha	*GATAD2A*	0.000468	0.050217
P19838	Nuclear factor NF-kappa-B p105 subunit	*NFKB1*	0.000781	0.076039
Q96PU5	E3 ubiquitin-protein ligase NEDD4-like	*NEDD4L*	0.00087	0.076039
Q6UVK1	Chondroitin sulfate proteoglycan 4	*CSPG4*	0.001209	0.089134

B

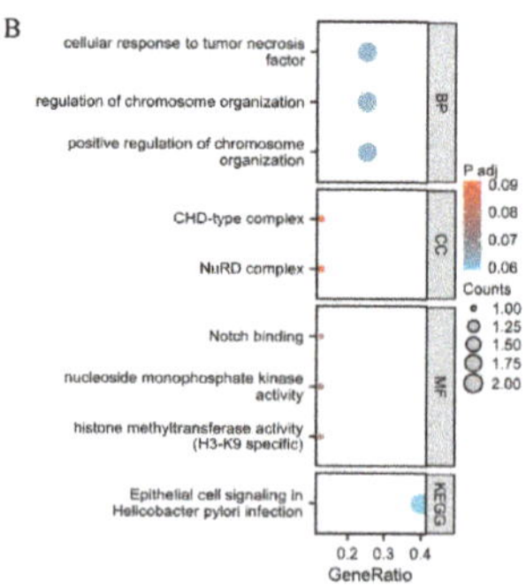

Figure 3. (**A**) The list of 10 prime targets with adjusted *p*-value < 0.1. Fstat computed with NPARC method quantifies the relative reduction in residuals from null to alternative model. *p* values were computed from the values of the Fstat, and the Benjamini–Hochberg procedure was used to adjust the *p* values for multiple hypothesis test. (**B**) GSEA of these 10 proteins.

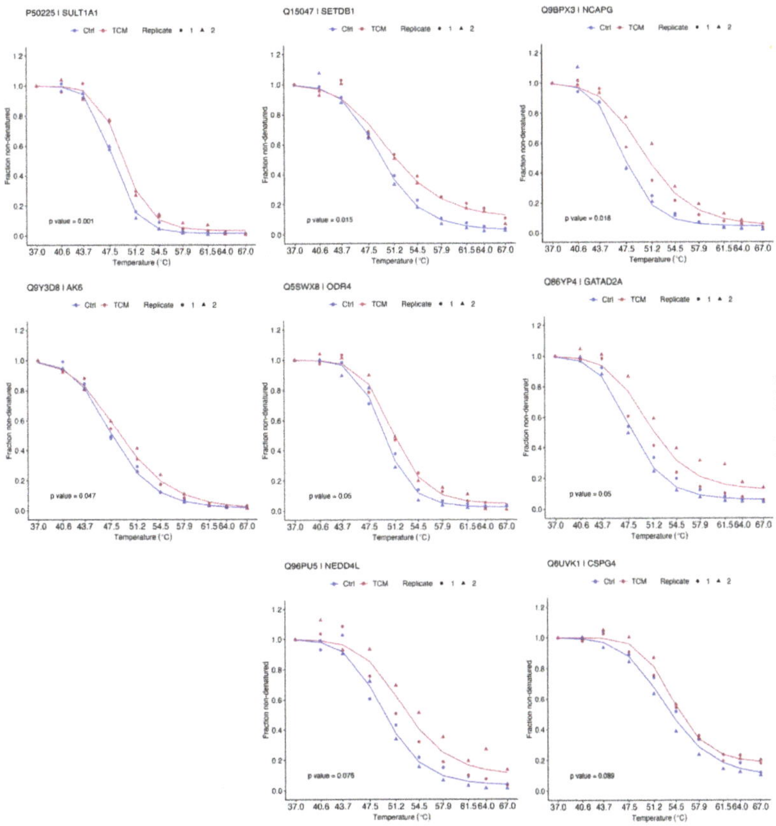

Figure 4. The melting curves of 10 prime targets with adjusted *p* values < 0.1. TCM stands for Traditional Chinese Medicine, specifically referring to the QLXP.

2.3. ADAM17 Is a Key Candidate Target Associated with CAG and GC

We conducted a joint analysis of the above network pharmacology and TPP results and integrated relevant literature reports to identify key targets for subsequent research. We combined the 86 targets derived from network pharmacology with the 115 significant QLXP-modulated proteins from TPP and imported them into STRING for Protein–Protein Interaction (PPI) analysis, specifying the *Homo* species. Following the elimination of proteins without connections, we rendered the network in Cytoscape 3.8.0, consisting of 177 nodes and 1702 edges (Figure 5A). By calculating the degree parameter, TNF was identified as the top target. Furthermore, we evaluated a prospective multicenter longitudinal cohort study [21], in which researchers analyzed 1256 gastric samples and identified 26 IM driver genes across different pathways, including 9 significant driver genes. We also performed a PPI analysis between the proteins of these nine significant IM driver genes and QLXP targets with adjusted $p < 0.1$ from TPP, revealing a notable interaction between ADAM17 and the driver genes, mediated by NF-κB1 (Figure 5B).

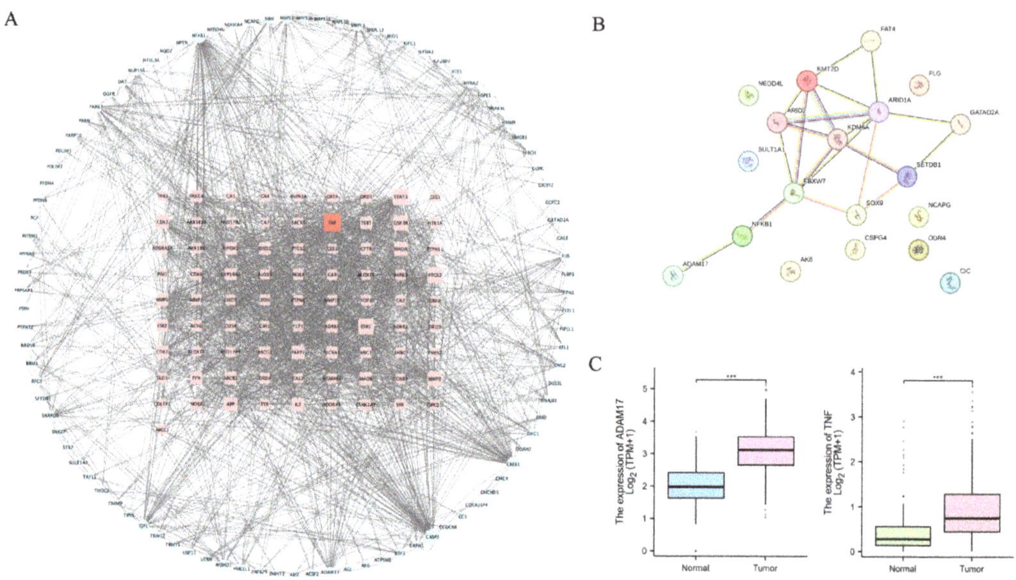

Figure 5. Bioinformatic analysis of predicted targets, binding targets, and public data. (**A**) Protein–protein interaction network of predicted targets and binding targets with QLXP. Blue circles represent binding targets with QLXP, pink round rectangles represent predicted targets. Node size indicates the degree of connectivity, with larger nodes representing higher connectivity. TNF is the top node. (**B**) Protein–protein interaction analysis between the proteins of nine IM driver genes and QLXP targets with adjust-$p < 0.1$. (**C**) The expression of ADAM17 and TNFα in GC and normal tissue of TPM-formatted RNA-seq data from TCGA and GTEx datasets, Statistical significance is indicated as follows: *** $p < 0.001$.

Chronic inflammation is closely related to CAG. Through the aforementioned combined analysis, it so happens that TNF, ADAM17, and NF-κB1 are all important molecules associated with chronic inflammation. ADAM17, also known as TNF-α-converting enzyme (TACE), is crucial for the cleavage and release of TNF-α from its membrane-bound precursor. This process allows TNF-α to bind to its receptors and initiate the classical NF-κB inflammatory pathway, leading to pro-inflammatory effects [22]. NF-κB transcription factors play a role in the regulation of ADAM17 expression [23]. Given this interplay between ADAM17 and the inflammatory cascade, selecting ADAM17 as a pivotal research target protein is strongly justified. Moreover, since NF-κB1 has been extensively studied in CAG, we intend to focus our research on ADAM17. To delve into the relationship between ADAM17 and gastric mucosal inflammation-related cancer, we analyzed public databases, including TPM-formatted RNA-seq data from the TCGA and GTEx datasets, to investigate the transcriptional variations between GC and normal tissues. These datasets were uniformly processed using the Toil pipeline (https://toil.ucsc-cgl.org/, accessed on 20 July 2023) [24] and obtained from the UCSC XENA database (https://xenabrowser.net/datapages/, accessed on 20 July 2023). Our analysis included 414 GC and 210 normal tissue samples. Upon comparing the transcriptional profiles, we found that ADAM17 and TNF-α mRNA levels were significantly increased in GC tissues compared to those in normal tissue (Figure 5C). We therefore considered ADAM17 to be a key candidate target associated with CAG and GC.

2.4. Validation of ADAM17 as a Target of QLXP

To confirm the interaction between QLXP and ADAM17, we conducted CETSA to assess the temperature-dependent alterations in ADAM17 stability. Under experimental conditions analogous to TPP, ADAM17 exhibited increased stability in the presence of QLXP, confirming its role as an QLXP-binding partner (Figure 6A).

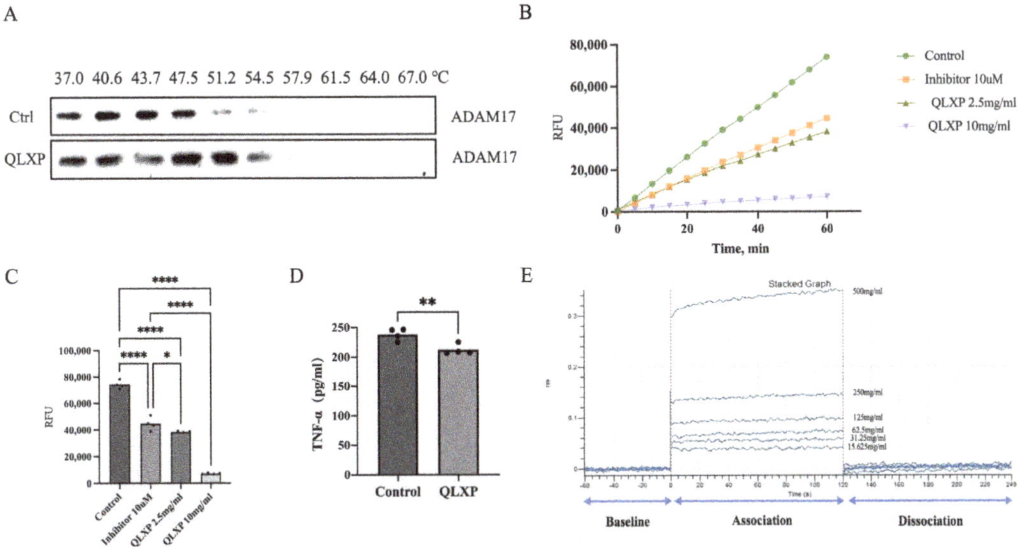

Figure 6. (**A**) CETSA of ADAM17 with escalating temperature by Western blotting. (**B**) Kinetics analysis of the inhibitory effect of QLXP on the enzymatic activity of ADAM17. (**C**) Endpoint analysis of the inhibitory effect of QLXP on the enzymatic activity of ADAM17. Statistical significance is indicated as follows: * $p < 0.05$, **** $p < 0.0001$. (**D**) Inhibitory effect of QLXP on the expression of TNF-α. ** $p < 0.01$. (**E**) Real-time kinetic binding sensorgrams of different concentrations of QLXP increasing from 15.625 to 500 mg/mL are shown. Response (nm) indicates the optical thickness on the SAA biosensor layer.

To investigate whether QLXP attenuates the enzymatic activity of ADAM17, we incubated GES-1 cell lysates with H_2O as negative control and ADAM17's inhibitor as positive control, subsequently assessing changes in ADAM17 activity using an ADAM17 activity assay kit (AnaSpec, Fremont, CA, USA; cat. #AS-72085). Following dual analysis of kinetic and endpoint data, we found that QLXP significantly inhibits the enzymatic activity of ADAM17 (Figure 6B,C).

As ADAM17 functions as TACE and AGS cells express abundant TNF-α, to assess whether QLXP inhibits the expression of TNF-α, we treated AGS cells with QLXP for 12 h, using H_2O as a negative control. We found that QLXP exerted an inhibitory effect on the release of TNF-α (Figure 6D). In summary, the integrated analysis of the interactions between QLXP and ADAM17, along with the assessment of its influence on TNF-α, elucidated the molecular basis of the therapeutic efficacy of QLXP.

2.5. BLI Analysis Identifies Components Binding to ADAM17 in QLXP

BLI provides a sensitive and label-free method for real-time analysis of biomolecular interactions. We initially employed BLI to evaluate the binding of QLXP to ADAM17, monitoring the real-time association and dissociation kinetics between QLXP (at concentrations from 15.625 to 500 μg/mL) and biotinylated ADAM17. The findings revealed a clear, concentration-responsive, and reversible interaction between the two molecules, as evidenced by the proportional increase in the optical thickness (nm) measured on the sensor surface (Figure 6E). In summary, using TPP, CETSA, and BLI analyses, we confirmed that ADAM17 is a binding partner of QLXP.

To identify the components in QLXP that interact with ADAM17, we collected the dissociation solutions from both the QLXP group and the blank control group for analysis using UPLC-Orbitrap MS. For the identification of ADAM17-binding components, we applied two specific criteria: (1) The "mzVault Best Match" score must have exceeded 70. (2) Not present in the dissociation solution of the blank control group. After the rigorous quality control of signal stability, we identified the components that bind to ADAM17 (Table 3). Among the screened components, alkaloids and flavonoids were most abundant, followed by isoflavones and organic acids. Alkaloids and flavonoids, two types of plant secondary metabolites, have various biological properties, including antioxidant, anti-inflammatory, antiviral, anticancer, antiplatelet, and antibacterial properties.

Table 3. Main components binding with ADAM17 in QLXP.

Name	Formula	*m/z*	RT [min]
Epiberberine	$C_{20}H_{17}NO_4$	336.12263	12.735
Palmatine	$C_{21}H_{21}NO_4$	352.15407	12.696
Jatrorrhizine	$C_{20}H_{19}NO_4$	338.13866	11.872
(+)-Magnoflorine	$C_{20}H_{23}NO_4$	342.16997	8.584
Berberrubine	$C_{19}H_{15}NO_4$	322.10752	10.559
Demethyleneberberine	$C_{19}H_{17}NO_4$	324.12316	10.732
Nobiletin	$C_{21}H_{22}O_8$	403.13876	15.267
Sinensetin	$C_{20}H_{20}O_7$	373.12831	14.714
Formononetin	$C_{16}H_{12}O_4$	269.08093	14.401
Dehydroglaucine	$C_{21}H_{23}NO_4$	354.16999	11.123
6-Demethoxytangeretin	$C_{19}H_{18}O_6$	343.11792	15.312
Quinic acid	$C_7H_{12}O_6$	191.05673	1.02
Oroxylin A-7-*O*-β-D-glucuronide	$C_{22}H_{20}O_{11}$	459.09442	13.101
TF-Hesperidin	$C_{28}H_{34}O_{15}$	609.184	11.383
Narirutin	$C_{27}H_{32}O_{14}$	579.17336	10.778

2.6. Molecular Docking Analysis of ADAM17 and Its Binding Components

Based on the binding component classification, we selected two alkaloids (jatrorrhizine and berberrubine) and two flavonoids (narirutin and sinensetin) for molecular docking analysis. The XP Gscore is commonly used as a reference metric. A binding free energy is considered low when the XP Gscore is below −6 or the MM-GBSA dG Bind value is less than −30 kcal/mol, signifying a stable interaction between the ligand and the protein [25]. Our analyses revealed that all four components exhibited significant binding affinity towards ADAM17. Notably, narirutin and berberrubine showed promising interactions with ADAM17, which exhibited the best docking performance, indicating particularly stable binding with ADAM17 (Table 4). In detail, narirutin formed hydrogen bonds with HIP709, SER711, ASN712, and MET715 (Figure 7A). Similarly, jatrorrhizine also bound to HIP709 via a hydrogen bond (Figure 7B). Berberrubine interacted with HIP709 via both a hydrogen bond and a π–cation bond (Figure 7C). Sinensetin formed two π–π bonds and two π–cation bonds with the same residue (Figure 7D). These findings offer critical insights into the molecular interactions, elucidating the specific binding modes and the potential for these components to modulate ADAM17 activity. The predominance of HIP709 in the binding events suggests that this histidine residue acts as a pivotal anchor point within the ADAM17 catalytic domain. Interactions between ligands and HIP709, such as hydrogen bonds and π–cation interactions, may inhibit enzyme activity. Adjacent residues, such as SER711, ASN712, and MET715, are likely involved in the stability of the binding pocket.

Table 4. Molecular docking result of components binding ADAM17.

ChemSpider ID	Compound	XP GScore	MM-GBSA dG Bind (kcal/mol)
390871	Narirutin	−6.114	−34.20
65269	Jatrorrhizine	−2.447	−22.11
402990	Berberrubine	−2.200	−31.28
128491	Sinensetin	−1.373	−30.91

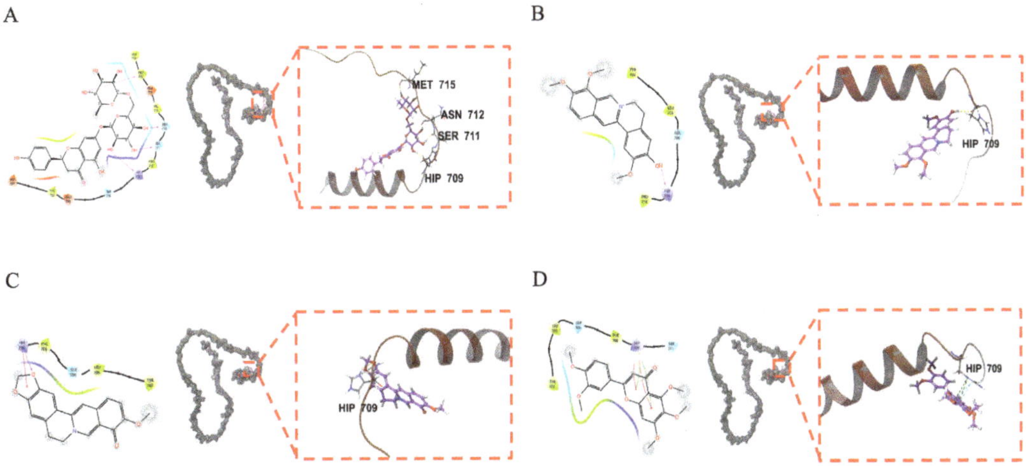

Figure 7. Molecular docking result of narirutin, jatrorrhizine, berberrubine, and sinensetin with ADAM17. (**A**) Docking diagrams of narirutin and ADAM17 protein. Narirutin binds to the surface of the active pocket in the intracellular domain of ADAM17 protein, forming a hydrogen bond with each of the residues HIP709, SER711, ASN712, and MET715 in the ADAM17 protein. Yellow represents hydrogen bonding. (**B**) Docking diagrams of jatrorrhizine and ADAM17 protein. Jatrorrhizine binds to the surface of the active pocket in the intracellular domain of the ADAM17 protein, forming a hydrogen bond with the residue HIP709 in the ADAM17 protein. Yellow represents hydrogen bonding. (**C**) Docking diagrams of berberrubine and ADAM17 protein. Berberrubine binds to the surface of the active pocket in the intracellular domain of the ADAM17 protein, forming a hydrogen bond and a π–cation bond with the residue HIP709 in the ADAM17 protein. Yellow represents hydrogen bonding, while green represents π–cation bonding. (**D**) Docking diagrams of sinensetin and ADAM17 protein. Sinensetin binds to the surface of the active pocket in the intracellular domain of the ADAM17 protein, forming two π–π bonds and two π–cation (π-positive ion) bonds with the residue HIP709 in the ADAM17 protein. Blue represents π –π bonds, while green represents π–cation (π-positive ion) bonds.

3. Discussion

CAG, a chronic inflammatory condition characterized by the progressive loss of gastric glandular cells, is considered a precancerous lesion and is strongly correlated with an increased risk of GC. Our prior RCT revealed that QLXP can alleviate gastric mucosal atrophy and IM, and it effectively inhibits the EMT process. However, the molecular targets of QLXP remained undefined. By integrating network pharmacology, TPP, BLI, and molecular docking, the target proteins and interacting compounds of QLXP were identified in the present study.

We utilized UPLC-Orbitrap MS to analyze the aqueous extract of QLXP, identifying 54 unique compounds after applying strict criteria. Targets for these compounds were predicted using the Swiss Target Prediction database, resulting in 86 targets linked to 38 components. Subsequently, we used TPP to identify 115 potential targets of QLXP. A PPI analysis of the 86 predicted targets and 115 significant QLXP-shifted proteins identified TNF as the top target among the predicted targets. Through the implementation of a rigorous data filter in TPP, 10 proteins, including ADAM17, were found to bind to QLXP with high confidence. After considering the relationship between ADAM17 and TNF, the association with IM driver genes, and differential expression in GC tissues, ADAM17 was determined to be a key candidate target of QLXP associated with CAG and GC. Therefore, we verified the binding of QLXP to ADAM17 using CETSA and BLI techniques.

ADAM17 belongs to the "A Disintegrin And Metalloproteinase" (ADAM) family of type I transmembrane proteins [26,27]. ADAM17 is primarily involved in the ectodomain shedding of membrane proteins, including cytokines, growth factors, receptors, and adhesion molecules, and plays a role in cell signaling, adhesion, migration, and other biological processes [7]. ADAM17 further plays a pivotal role in inflammation and cancer, as ADAM17-mediated shedding events have been implicated in regulating inflammatory responses and promoting tumor growth, invasion, and metastasis [27–30]. ADAM17 mediates the proteolytic cleavage and release of inflammatory mediators, such as TNF-α and IL-6R, in gastric mucosal inflammation. During *H. pylori* infection, CagL dissociates ADAM17 from integrin α5β1, activating the ADAM17-dependent and NF-κB-mediated repression of HKα, intensifying the inflammatory process [31,32]. Furthermore, ADAM17 facilitates EMT in gastric cancer cells by activating the TGF-β/Smad signaling pathway, thereby contributing to tumor progression and metastasis [33]. Beyond inflammation and cancer, ADAM17 has been implicated in the pathogenesis of other diseases. In cardiovascular diseases, it may contribute to atherosclerosis and heart failure through the shedding of cell adhesion molecules [34]. In neurological disorders, ADAM17 could be involved in the cleavage of neuregulin, affecting synaptic function and contributing to diseases like Alzheimer's and Parkinson's [35]. In autoimmune diseases, the dysregulation of ADAM17 activity may lead to an imbalance in immune responses, exacerbating conditions such as rheumatoid arthritis and multiple sclerosis [36]. ADAM17 is a pivotal enzyme in the elucidation of disease pathogenesis and serves as a promiscuous therapeutic target in pharmacological research. Our findings reveal that QLXP effectively inhibits the enzymatic activity of ADAM17, thereby decreasing the secretion of TNF-α. This mechanism of action clarifies QLXP's inhibitory effect on gastric mucosal inflammation. These results provide preliminary evidence supporting the potential development of QLXP as an ADAM17 inhibitor. However, the development of ADAM17 inhibitors requires addressing challenges such as precise delivery, dynamic monitoring, and combination therapy to overcome issues of toxicity and resistance, thereby facilitating their transition to clinical application [37].

Other potential targets of QLXP include enzymes (SULT1A1 and AK6), transcription factors (SETDB1 and GATAD2A), signal transduction proteins (ODR4), cell surface proteoglycans (CSPG4), chromatin remodeling complex components (NCAPG), and ubiquitin ligases (NEDD4L). While these targets were identified, the current study did not focus on their specific interactions with QLXP. Nonetheless, the potential involvement of these molecules warrants further discussion. SETDB1's role in epigenetic regulation and its association with GC suggest that it could be a significant player in the therapeutic response to QLXP. Future work could explore the extent to which QLXP modulates SETDB1 activity and its downstream effects on gene expression in the context of gastric mucosal inflammation and cancer.

BLI has played a crucial role in screening and validating the binding affinities of small molecules from TCM to Aβ peptides, which are key pathological features of Alzheimer's disease [38,39]. Through BLI technology and affinity-fish compounds binding ADAM17 in QLXP, we identified a range of bioactive compounds, including alkaloids, flavonoids, isoflavones (formononetin and dehydroglaucine), and organic acids. After a molecular docking analysis, we found that narirutin exhibited the best docking performance with ADAM17, indicating stable binding between this compound and the intracellular domain of ADAM17. Narirutin is a flavonoid compound commonly found in citrus peels, such as the *Citrus × aurantium* L. in QLXP. Studies have demonstrated that narirutin has diverse pharmacological properties, such as antioxidant, anti-inflammatory, anticancer, and neuroprotective properties [40]. Further studies should be conducted to investigate the anti-inflammatory and anticancer effects of narirutin. In present study, narirutin may directly affect enzyme activity through HIP709. Adjacent residues, such as SER711, ASN712, and MET715, are likely involved in substrate recognition and the stability of the binding pocket. In future studies, we intend to utilize site-directed mutagenesis and other techniques to further validate these interactions and their impact on ADAM17 function. Additionally, berberrubine and sinensetin exhibited promising binding affinities. Berberrubine, the major metabolite of berberine, originates from *Coptis chinensis Franch* in QLXP. Previous studies have shown that berberrubine has pharmacological properties, including anti-tumor, anti-inflammatory, and lipid-lowering functions [41]. Sinensetin is a plant-derived polymethoxylated flavonoid found in citrus fruits, such as the *Citrus × aurantium* L. In vitro and in vivo studies have confirmed the potent anticancer effects of sinensetin, along with its broad pharmacological profile, which includes anti-inflammatory, antioxidant, anti-obesity, anti-dementia, and vasorelaxant activities [42].

In summary, the synergistic application of network pharmacology, TPP, BLI, and molecular docking provides a comprehensive framework for investigating the target proteins of QLXP. To date, the application of such a systematic methodological combination in the research of TCM is relatively rare. We are hopeful that our research methodology will gain recognition and be broadly applied in the field. However, it is crucial to acknowledge the limitations inherent in the current research design. The primary limitation of this study is its restriction to in vitro cellular experiments, which may not entirely reflect the intricate physiological and pathological dynamics within a living organism. To address this, we intend to confirm the anti-inflammatory properties of QLXP in a murine model of CAG, with a particular emphasis on the suppression of TNF-α and the modulation of ADAM17 activity in a systemic inflammatory context. Our investigation has been focused on the interaction between ADAM17 and narirutin, a single target and component of QLXP. However, QLXP's therapeutic effects are likely multifaceted, involving multiple targets and constituents. The impact of narirutin on proteins other than ADAM17 remains to be explored. Consequently, further in vivo studies are necessary to corroborate our in vitro findings and to identify additional potential targets and active components of QLXP. Such research will deepen our understanding of QLXP's therapeutic promise and its utility in the management of CAG and IM.Additionally, the study may be influenced by confounding factors, including the complexity of the herbal formulation, inter-individual variability, and dose-related effects, all of which can affect the medication's efficacy. To overcome these challenges, a systems pharmacology approach is advocated, which incorporates AI for mapping component interactions, multi-omics for patient stratification, and physiologically-based pharmacokinetic modeling. This approach will not only enhance the robustness of our findings but also provide a more comprehensive understanding of QLXP's mechanism of action and its potential clinical application. Ultimately, this method holds the potential to transform traditional herbal practices to a modern, mechanism-guided approach within the realm of Traditional Chinese Medicine.

4. Materials and Methods

4.1. Network Pharmacology

4.1.1. Aqueous Extraction and Preparation of QLXP

QLXP granules were sourced from Guangdong Yifang Pharmaceutical Co., Ltd. (Foshan, China). The active ingredients in QLXP were extracted using the aqueous extraction method. One gram of QLXP granules was dissolved in 10 mL of distilled water, heated to 100 °C in a water bath for 1 h, and centrifuged to collect the supernatant. The supernatant was then filtered through a 0.22 μm filter in a sterile environment and stored at 4 °C for future use.

4.1.2. LC-MS/MS Analysis

The aqueous extract of QLXP was analyzed using UPLC-Orbitrap MS. Separation was achieved on an ethylene bridged hybrid C18 column (Waters, Milford, MA, USA) with a binary solvent system (A: H_2O + 0.1% formic acid; B: CAN + 0.1% formic acid) at 250 μL/min over 25 min. Data were acquired in both positive and negative ion modes with MS/MS and subsequently processed and identified using the Compound Discoverer 3.3 software.

4.1.3. Prediction of the Potential Targets of the Major Compounds in QLXP

The major components were converted into standard SMILES files using ChemSpider (https://www.chemspider.com/, accessed on 5 May 2023) [43]. The potential targets of the major compounds in QLXP were obtained from the Swiss Target Prediction database (http://swisstargetprediction.ch/, accessed on 12 May 2023) [44].

4.1.4. Construction and Analysis of the "Component-Target" Network

The "component-target" network of QLXP was constructed using Cytoscape 3.8.0. The Network analyzer plugin in the Cytoscape software was used to calculate parameters, such as degree centrality.

4.2. Thermal Proteome Profiling

4.2.1. Cell Culture

GES-1 and AGS cell lines, obtained from the cell bank of the Chinese Academy of Sciences, were cultured in DMEM and RPMI-1640 media (Wisent, Montreal, QC, Canada). The culture media were supplemented with 10% fetal bovine serum (PAN-Biotech, Aidenbach, Bavaria, Germany) and 1% penicillin/streptomycin (Wisent, Montreal, QC, Canada). The cells were maintained in an incubator set to 37 °C with 5% CO_2.

4.2.2. Sample Preparation for Thermal Proteome Profiling

The GES-1 cells were collected, washed thrice with phosphate-buffered saline (PBS, pH 7.4), and resuspended in lysis buffer (PBS containing a protease inhibitor cocktail and 1.5 mM $MgCl_2$). The cell suspension was then mechanically disrupted using a glass grinding rod (50 strokes). The methodology employed for the TPP used an established protocol with multiplexed quantitative mass spectrometry-based proteomics to evaluate the thermal stability of proteins across the proteome [45]. In brief, two groups of crude cellular extracts were incubated with 5 mg/mL QLXP and water for 15 min, respectively, with water serving as the negative control. Following this, aliquots of the treated lysates were subjected to a temperature range of 37–67 °C for 3 min, followed by incubation at

25 °C for 3 min. Membrane- and DNA-bound proteins were extracted using 0.8% NP40 (Biodee, Beijing, China; cat. #74385) and 250 U/mL benzonase (Sigma, St. Louis, MO, USA; cat. #E1014) and protein aggregates were removed via ultracentrifugation. The protein pellet was air-dried after removing the supernatant and acetone, then redissolved in 200 µL of 8 M urea in PBS. Reduction/alkylation was conducted with 5 mM DTT at 55 °C for 45 min, followed by 12.5 mM IAM at room temperature in the dark for 30 min. Samples were diluted to 1.5 M urea in PBS, trypsin was added at a 1:40 ratio, and digestion was performed overnight at 37 °C. Digestion was terminated by adding 10% TFA to acidify to pH 2. Desalting was carried out using a Sep-Pak C18 cartridge. Peptides were dried with SpeedVac (Thermo Scientific, Waltham, MA, USA) and resuspended in 50 µL of 100 mM TEAB before TMT labeling for 1 h at room temperature. The labeling reaction was quenched with 5% hydroxylamine, and mixed peptide samples were diluted, acidified, and desalted. The samples were dried to less than 300 µL and fractionated by high-pH reverse-phase HPLC. Fractions were concatenated into 12 samples, dried, and resuspended in 40 µL of 0.1% formic acid for LC-MS/MS analysis.

4.2.3. LC-MS/MS Analysis and Protein Identification and Quantification

The LC-MS/MS analysis was conducted using a previously described method [45]. The labeled peptides were subjected to LC-MS/MS on a UHPLC3000 system coupled to a Q Exactive HF-X MS (Thermo Scientific, Waltham, MA, USA) with a procolumn connected to a C18 column (Waters, Milford, MA, USA). Protein identification and quantification were performed using Proteome Discoverer 2.3 and the Homo sapiens database.

4.2.4. Bioinformatic Analysis

Gene Ontology (GO) enrichment analysis was conducted using the R package clusterProfiler 4.1.1 to categorize and annotate the functional properties of the target genes, highlighting significant GO terms. Using the KEGG API, we retrieved the background gene set and performed enrichment analysis using clusterProfiler 4.1.1 to further uncover the enriched pathways in our target gene set, offering insights into their biological roles. Additionally, we constructed a protein–protein interaction (PPI) network using the STRING database (https://string-db.org/, accessed on 1 July 2023) and visualized it using Cytoscape 3.8.0, revealing key interaction hubs and pathways.

4.3. Western Blotting

The cells were lysed using RIPA lysis buffer (Beyotime, Shanghai, China, cat. #P0013K) supplemented with a protease inhibitor cocktail. Equal protein volumes were separated on a 12% sodium dodecyl sulfate-polyacrylamide gel and electroblotted onto a polyvinylidene difluoride membrane. Immunoblotting was performed using the primary antibody anti-ADAM17 (Abcam, Cambridge, UK; cat. #ab291073) and secondary antibody anti-rabbit horseradish peroxidase (HRP)-IgG (Cell Signaling Technology, Danvers, MA, USA;cat. #7074).

4.4. ADAM17 Activity Assay

The effects of QLXP on ADAM17 activity were determined using the ADAM17 activity assay kit (AnaSpec, Fremont, CA, USA; cat. #AS-72085) with H_2O as negative control and ADAM17's inhibitor as positive control, according to the manufacturer's protocol. In brief, GES-1 cells were washed with PBS, lysed using assay buffer containing Triton-X 100, and centrifuged to collect the cell lysate in the supernatant. The TACE substrate was diluted in assay buffer to create a working solution. The TACE-containing samples were then added to a microplate, followed by a TACE substrate solution, and the plate was gently shaken to mix the reagents. Fluorescence was measured at Ex/Em = 490 nm/520 nm, either continuously over time or as an endpoint reading after a specified incubation period. The experiments were repeated four times.

4.5. Enzyme-Linked Immunosorbent Assay of TNF-α

The effects of QLXP on the secretion of TNF-α were assayed using the Human TNF-α enzyme-linked immunosorbent assay (ELISA) Kit (Proteinch, Rosemont, IL, USA; cat. #KE00154), according to the manufacturer's guidelines. In brief, the supernatant from AGS cell culture media, after a 12 h QLXP treatment, was harvested and centrifuged at 500× *g* for 5 min. Standards or samples were then gradient-diluted and sequentially incubated with detection antibody and HRP-conjugated secondary antibody. The optical density (OD) of each well was measured at 450 nm using an ELISA reader with a correction wavelength of 630 nm, if available, to ensure accurate readings.

4.6. BLI Analysis

The BLI analysis was performed using the ForteBio Octet® RED96e system (Göttingen, Germany). The ADAM17 fusion protein (Proteintech, Rosemont, IL, USA; cat. #Ag32418) was prepared in PBS and at a concentration of 50 µg/mL and subjected to biotinylating with EZ-Link NHS-LC-LC-Biotin. Prior to immobilizing the biotinylated ADAM17 onto the SSA biosensor, the biosensor was pre-wetted with PBS to establish a baseline. The extracts of QLXP were meticulously diluted within a PBS solution that was fortified with 15% DMSO and 0.02% Tween 20, with a final volume of 200 µL per well. An equivalent volume of the same PBS solution was dispensed into separate wells to constitute the control group of without QLXP or without ADAM17 fusion protein. The experiment proceeded in a cyclic fashion with four basic steps: loading for 300 s, establishing a baseline for 60 s, association for 120 s, and dissociation for 120 s. Data acquisition and analysis were performed using the ForteBio Octet Data Acquisition and Analysis software, with background subtraction performed using a double-negative control for interaction signals. Using UPLC-Orbitrap MS, the dissociation and control buffers for the BLI analysis were analyzed as described in Section 4.1.2 to identify components that interact with ADAM17.

4.7. Molecular Docking Analysis

Given that our study focused on the intracellular region of ADAM17 involved in the BLI analysis, we utilized AlphaFold2 to predict the crystal structure of the intracellular domain of ADAM17 [46]. The predicted protein structures were processed using the Protein Preparation Wizard module in Schrödinger software 2024-2. The 2D SDF structure files of the compounds were processed using the LigPrep module in the Schrödinger software to generate all the possible 3D chiral conformations. In molecular docking, the XP mode incorporated flexible docking, enabling both the protein and ligand to adapt to their conformations, thereby offering the most sophisticated computational approach. A subsequent analysis using MM-GBSA served as a robust validation step, reinforcing the XP docking findings.

4.8. Statistical Analysis

R (version 4.3) and GraphPad Prism software (version 9.0) were used for statistical analysis and plotting. Specifically, TPP data were fitted with two competing models in the NPARC method: a null model which analyzed the relative protein abundances changes with temperature by using a single smooth function of temperature irrespective of the ligand treatment, and an alternative model that analyzed the relative protein abundances changes for the vehicle and treatment group, respectively. The sum of squared residuals (RSS), which was calculated as the deviations between the fitted model and observed data, were used to calculate the F-statistic to estimate the variability between groups and within groups. For each protein, a p-value was computed from the F-statistic based on the cumulative F-distribution. To account for multiple hypothesis testing, the Benjamini and Hochberg method was applied to adjust the p-values across all proteins. Differences were considered statistically significant if Student's t-test yielded p-values less than 0.05. Other data are presented as mean $\pm$ standard error of the mean (SEM). Statistical comparisons across all groups were performed using either a one-way analysis of variance (ANOVA) test or an unpaired Student's t-test.

5. Conclusions

Utilizing network pharmacology and TPP, we pinpointed ADAM17 as a target of QLXP, where QLXP inhibits the enzymatic activity of ADAM17, thereby suppressing TNF-α secretion and exerting anti-inflammatory effects. BLI confirmed the direct and reversible binding of QLXP to ADAM17, with narirutin exhibiting the highest binding affinity. Our findings demonstrate that the "network pharmacology—TPP—BLI—molecular docking" method is a powerful tool to reveal the mechanisms of action of traditional Chinese herbal formulae.

Author Contributions: S.D.: Conceptualization, data curation, formal analysis, methodology, writing original draft. T.W.: conceptualization, data curation, methodology, writing—review and editing. Z.L.: conceptualization, formal analysis, methodology, writing—review and editing. T.L.: investigation, methodology. Z.M.: investigation, methodology. Y.C.: data curation. S.Z.: formal analysis. W.W.: funding acquisition, project administration, supervision. H.D.: conceptualization, methodology, funding acquisition, project administration, supervision, writing—review and editing. All authors have read and agreed to the published version of the manuscript.

Funding: This study was supported by the Innovation Team and Talents Cultivation Program of National Administration of Traditional Chinese Medicine (Grant No. ZYYCXTD-C-202210), the National Natural Science Foundation of China (Grant No. T2293763 and Grant No. 82172556), and Beijing Natural Science Foundation (IS24040).

Institutional Review Board Statement: Not applicable.

Informed Consent Statement: Not applicable.

Data Availability Statement: The data presented in this study are available on request from the corresponding author. The data are not publicly available due to intellectual property protection.

Acknowledgments: We greatly appreciate the Facility for Protein Chemistry and Proteomics, Metabolomics Facility Center of Metabolomics and Lipidomics at Tsinghua University, for the sample analysis.

Conflicts of Interest: The authors declare no conflicts of interest.

Abbreviations

GC	Gastric cancer
CAG	Chronic atrophic gastritis
IM	Intestinal metaplasia
TCM	Traditional Chinese medicine
RCT	Randomized controlled trial
QLXP	Qilianxiaopi formula
EMT	Epithelial–mesenchymal transition
TPP	Thermal proteome profiling
CETSA	Cellular thermal shift assay
BLI	Bio-layer interferometry
HPLC	High-performance liquid chromatography

LC-MS	Liquid chromatography-tandem mass spectrometry
NPARC	Nonparametric analysis of response curves
GO	Gene Ontology
PPI	Protein–protein interaction
HRP	Horseradish peroxidase
OD	Optical density
TMT	Tandem mass tag
Tm	Melting temperature
GSEA	Gene Set Enrichment Analysis
TACE	TNF-α-converting enzyme
ADAM	A Disintegrin And Metalloproteinase

References

1. Sung, H.; Ferlay, J.; Siegel, R.L.; Laversanne, M.; Soerjomataram, I.; Jemal, A.; Bray, F. Global Cancer Statistics 2020: GLOBOCAN Estimates of Incidence and Mortality Worldwide for 36 Cancers in 185 Countries. *CA Cancer J. Clin.* **2021**, *71*, 209–249. [CrossRef]
2. GBD 2017 Stomach Cancer Collaborators. The Global, Regional, and National Burden of Stomach Cancer in 195 Countries, 1990-2017: A Systematic Analysis for the Global Burden of Disease Study 2017. *Lancet Gastroenterol. Hepatol.* **2020**, *5*, 42–54. [CrossRef]
3. Pimentel-Nunes, P.; Libânio, D.; Marcos-Pinto, R.; Areia, M.; Leja, M.; Esposito, G.; Garrido, M.; Kikuste, I.; Megraud, F.; Matysiak-Budnik, T.; et al. Management of Epithelial Precancerous Conditions and Lesions in the Stomach (MAPS II): European Society of Gastrointestinal Endoscopy (ESGE), European Helicobacter and Microbiota Study Group (EHMSG), European Society of Pathology (ESP), and Sociedade Portuguesa de Endoscopia Digestiva (SPED) Guideline Update 2019. *Endoscopy* **2019**, *51*, 365–388. [CrossRef]
4. Song, H.; Ekheden, I.G.; Zheng, Z.; Ericsson, J.; Nyrén, O.; Ye, W. Incidence of Gastric Cancer among Patients with Gastric Precancerous Lesions: Observational Cohort Study in a Low Risk Western Population. *BMJ* **2015**, *351*, h3867. [CrossRef]
5. Shichijo, S.; Hirata, Y.; Niikura, R.; Hayakawa, Y.; Yamada, A.; Ushiku, T.; Fukayama, M.; Koike, K. Histologic Intestinal Metaplasia and Endoscopic Atrophy Are Predictors of Gastric Cancer Development after *Helicobacter pylori* Eradication. *Gastrointest. Endosc.* **2016**, *84*, 618–624. [CrossRef]
6. Ortigão, R.; Figueirôa, G.; Frazzoni, L.; Pimentel-Nunes, P.; Hassan, C.; Dinis-Ribeiro, M.; Fuccio, L.; Libânio, D. Risk Factors for Gastric Metachronous Lesions after Endoscopic or Surgical Resection: A Systematic Review and Meta-Analysis. *Endoscopy* **2022**, *54*, 892–901. [CrossRef]
7. Scheller, J.; Chalaris, A.; Garbers, C.; Rose-John, S. ADAM17: A Molecular Switch to Control Inflammation and Tissue Regeneration. *Trends Immunol.* **2011**, *32*, 380–387. [CrossRef]
8. Li, X.; Feng, M.; Yuan, G. Clinical Efficacy of Weisu Granule Combined with Weifuchun Tablet in the Treatment of Chronic Atrophic Gastritis and Its Effect on Serum G-17, PG I and PG II Levels. *Am. J. Transl. Res.* **2022**, *14*, 275–284.
9. Dai, Y.-K.; Zhang, Y.-Z.; Li, D.-Y.; Ye, J.-T.; Zeng, L.-F.; Wang, Q.; Hu, L. The Efficacy of Jianpi Yiqi Therapy for Chronic Atrophic Gastritis: A Systematic Review and Meta-Analysis. *PLoS ONE* **2017**, *12*, e0181906. [CrossRef]
10. Cao, Y.; Zheng, Y.; Niu, J.; Zhu, C.; Yang, D.; Rong, F.; Liu, G. Efficacy of Banxia Xiexin Decoction for Chronic Atrophic Gastritis: A Systematic Review and Meta-Analysis. *PLoS ONE* **2020**, *15*, e0241202. [CrossRef]
11. Zeng, J.; Yan, R.; Pan, H.; You, F.; Cai, T.; Liu, W.; Zheng, C.; Zhao, Z.; Gong, D.; Chen, L.; et al. Weipixiao Attenuate Early Angiogenesis in Rats with Gastric Precancerous Lesions. *BMC Complement. Altern. Med.* **2018**, *18*, 250. [CrossRef] [PubMed]
12. Hu, J.; Qiao, J.; Kang, D.; Liu, B. Analysis on the Distinguishing Features of Traditional Chinese Therapeutics and Related Statistical Issues. *Front. Med.* **2011**, *5*, 203–207. [CrossRef] [PubMed]
13. Zhao, L.; Zhang, H.; Li, N.; Chen, J.; Xu, H.; Wang, Y.; Liang, Q. Network Pharmacology, a Promising Approach to Reveal the Pharmacology Mechanism of Chinese Medicine Formula. *J. Ethnopharmacol.* **2023**, *309*, 116306. [CrossRef] [PubMed]
14. Zhang, P.; Zhang, D.; Zhou, W.; Wang, L.; Wang, B.; Zhang, T.; Li, S. Network Pharmacology: Towards the Artificial Intelligence-Based Precision Traditional Chinese Medicine. *Brief. Bioinform.* **2023**, *25*, bbad518. [CrossRef]
15. Martinez Molina, D.; Jafari, R.; Ignatushchenko, M.; Seki, T.; Larsson, E.A.; Dan, C.; Sreekumar, L.; Cao, Y.; Nordlund, P. Monitoring Drug Target Engagement in Cells and Tissues Using the Cellular Thermal Shift Assay. *Science* **2013**, *341*, 84–87. [CrossRef]
16. Leijten, N.M.; Bakker, P.; Spaink, H.P.; den Hertog, J.; Lemeer, S. Thermal Proteome Profiling in Zebrafish Reveals Effects of Napabucasin on Retinoic Acid Metabolism. *Mol. Cell. Proteom.* **2021**, *20*, 100033. [CrossRef]
17. Al-Amin, R.A.; Gallant, C.J.; Muthelo, P.M.; Landegren, U. Sensitive Measurement of Drug-Target Engagement by a Cellular Thermal Shift Assay with Multiplex Proximity Extension Readout. *Anal. Chem.* **2021**, *93*, 10999–11009. [CrossRef]

18. Tu, Y.; Tan, L.; Tao, H.; Li, Y.; Liu, H. CETSA and Thermal Proteome Profiling Strategies for Target Identification and Drug Discovery of Natural Products. *Phytomedicine* **2023**, *116*, 154862. [CrossRef]
19. Petersen, R.L. Strategies Using Bio-Layer Interferometry Biosensor Technology for Vaccine Research and Development. *Biosensors* **2017**, *7*, 49. [CrossRef]
20. Pinzi, L.; Rastelli, G. Molecular Docking: Shifting Paradigms in Drug Discovery. *Int. J. Mol. Sci.* **2019**, *20*, 4331. [CrossRef]
21. Huang, K.K.; Ma, H.; Chong, R.H.H.; Uchihara, T.; Lian, B.S.X.; Zhu, F.; Sheng, T.; Srivastava, S.; Tay, S.T.; Sundar, R.; et al. Spatiotemporal Genomic Profiling of Intestinal Metaplasia Reveals Clonal Dynamics of Gastric Cancer Progression. *Cancer Cell* **2023**, *41*, 2019–2037.e8. [CrossRef] [PubMed]
22. Yu, H.; Lin, L.; Zhang, Z.; Zhang, H.; Hu, H. Targeting NF-κB Pathway for the Therapy of Diseases: Mechanism and Clinical Study. *Signal Transduct. Target Ther.* **2020**, *5*, 209. [CrossRef] [PubMed]
23. Wawro, K.; Wawro, M.; Strzelecka, M.; Czarnek, M.; Bereta, J. The Role of NF-κB and Elk-1 in the Regulation of Mouse ADAM17 Expression. *Biol. Open* **2019**, *8*, bio039420. [CrossRef] [PubMed]
24. Vivian, J.; Rao, A.A.; Nothaft, F.A.; Ketchum, C.; Armstrong, J.; Novak, A.; Pfeil, J.; Narkizian, J.; Deran, A.D.; Musselman-Brown, A.; et al. Toil Enables Reproducible, Open Source, Big Biomedical Data Analyses. *Nat. Biotechnol.* **2017**, *35*, 314–316. [CrossRef]
25. Wang, W.; Di, T.; Wang, W.; Jiang, H. EGCG, GCG, TFDG, or TSA Inhibiting Melanin Synthesis by Downregulating MC1R Expression. *Int. J. Mol. Sci.* **2023**, *24*, 11017. [CrossRef]
26. Black, R.A.; Rauch, C.T.; Kozlosky, C.J.; Peschon, J.J.; Slack, J.L.; Wolfson, M.F.; Castner, B.J.; Stocking, K.L.; Reddy, P.; Srinivasan, S.; et al. A Metalloproteinase Disintegrin That Releases Tumour-Necrosis Factor-Alpha from Cells. *Nature* **1997**, *385*, 729–733. [CrossRef]
27. Moss, M.L.; Jin, S.L.; Milla, M.E.; Bickett, D.M.; Burkhart, W.; Carter, H.L.; Chen, W.J.; Clay, W.C.; Didsbury, J.R.; Hassler, D.; et al. Cloning of a Disintegrin Metalloproteinase That Processes Precursor Tumour-Necrosis Factor-Alpha. *Nature* **1997**, *385*, 733–736. [CrossRef]
28. Zunke, F.; Rose-John, S. The Shedding Protease ADAM17: Physiology and Pathophysiology. *Biochim. Biophys. Acta (BBA) Mol. Cell Res.* **2017**, *1864*, 2059–2070. [CrossRef]
29. Schumacher, N.; Rose-John, S. ADAM17 Activity and IL-6 Trans-Signaling in Inflammation and Cancer. *Cancers* **2019**, *11*, 1736. [CrossRef]
30. Schumacher, N.; Rose-John, S. ADAM17 Orchestrates Interleukin-6, TNFα and EGF-R Signaling in Inflammation and Cancer. *Biochim. Biophys. Acta (BBA) Mol. Cell Res.* **2022**, *1869*, 119141. [CrossRef]
31. Saha, A.; Backert, S.; Hammond, C.E.; Gooz, M.; Smolka, A.J. *Helicobacter pylori* CagL Activates ADAM17 to Induce Repression of the Gastric H, K-ATPase α Subunit. *Gastroenterology* **2010**, *139*, 239–248. [CrossRef] [PubMed]
32. Gebremariam, H.G.; Qazi, K.R.; Somiah, T.; Pathak, S.K.; Sjölinder, H.; Sverremark Ekström, E.; Jonsson, A.-B. Lactobacillus Gasseri Suppresses the Production of Proinflammatory Cytokines in *Helicobacter pylori*-Infected Macrophages by Inhibiting the Expression of ADAM17. *Front. Immunol.* **2019**, *10*, 2326. [CrossRef]
33. Xu, M.; Zhou, H.; Zhang, C.; He, J.; Wei, H.; Zhou, M.; Lu, Y.; Sun, Y.; Ding, J.W.; Zeng, J.; et al. ADAM17 Promotes Epithelial-Mesenchymal Transition via TGF-β/Smad Pathway in Gastric Carcinoma Cells. *Int. J. Oncol.* **2016**, *49*, 2520–2528. [CrossRef]
34. Satoh, M.; Nakamura, M.; Satoh, H.; Saitoh, H.; Segawa, I.; Hiramori, K. Expression of Tumor Necrosis Factor-Alpha--Converting Enzyme and Tumor Necrosis Factor-Alpha in Human Myocarditis. *J. Am. Coll. Cardiol.* **2000**, *36*, 1288–1294. [CrossRef]
35. Hooper, N.M.; Turner, A.J. The Search for Alpha-Secretase and Its Potential as a Therapeutic Approach to Alzheimer s Disease. *Curr. Med. Chem.* **2002**, *9*, 1107–1119. [CrossRef]
36. Moss, M.L.; Sklair-Tavron, L.; Nudelman, R. Drug Insight: Tumor Necrosis Factor-Converting Enzyme as a Pharmaceutical Target for Rheumatoid Arthritis. *Nat. Clin. Pract. Rheumatol.* **2008**, *4*, 300–309. [CrossRef]
37. Calligaris, M.; Cuffaro, D.; Bonelli, S.; Spanò, D.P.; Rossello, A.; Nuti, E.; Scilabra, S.D. Strategies to Target ADAM17 in Disease: From Its Discovery to the iRhom Revolution. *Molecules* **2021**, *26*, 944. [CrossRef]
38. Yu, L.; Wu, A.-G.; Wong, V.K.-W.; Qu, L.-Q.; Zhang, N.; Qin, D.-L.; Zeng, W.; Tang, B.; Wang, H.-M.; Wang, Q.; et al. The New Application of UHPLC-DAD-TOF/MS in Identification of Inhibitors on β-Amyloid Fibrillation From Scutellaria Baicalensis. *Front. Pharmacol.* **2019**, *10*, 194. [CrossRef]
39. Guo, M.; Zhu, F.; Qiu, W.; Qiao, G.; Law, B.Y.-K.; Yu, L.; Wu, J.; Tang, Y.; Yu, C.; Qin, D.; et al. High-Throughput Screening for Amyloid-β Binding Natural Small-Molecules Based on the Combinational Use of Biolayer Interferometry and UHPLC-DAD-Q/TOF-MS/MS. *Acta Pharm. Sin B* **2022**, *12*, 1723–1739. [CrossRef]
40. Mitra, S.; Lami, M.S.; Uddin, T.M.; Das, R.; Islam, F.; Anjum, J.; Hossain, M.J.; Emran, T.B. Prospective Multifunctional Roles and Pharmacological Potential of Dietary Flavonoid Narirutin. *Biomed. Pharmacother.* **2022**, *150*, 112932. [CrossRef]
41. Zhang, Y.-T.; Yu, Y.-Q.; Yan, X.-X.; Wang, W.-J.; Tian, X.-T.; Wang, L.; Zhu, W.-L.; Gong, L.-K.; Pan, G.-Y. Different Structures of Berberine and Five Other Protoberberine Alkaloids That Affect P-Glycoprotein-Mediated Efflux Capacity. *Acta Pharmacol. Sin.* **2019**, *40*, 133–142. [CrossRef] [PubMed]

42. Han Jie, L.; Jantan, I.; Yusoff, S.D.; Jalil, J.; Husain, K. Sinensetin: An Insight on Its Pharmacological Activities, Mechanisms of Action and Toxicity. *Front. Pharmacol.* **2021**, *11*, 553404. [CrossRef] [PubMed]
43. Editorial: ChemSpider—A Tool for Natural Products Research. *Nat. Prod. Rep.* **2015**, *32*, 1163–1164. [CrossRef] [PubMed]
44. Daina, A.; Michielin, O.; Zoete, V. SwissTargetPrediction: Updated Data and New Features for Efficient Prediction of Protein Targets of Small Molecules. *Nucleic Acids Res.* **2019**, *47*, W357–W364. [CrossRef]
45. Yang, C. Flavonoid 4,4′-Dimethoxychalcone Suppresses Cell Proliferation via Dehydrogenase Inhibition and Oxidative Stress Aggravation. *Free Radic. Biol. Med.* **2021**, *175*, 206–215. [CrossRef]
46. Jumper, J.; Evans, R.; Pritzel, A.; Green, T.; Figurnov, M.; Ronneberger, O.; Tunyasuvunakool, K.; Bates, R.; Žídek, A.; Potapenko, A.; et al. Highly Accurate Protein Structure Prediction with AlphaFold. *Nature* **2021**, *596*, 583–589. [CrossRef]

pharmaceuticals

MDPI

Article

Anti-Inflammatory and Anti-Adipocyte Dysfunction Effects of *Ficus lindsayana* Latex and Root Extracts

Jirarat Karinchai [1,†], Pensiri Buacheen [1,†], Daraphan Rodthayoy [1], Tanpitcha Yodweerapong [1], Arisa Imsumran [1], Ariyaphong Wongnoppavich [1], Bhanumas Chantarasuwan [2], Uthaiwan Suttisansanee [3], Piya Temviriyanukul [3] and Pornsiri Pitchakarn [1,*]

[1] Department of Biochemistry, Faculty of Medicine, Chiang Mai University, Muang Chiang Mai, Chiang Mai 50200, Thailand; jirarat.ka@cmu.ac.th (J.K.); pensiri.bc@gmail.com (P.B.); daraphanr@gmail.com (D.R.); tanpitcha.y@hotmail.com (T.Y.); arisa.bonness@cmu.ac.th (A.I.); ariyaphong.w@cmu.ac.th (A.W.)

[2] Thailand Natural History Museum, National Science Museum, Khlong 5, Khlong Laung, Pathum Thani 12120, Thailand; b.chantarasuwan@gmail.com

[3] Institute of Nutrition, Mahidol University, Salaya, Nakhon Pathom 73170, Thailand; uthaiwan.sut@mahidol.ac.th (U.S.); piya.tem@mahidol.ac.th (P.T.)

* Correspondence: pornsiri.p@cmu.ac.th; Tel.: +66-53-935325

† These authors contributed equally to this work.

Abstract: Low-grade chronic inflammation and adipocyte dysfunction are prominent risk factors of insulin resistance and type 2 diabetes mellitus (T2DM) in obesity. Thus, prevention of inflammation and adipocyte dysfunction could be one possible approach to mitigate T2DM development. Several *Ficus* species have been used in traditional medicine for ameliorating inflammation and T2DM. Our previous studies reported biological effects of *Ficus lindsayana* including antioxidant, anti-cancer, and anti-α-glucosidase activities. Further, this study therefore investigated whether *F. lindsayana* latex (FLLE) and root (FLRE) extracts inhibit inflammation-stimulated insulin resistance in adipocytes and inflammation in macrophages. FLLE and FLRE (200 μg/mL) had no significant cytotoxicity for macrophages, adipocytes, and blood cells (PBMCs and RBCs). FLRE had a total flavonoid content about three times higher than FLLE, while both had similar levels of total phenolic content. FLRE showed higher abilities than FLLE in suppressing inflammation in both macrophages and adipocytes and reversing the inflammation-induced insulin resistance in adipocytes. In TNF-α-induced adipocytes, FLRE significantly improved insulin-induced glucose uptake and insulin-suppressed lipolysis, while FLLE only significantly improved glucose uptake. Moreover, FLRE and FLLE remarkably reduced chemoattractant (MCP-1) but improved adipogenic (PPARγ and CEBPα) gene expression, leading to the promotion of adipogenesis and the suppression of insulin resistance. In LPS-induced macrophages, FLRE, but not FLLE, significantly inhibited LPS-induced NO production. Moreover, FLRE significantly reduced LPS-stimulated iNOS, COX-2, IL-1β, IL-6, and TNF-α gene expression. These results may provide the potential data for the development of this plant, especially the root part, as an alternative medicine, functional ingredient, or food supplement for the prevention of inflammation and obesity-associated insulin resistance, as well as T2DM.

Keywords: *Ficus lindsayana*; adipogenesis; insulin resistance; chronic inflammation; metabolic diseases

1. Introduction

Insulin resistance generally refers to a condition in which the body does not respond properly to insulin, affecting glucose transport and metabolism in adipocytes and skeletal muscle, as well as decreasing the ability to suppress glucose production in the liver. Normally, insulin promotes the development of preadipocytes into adipocytes and stimulates glucose transport and facilitates the production of triglycerides (lipogenesis) in mature adipocytes, while also preventing the breakdown of triglycerides (lipolysis). Recently, it has been well-established that adipocyte dysfunction plays a central role in linking insulin resistance to obesity. An imbalance of hypertrophy/hyperplasia, where adipogenesis is suppressed, can cause the over-expansion of adipocytes (hypertrophic adipocytes). The adipocyte hypertrophy prevalence induces hypoxia and cellular stress that promote chronic inflammation by secreted chemokines, especially monocyte chemoattractant protein-1 (MCP-1) from adipocytes, leading to the recruitment of pro-inflammatory macrophages into the adipose tissue [1]. The macrophages then generate several pro-inflammatory cytokines, including tumor necrotic factor α (TNF-α), interleukin-1β (IL-1β), and interleukin-6 (IL-6) [2]. The increase in these cytokines causes adipocyte dysfunction and inhibits insulin signaling, leading to insulin resistance [1,3,4]. Thus, obesity could cause chronic low-grade systemic and local inflammation that leads to the emergence of insulin resistance and type 2 diabetes mellitus (T2DM).

Chronic inflammation is a prolonged inflammatory response that follows an acute inflammation or long-term exposure to low-grade inflammation. It involves a progressive change in the type of cells present at the inflammatory site. In chronic inflammation conditions, many chemotactic and activating factors are continually released from immune cells to stimulate immune and stromal cells. A variety of inflammatory cytokines, such as TNF-α, IL-1β, IL-6, inducible nitric oxide synthase (iNOS), and cyclooxygenase 2 (COX-2) secreted from the macrophages are further involved in various inflammation-related diseases [5]. Moreover, chronic inflammation is usually associated with free radical damage and oxidative stress, which can cause cancer by mutation and DNA damage [6,7]. Therefore, the prevention of inflammation could protect people from inflammation-induced disorders including insulin resistance in obesity and T2DM. Anti-inflammation agents have been demonstrated to improve the sensitivity and secretion of insulin in patients with T2DM [8,9]. However, these medications, especially non-steroidal anti-inflammatory drugs (NSAIDs), which block the COX enzyme and reduce prostaglandins [10] usually cause multiple adverse effects on the gastrointestinal tract, cardiovascular, and kidney function [11]. So, the usage of existing natural products for inflammation prevention is one of the alternative ways to treat inflammation-induced chronic diseases. Many phytochemicals have been reported for their pharmacological activities such as anti-diabetes type 2 [12], anti-cancer [13], and anti-arthritic properties [14] via mechanisms involving the suppression of oxidative stress, inflammation, and tissue damage [15].

Plants in the *Ficus* genus include over 800 species that have been consumed as food and utilized for medicinal properties in Ayurvedic and traditional Chinese medicine for centuries [16,17]. *Ficus* spp. are distributed in tropical and subtropical regions of India, China, Sri Lanka, Australia, and Myanmar. Various parts, such as tree bark, fruits, latex, leaves, roots, and twigs of *Ficus* spp. have been reported to be used in traditional medicine for treating conditions like diarrhea, stomach problems, cancer, inflammation and diabetes [18–20]. For example, *Ficus carica* Linn has antioxidant and antimicrobial activities [21] and remarkable curative effects for chronic diseases [19]. *Ficus sycomorus* Linn (bark), *Ficus racemosa* Linn (bark), *Ficus lutea* Vahl (leaf), and *Ficus deltoidei* Jack(fruit) exhibit anti-diabetic effects [19,22–24]. Moreover, flavonoids in the *Ficus* sp. extracts are associated with their blood glucose-reducing activity, anti-cancer, antioxidant, antihistaminic, and anti-inflammation [20,25,26].

Ficus lindsayana (FL) Beentje, previously named *Ficus dubia* Wall. ex King [27] is another species found in the tropical evergreen rain forests of Southern Thailand, Malaysia, and Brunei [28] (The plant name has been checked with WFO (http://www.worldfloraonline.org/taxon/wfo-1000027124, accessed on 25 December 2023)). The tree can grow to be 30–35 m tall, with auxiliary aerial roots that extend to the ground from branches or the trunk. Due to its unique red latex after exposure to the air, local people believe that this plant may offer health benefits, similar to Dragon's blood, an acclaimed traditional medicine obtained from different plants such as *Croton* spp., *Daemonorops* spp., *Dracaena* spp., and *Pterocarpus* spp. [29]. Previous studies reported several biological activities of various parts of FL. The extract from stems and twigs showed anti-HIV and anti-bacterial activities [30]. The root and latex extracts of FL exhibited strong antioxidant activity correlated with the high amount of total phenolics and flavonoids [31,32]. In addition, the root ethanolic extract displays potent antidiabetic effects through the inhibition of α-glucosidase, one of the drug targets for diabetes, and anticancer activity against lung- and ovarian-cancer cell lines with genome-safe [31]. Moreover, it was found that the latex extract has the potential for the prevention and treatment of human colorectal cancer through the regulation of the inflammatory pathway [33,34]. Although FL has been reported to have the potential against inflammation and diabetes, there is no scientific information of its bioactive compounds and biological activity on inflammation-associated adipocyte dysfunction, which is a major cause of insulin resistance and diabetes (T2DM).

In this study, we determined whether *Ficus lindsayana* latex and root extracts affect adipogenesis, insulin resistance in 3T3-L1 adipocytes, and inflammation in RAW 264.7 macrophages. The knowledge gained from this study will support evidence of the health benefits of this plant for further development as an alternative medicine, functional ingredient, or food supplement in preventing obesity-related and inflammation-involved metabolic disorders, especially insulin resistance and T2DM.

2. Results

2.1. Phenolic and Flavonoid Composition of the FLLE and FLRE

The yield of FLLE and FLRE was 47% and 5%, respectively. The total phenolic content of FLRE and FLLE was 208.31 ± 9.90 and 248.53 ± 1.46 mg GAE/g extract, respectively (Table 1). The total flavonoid content of FLRE and FLLE was 157.33 ± 1.36 and 55.78 ± 4.00 mg CE/g extract, respectively (Table 1). The result showed that FLLE contained a higher amount of phenolic content, whereas FLRE contained a higher level of total flavonoid content than the other extract.

Table 1. Total Phenolic and Total Flavonoid Contents and DPPH or ABTS Free-Radical Scavenging Activities (SC50) of FLLE and FLRE.

FL Extracts	Total Phenolic (mg GAE/g Extract)	Total Flavonoid (mg CE/g Extract)	DPPH Assay SC50 [1] (μg/mL)	ABTS Assay SC50 (μg/mL)
FLLE	248.53 ± 1.46 **	55.78 ± 4.00	210.59 ± 6.13	33.59 ± 6.26
FLRE	208.31 ± 9.90	157.33 ± 1.36 ***	83.12 ± 8.86 ***	9.44 ± 3.26 **

[1] SC50 = the concentration of the extracts that scavenge 50% of DPPH or ABTS free radicals. FL, *Ficus lindsayana*; GAE, gallic acid equivalent; CE, catechin equivalent. Each value is represented as mean ± SD, $n = 3$ ** $p < 0.01$ and *** $p < 0.001$ in FLRE vs FLLE.

Compared to the known standard phenolics and flavonoids, chlorogenic acids (CGAs) and apigenin were detectable in FLRE, while only CGAs were detectable in FLLE by HPLC analysis (Table 2). Determination of chlorogenic derivatives including 3-, 4-, and 5-CQA showed 3-CQA was the most abundant in FLLE and FLRE. The content of CGAs and the derivatives were much greater in FLLE than in FLRE.

Table 2. Total Phenolic Contents Using Chlorogenic Acid and Total Flavonoid Contents Using Apigenin Equivalent and Quantification of Chlorogenic Acid Derivatives and Apigenin Using HPLC in FLLE and FLRE.

			Chlorogenic Acid (CGAs) (mg/g Extract)			Apigenin (AP) (mg/g Extract)
FL Extracts	Total Phenolic (mg CGAE/g Extract)	Total Flavonoid (mg APE/g Extract)	3-CQA	4-CQA	5-CQA	Apigenin
FLLE	517.28 ± 2.72	33.55 ± 1.20	39.85 ± 0.88	19.80 ± 0.52	26.00 ± 0.93	ND [1]
FLRE	111.96 ± 0.67	51.81 ± 2.88	4.98 ± 0.10	1.08 ± 0.06	0.46 ± 0.08	0.93 ± 0.09

FL, *Ficus lindsayana*; CGAE, chlorogenic acid equivalent; APE, apigenin equivalent; 3-CQA, neochlorogenic acid; 4-CQA, cryptochlorogenic acid; 5-CQA, chlorogenic acid. Each value is represented as mean ± SD, $n = 3$. [1] ND not detectable.

Consistent with the results from the HPLC analysis, the LC-MS analysis revealed that CGAs found in FLLE were higher than in FLRE. Moreover, caffeic acid was detectable in FLLE and FLRE. Apigenin, genistein, 3,4-dihydroxybenzoic acid, naringenin, luteolin, and gallic acid were detected in FLRE, but not in FLLE (Table 3). These results demonstrated that FLLE and FLRE contained different phytochemical patterns which may influence their biological activities.

Table 3. Quantification of Phenolic Contents Using LC-MS/MS.

	FLLE	FLRE
Compounds	**mg/g Extract**	**Mg/G Extract**
Gallic acid	ND [1]	0.08
Chlorogenic acid (5-CQA)	3.34	0.74
3,4-Dihydroxybenzoic acid	ND	0.56
Caffeic acid	0.40	0.21
Luteolin	ND	0.24
Genistein	ND	1.40
Apigenin	ND	0.88
Naringenin	ND	0.53

[1] ND not detectable.

2.2. *DPPH• and ABTS•+ Scavenging Activities of FLLE and FLRE*

This experiment investigated the antioxidant activity of the extracts using DPPH and ABTS assays. The result showed that FLLE and FLRE significantly scavenged DPPH$^{\bullet}$ and ABTS$^{\bullet+}$ free radicals, as shown in Table 1. The results from the DPPH assay showed that SC50 of FLLE and FLRE was 210.59 ± 6.13 and 83.12 ± 8.86 µg/mL, respectively, while the SC50 of FLLE and FLRE was 33.59 ± 6.26 and 9.44 ± 3.26 µg/mL, respectively, determined by the ABTS assay. In addition, the SC50 of the extracts determined by the ABTS assay was lower than that of the DPPH assay, possibly due to the solvent used in each assay (DPPH; EtOH, ABTS; water). The major antioxidants in the extracts are probably water-soluble compounds.

2.3. *Cytotoxicity of FLLE and FLRE on RAW 264.7 Macrophages, Human PBMCs, Human RBCs, and Mature 3T3-L1 Adipocytes*

FLLE and FLRE at doses up to 200 µg/mL slightly decreased the cell viability of RAW 264.7 macrophages (Figure 1A). The inhibitory concentration of 20 (IC20) of FLLE and FLRE was 244 and 331 µg/mL, respectively. The half-maximal inhibitory concentration (IC50) of FLLE and FLRE was >800 and 506 µg/mL, respectively.

Figure 1B shows that FLLE and FLRE at doses up to 800 µg/mL did not show any toxicity to human PBMCs. Table 4 shows that FLRE at the dose of up to 400 µg/mL induced hemolysis at less than 10%, while 600 and 800 µg/mL of the extract caused hemolysis of approximately 10–13%. FLLE at the dose of up to 800 µg/mL slightly induced hemolysis of approximately 3–6% when compared with 0.05% triton x-100, which was used as a positive control (100% hemolysis). Normal saline was used as a negative control (0% hemolysis). Thus, the results can be interpreted as showing that FLRE at the concentration of up to 400 µg/mL was not toxic to human RBCs, while the concentration of up to 800 µg/mL slightly induced hemolysis. FLLE (at up to 800 µg/mL) was a non-hemolytic induction agent.

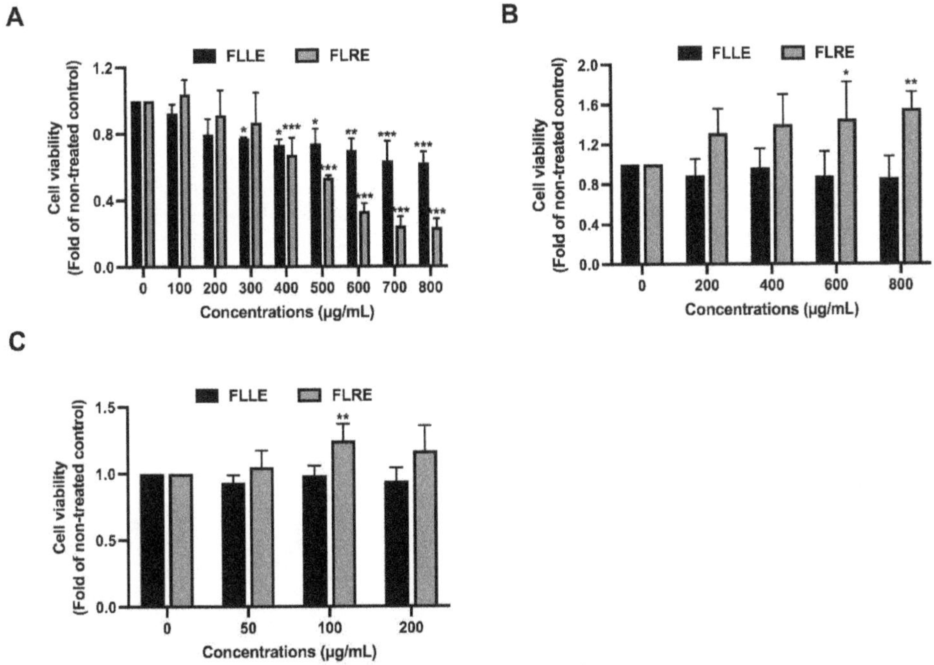

Figure 1. Cytotoxicity effect of FLLE and FLRE. Cell viability of RAW 264.7 macrophages (**A**), normal human PBMCs (**B**), and 3T3-L1 mature adipocytes (**C**). RAW 264.7 cells and PBMCs were treated with various concentrations of the extracts (0–800 μg/mL) for 48 h. Cell viability was determined by MTT assay. 3T3-L1 mature adipocytes were treated with 0–200 μg/mL of the extracts for 48 h, and cell viability was then examined by SRB assay. Each value represents mean ± SD (n = 3) * $p < 0.05$, ** $p < 0.01$ and *** $p < 0.001$ vs. non-treated control.

Table 4. Hemolysis Effect of FLLE and FLRE.

Extracts (μg/mL)	% Hemolysis (n = 5)
0.05% Triton x-100 [1]	100 ± 0.00
FLLE	
200	4.55 ± 0.70
400	4.90 ± 0.79
600	5.41 ± 0.73
800	5.95 ± 0.65
FLRE	
200	5.59 ± 0.43
400	8.12 ± 1.36
600	10.70 ± 2.22
800	12.70 ± 3.19

[1] 0.05% triton x-100 was used as a positive control. The results were expressed as mean ± SD, n = 5 (hemolysis, (0–10% hemolysis is non-hemolysis, 10–25% hemolysis is a slight hemolysis induction, and >25% hemolysis is a high hemolysis induction.).

In mature 3T3-L1 adipocytes, the concentration of extracts at 200 μg/mL did not show any significant cytotoxicity, which is shown in Figure 1C.

These results suggested that FLRE at high concentration was more cytotoxic to the cells than FLLE. The non-toxic concentrations (0–200 μg/mL) were used for further experiments.

2.4. Effect of FLLE and FLRE on TNF-α-Induced Insulin Resistance and Adipogenesis in 3T3-L1 Cells

To evaluate the anti-insulin resistance activity of FLLE and FLRE, insulin-induced glucose uptake ability was measured in TNF-α-induced 3T3-L1 adipocytes. Treatment of the cells with TNF-α 50 ng/mL significantly decreased glucose uptake ability induced by insulin at approximately 19% when compared with the control group (Figure 2A). In contrast, co-treatment of FLLE (100 and 200 μg/mL) and FLRE (200 μg/mL) in TNF-α-treated cells at 100 and 200 μg/mL significantly enhanced the insulin-stimulated glucose uptake (Figure 2A).

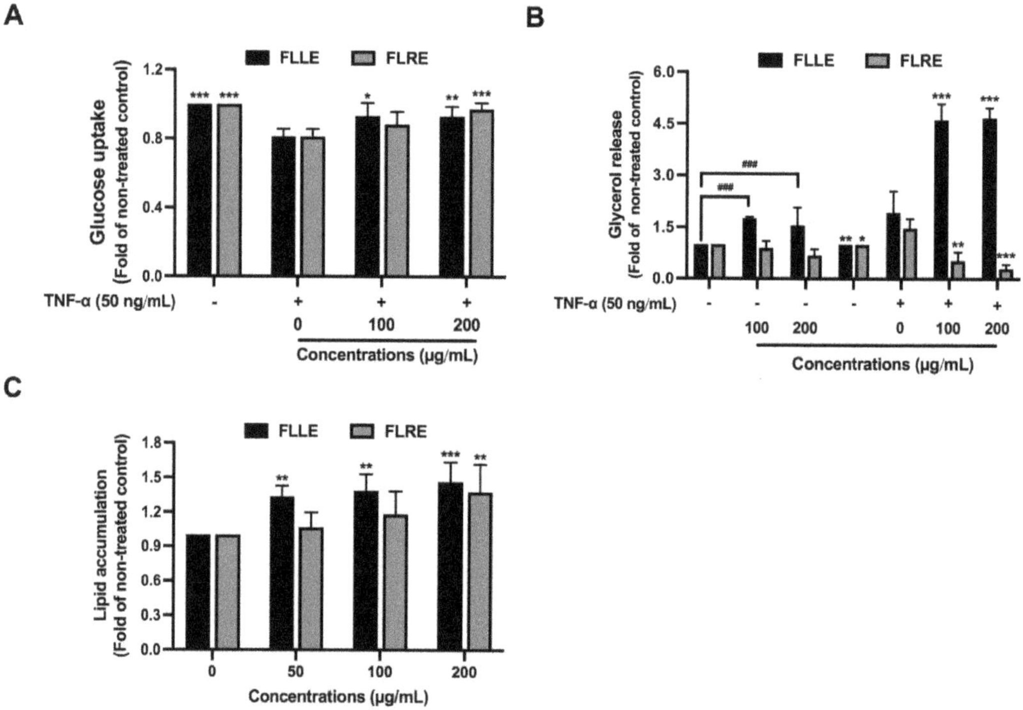

Figure 2. Effect of FLLE and FLRE on TNF-α-induced insulin resistance in 3T3-L1 adipocytes. Anti-insulin resistance effects of the extracts on glucose uptake (**A**) and lipolysis (**B**). Mature 3T3—L1 adipocytes were co-treated with TNF-α (50 ng/mL) and various concentrations of FLLE or FLRE for 24 h. The treated cells were subjected to determined insulin-stimulated glucose uptake using 2-NBDG, a glucose fluorescence analog. The conditioned medium was collected to measure the glycerol level indicating lipolysis activity using a glycerol detection kit. The effect of FLLE and FLRE on adipogenesis in 3T3-L1 adipocyte is shown in (**C**). To determine the effect of FLLE and FLRE on lipid accumulation in 3T3-L1 adipocytes, cells were treated with the extracts during cell differentiation for 12 days. Lipid accumulation was performed using Oil Red O assay. Each value represents mean ± SD (n = 3) * $p < 0.05$, ** $p < 0.01$, and *** $p < 0.001$ vs. TNF-α-treated group (**A**,**B**) or vs. non-treated control (**C**), ### $p < 0.001$ vs. non-treated control.

To confirm insulin resistance in adipocytes, lipolysis was also determined by measuring glycerol release. TNF-α 50 ng/mL treatment significantly increased the glycerol level in the culture supernatant by 20%, even in the presence of insulin. FLRE (100, 200 μg/mL) significantly suppressed the glycerol release; on the other hand, FLLE (100, 200 μg/mL) dramatically induced the release in TNFα-treated adipocytes (Figure 2B). Treatment of

FLLE in the absence of TNF-α significantly induced the release of glycerol, suggesting the lipolytic effect of this extract.

FLLE (50, 100, 200 μg/mL) and FLRE (200 μg/mL) treatment during differentiation for 12 days significantly increased lipid accumulation in the adipocytes (Figure 2C), suggesting that the extracts significantly promoted adipogenesis, which may either lead to the expansion of adipose tissue (induce obesity) or the prevention of insulin resistance (improved adipocyte function) [35,36].

2.5. Effect of FLLE and FLRE on the mRNA Expression of Inflammatory-Associated and Adipogenesis-Related Molecules in TNF-α-Induced 3T3-L1 Adipocytes

The next experiments investigated the effect of FLLE and FLRE on adipocyte inflammation and dysfunction. MCP-1 and IL-6 mRNA expressions were measured to observe the inflammatory condition in the cells. TNFα-treated 3T3-L1 adipocytes showed the significant upregulation of IL-6 and MCP-1 mRNA, whereas FLRE (200 μg/mL) significantly suppressed the TNFα-stimulated IL-6 and MCP-1 mRNA expressions (Figure 3A,B). FLLE (100, 200 μg/mL) significantly reduced MCP-1 mRNA expression but markedly induced IL-6 mRNA expression in the TNFα-treated cells (Figure 3A,B). The result suggested that FLRE may inhibit the transcription of MCP-1 and IL-6, while FLLE may inhibit the transcription and reduce the protein level of MCP-1 but induce mRNA and protein levels of IL-6.

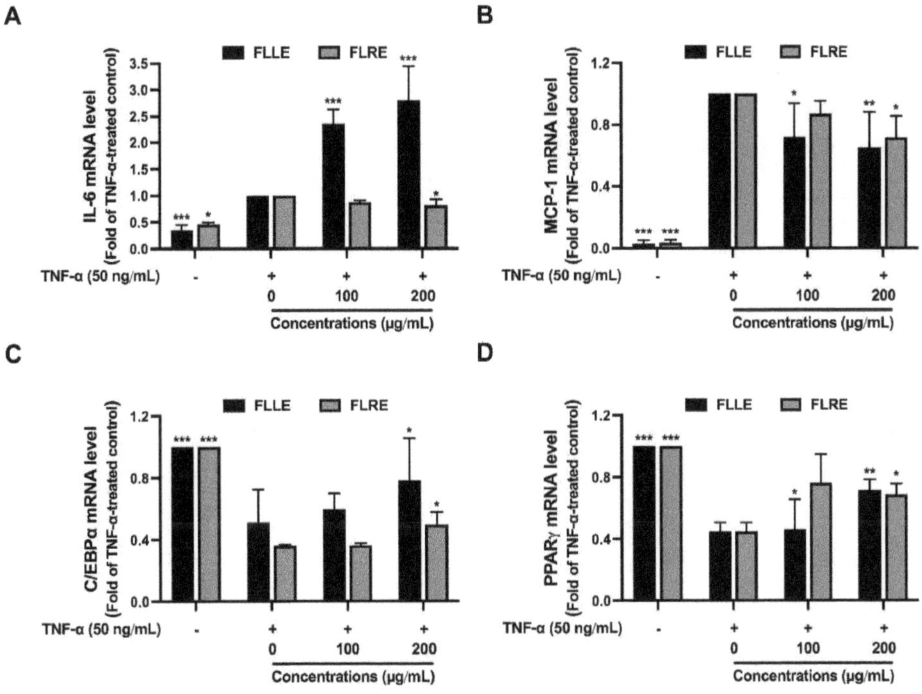

Figure 3. Effect of FLLE and FLRE on TNF–α–induced adipocyte inflammation and dysfunction. Effect of FLLE and FLRE on the mRNA expression of an inflammatory–associated molecule including IL–6 (**A**) and MCP–1 (**B**), and adipogenesis–related molecules including CEBPα (**C**) and PPARγ (**D**). Total RNA was extracted from the treated cells and subjected to RT–qPCR with specific primers for IL–6, MCP–1, CEBPα, and PPARγ. Each value represents mean ± SD (n = 3) * $p < 0.05$, ** $p < 0.01$, and *** $p < 0.001$ vs. TNF–α–treated group.

We further determined the expression of PPARγ and CEBPα, adipogenic genes which normally express in mature adipocytes, to observe adipocyte dysfunction in TNFα-treated

3T3-L1. Both CEBPα and PPARγ mRNA expressions were significantly suppressed by TNFα treatment. Interestingly, FLLE and FLRE (200 μg/mL) significantly improved CEBPα and PPARγ mRNA expressions when compared with the TNFα-treated group (Figure 3C,D).

These results suggested that TNFα induced inflammation and dysfunction of adipocytes, whereas FLLE and FLRE abrogated these effects. It could be confirmed that FLLE and FLRE rescued insulin resistance via adipogenesis induction and inflammation suppression, leading to an enhancement of adipocyte function and insulin sensitivity.

2.6. Anti-Inflammatory Activity of FLLE and FLRE in LPS-Stimulated RAW 264.7 Macrophages

As an indicator of an inflammatory response, LPS (1 μg/mL) significantly induced NO production in macrophages as measured by the accumulation of nitrite level in the culture supernatant. The treatment of FLRE significantly reduced the NO level in a dose-dependent manner, whereas FLLE significantly induced the NO level in a dose-dependent manner (Figure 4A). Since FLRE also contained higher flavonoid content and exhibited higher antioxidant efficacy, we further investigated only FLRE on the anti-inflammatory mechanism.

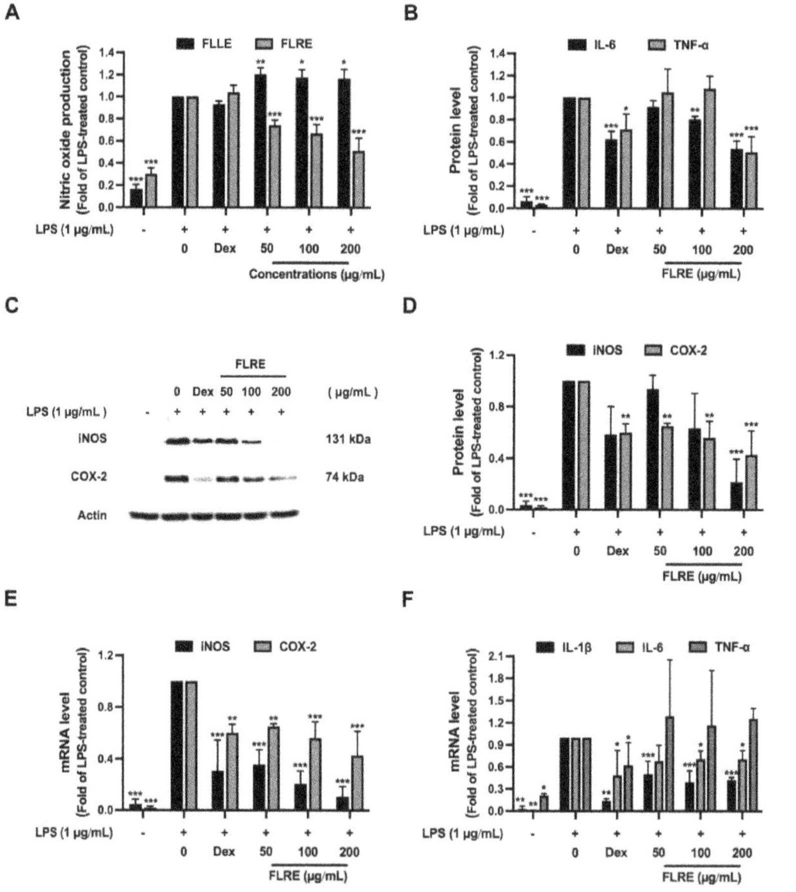

Figure 4. Anti–inflammation activity of FLLE and FLRE in LPS–stimulated RAW 264.7 macrophage. Effect of the extracts on NO production (**A**). Effect of FLRE on LPS–stimulated pro–inflammatory cytokine secretions including IL–6 and TNF–α (**B**). Effect of FLRE on inflammatory key enzymes protein level and mRNA expression. Immunoblotting of iNOS and COX–2 protein (**C**), the quantitative protein

level of iNOS and COX–2 normalized with β–actin (**D**). iNOS and COX–2 mRNA expression by qRT–PCR (**E**). Effect of FLRE on pro-inflammatory cytokine mRNA expression including IL–1β, IL–6, and TNF–α (**F**). RAW 264.7 macrophages were pre–treated with FLRE or FLLE (0–200 μg/mL) for 1 h followed by 1 μg/mL LPS for 24 h. The supernatant was collected to examine the nitrite level by Griess reagent assay and pro–inflammatory cytokine secretion level ELISA. The treated cells were collected to determine protein and mRNA expression of iNOS, and COX–2 by Western blotting and RT–qPCR, respectively. Each value represents mean ± SD (n = 3), * $p < 0.05$, ** $p < 0.01$ and *** $p < 0.001$ vs. LPS-treated group.

In chronic inflammation, many activating factors and pro-inflammatory cytokines are released from immune cells to stimulate the immune system and further involve various inflammation circumstances. To investigate whether FLRE suppressed pro-inflammatory cytokine secretion from LPS-induced RAW 264.7 macrophages, the protein levels of IL-6 and TNF-α were measured by ELISA. FLRE significantly decreased IL-6 (100 and 200 μg/mL) and TNF-α (200 μg/mL) proteins secreted in the culture supernatant when compared to the LPS-treated group (Figure 4B). The result suggested that the reduction in IL-6 and TNF-α protein secretion may be caused by the inhibition effect of the protein expression or the protein secretion.

LPS stimulates the expression of pro-inflammatory cytokines and mediators such as iNOS and COX-2. We further determined whether FLRE inhibited LPS-stimulated iNOS and COX-2 protein levels. The expression of iNOS and COX-2 proteins was strongly induced in the LPS-treated group but was significantly suppressed after the treatment of 200 μg/mL FLRE (Figure 4C,D). The result suggested that FLRE might inhibit the production of NO via the downregulation of iNOS protein, which may in turn reduce the PGE2 production due to the suppression of COX-2 level.

The next experiment investigated the effect of FLRE on mRNA expression of iNOS, COX-2, IL-1β, IL-6, and TNF-α by reverse transcription–quantitative real-time PCR. FLRE (50, 100, 200 μg/mL) significantly suppressed iNOS, COX-2, IL-1β and IL-6, and mRNA expressions in LPS-treated RAW 264.7 macrophages (Figure 4E,F), indicating that FLRE may inhibit the transcription of IL-6, leading to the reduction in its secretion. However, TNF-α mRNA expression was not altered (Figure 4F) by FLRE, suggesting that FLRE may inhibit the translation or the secretion of TNF-α in LPS-induced macrophages. Moreover, FLRE decreased iNOS, and COX-2 protein levels via the inhibition of their mRNA expression. It could be summarized that FLRE altered the gene expression of pro-inflammatory cytokines, IL-1β, and IL-6, and inflammation-related proteins iNOS, and COX-2, whereas it probably decreased the TNF-α level at the translation or secretion step.

3. Discussion

In this study, our *Ficus lindsayana* root extract (FLRE) had higher total flavonoid content, whereas the latex (FLLE) had a similar amount of total flavonoid content when compared to other previous studies in the same parts of other *Ficus* spp. The total flavonoid content of *Ficus benghalensis* Linn root extracted with ethyl acetate was 6.00 ± 0.55 mg QE/g extract [37]. Meanwhile, the total flavonoid of *Ficus carica* latex extract with water was 43.23 ± 3.35 mg QE/g extract [38]. We found the total flavonoid of FLLE and FLRE was 55.78 ± 4.00 and 157.33 ± 1.36 mg CE/g extract, respectively. FLRE contained a similar amount of phenolic content as FLLE, but showed higher flavonoid content with exhibited higher efficacy of scavenging DPPH$^{\bullet}$ and ABTS$^{\bullet+}$ radicals than FLLE. These data suggest that the antioxidant capacity of the extracts likely depends on their flavonoid contents. The consistency with previous studies of other *Ficus* spp. showed that the flavonoid contents of *Ficus pyriformis* Hook. & Arn. [39] and *Ficus carica* [40] were related to their efficiency in scavenging free radicals and suppressing NO production, a sign of inflammation. Phytochemical analysis revealed that CQA and caffeic acid content found in FLLE was higher than in FLRE, while apigenin, genistein, 3,4-dihydroxybenzoic acid, naringenin, luteolin, and gallic acid were detectable in FLRE, but not in FLLE.

Chlorogenic acids (CGAs) are ester forms of caffeic acid conjugated with quinic acids. Numerous studies showed several biological properties including antioxidant and anti-inflammation, anti-insulin resistance, and anti-obesity of CGAs, caffeic acid, and also their derivatives through the reduction in iNOS and COX-2 expressions, and also diminished pro-inflammatory cytokine including IL-1β and TNF-α in LPS-induced RAW 264.7 macrophage [41–45]. Likewise, apigenin, genistein, luteolin, and gallic acid have been reported to have an anti-inflammatory effect in LPS-induced RAW 264.7 through the inhibition of NO production, pro-inflammatory cytokines, and the NF-kB pathway. Moreover, apigenin, luteolin, 3,4-dihydroxybenzoic acid, CGAs, and caffeic acid attenuated obesity- and inflammation-induced insulin resistance [42,46–53]. Moreover, previous studies reported that CGAs and gallic acid induce the expression of GLUT4 which promotes the glucose uptake activity in 3T3-L1 cells [52,54]. This evidence can suggest that phenolic and flavonoid compounds found in FLRE and FLLE may play an important role in anti-inflammation and anti-insulin resistance.

Adipocyte inflammation and dysfunction cause abnormal lipid metabolism in adipose tissue, leading to a high blood level of free fatty acids (FFAs) and dysregulation of adipokines [1]. Furthermore, released chemokines and pro-inflammatory cytokines from adipocytes and macrophages constantly induce chronic inflammation surrounding the tissue. Signaling from the cytokines then disturbs insulin signaling by stimulating serine phosphorylation of insulin receptor substrate-1 and 2, leading to the inhibition of insulin receptor autophosphorylation activity. Then, GLUT4 translocation and the blood glucose clearance ability of adipocytes are decreased [1]. Persistence of these conditions can stimulate systemic insulin resistance and beta-cell dysfunction, which would increase the risk of T2DM. It is known that the blockage or reversion of insulin resistance is a promising strategy for the prevention of T2DM and other related metabolic diseases. This study has attempted to prove that FLLE and FLRE prevent inflammation both in adipocytes and macrophages, a major cascade of insulin-resistance progression.

Pro-inflammatory cytokines showed a correlation with insulin resistance in adipocytes, especially TNF-α, a major mediator in the development of chronic inflammation that leads to a reduction in insulin-induced glucose uptake ability [2]. TNF-α initiates an inflammatory signaling cascade via the NF-κB and MAPK pathways, which promotes the release of further inflammatory mediators such as IL-6, IL-10, IL-1β, and MCP-1 [1]. Both FLLE and FLRE treatment could reduce insulin resistance in TNF-α-induced adipocytes, which is consistent with a previous study in which ethanolic and methanolic extracts of *Ficus deltoidei* increased insulin-mediated glucose uptake [55]. FLRE could improve insulin function to induce glucose uptake and suppress lipolysis in the inflammation-induced insulin-resistance model. Although FLLE also enhanced insulin-induced glucose uptake, it failed to improve insulin-suppressed lipolysis in the insulin-resistant cells. FLLE and FLRE may promote insulin function in the insulin-resistant cells via an underlining mechanism(s) by which the adipogenesis is induced and/or the inflammation is suppressed, leading to an improvement in adipocyte function and insulin sensitivity. Furthermore, FLRE significantly decreased MCP-1 and IL-6 mRNA expression. Interestingly, FLLE could suppress only MCP-1, while increasing IL-6 expression by which lipolysis was induced. MCP-1 released from adipocytes is a chemoattractant that activates and recruits macrophages to the area. Moreover, it has a dedifferentiation effect, by altering adipocyte function and metabolism [56]. Previous studies showed that the expression of several adipogenic genes in differentiated 3T3-L1 adipocytes including GLUT-4 and PPARγ was considerably reduced after treatment with MCP-1 [57,58]. Although IL-6 is required for adipose-tissue macrophage accumulation, it causes weak changes in insulin sensitivity. FLRE showed an anti-lipolytic effect in TNF-α-induced adipocytes, whereas FLLE induced adipocyte lipolysis, which is consistent with the result of IL-6 expression, assuming that the increase in IL-6 by FLLE might induce lipolysis in adipocytes. It was previously known that IL-6 exerts a lipolytic effect but did not interfere with insulin sensitivity in adipocytes [59]. This could suggest that FLRE and FLLE might reduce inflammation in adipocytes and then suppress insulin resistance in TNF-α-induced adipocytes. Pro-inflammatory factors of adipocytes were activated via various pathways such as NF-κB and MAPK pathways, including ERK, JNK, and p38 [60]. FLRE and FLLE may exert their effects on adipocyte inflammation by different signaling pathways, which should be further investigated.

TNF-α has anti-adipogenic effects which down-regulate PPARγ and suppress other adipogenic genes, leading to loss of GLUT4 expression and insulin-stimulated activity [61]. PPARγ or CEBPα deficiency in adipocytes caused an absence of insulin-stimulated glucose transport by reducing tyrosine phosphorylation and expression of insulin receptors [62,63]. In our study, TNF-α inhibited mRNA expression of PPARγ and CEBPα, whereas FLRE and FLLE significantly improved their expressions, suggesting that the extracts abrogated TNF-α-interfered insulin signaling, reduced further inflammatory cytokine production and improved adipogenic gene expression, leading to the reduction in insulin resistance and dysfunction of adipocytes.

Adipocyte inflammation is related to macrophage recruitment and proinflammatory cytokine release from both cell types, leading to chronic inflammation surrounding adipose tissue [1]. As FLLE and FLRE showed anti-insulin resistance induced by TNF-α in adipocytes, the anti-inflammation ability of the extracts was further investigated in macrophages. FLRE, but not FLLE, significantly reduced NO production in LPS-induced RAW 264.7 macrophages. Our finding is similar to a previous study, which reported the anti-inflammation effect of *Ficus nota* (Blanco) Merr., which inhibited the production of NO depending on its total flavonoid content [64]. FLRE significantly decreased both iNOS mRNA and protein levels, which may contribute to the reduction in NO production. Moreover, COX-2 mRNA and protein, an inflammatory mediator which can be stimulated by NO [65], was significantly decreased by FLRE in LPS-induced macrophages. The inhibition of COX-2 expression may lead to the suppression of PGE2 production, which reduces the pathogenesis of inflammation such as pain and vasodilation [65] and prevents inflammation-induced diseases [66]. iNOS and COX-2 are stimulated via IKK and MAPK signaling by the group of pro-inflammatory cytokines including TNF- α, IL-1β, and IL-6 [67]. FLRE significantly decreased TNF-α (protein), IL-1β (mRNA) expression, and IL-6 (protein and mRNA) in LPS-induced macrophages. Likewise, *Ficus exasperata* Vahl significantly inhibited NO levels and inflammatory mediators (TNF-α and IL-1β) [68]. Additionally, *Ficus religiosa* Linn significantly inhibited the production of many inflammatory mediators (TNF-α, IL-1β, IL-6, iNOS, and COX-2) via down-regulation of MAPK and NF-κB signaling pathways [69]. Several data support the fact that ERK1/2 predominantly triggers the expression of IL-1β and IL-6, whereas JNK is the main transduction pathway of TNF-α, after LPS stimulation [70]. Furthermore, Fengying Huang et al. (2013) reported that IL-1β up-regulated the COX-2 expression through the activation of the p38 MAPK signaling pathway [71]. Therefore, it might be suggested that FLRE may inhibit LPS-stimulated signaling pathways via MAPK, leading to the reduction in inflammatory-related molecules.

In summary, we have shown that *Ficus lindsayana*, especially the root extracts, could effectively alleviate the inflammation-induced insulin resistance in 3T3-L1 adipocytes. Moreover, it can inhibit inflammation in both adipocytes and RAW 264.7 macrophages. These results may provide scientific data for the utilization and development of this plant as an alternative medicine or functional food for the prevention of inflammation and inflammation-related diseases including obesity, as well as type 2 diabetes mellitus.

4. Materials and Methods

All methods were performed in accordance with the relevant guidelines and regulations.

4.1. Chemicals and Reagents

TNF-alpha was purchased from PeproTech (Rehovot, Israel). Dexamethasone (Dex), 3-isobutyl-1-methylxanthine (IBMX), insulin, and lipopolysaccharide (LPS) were purchased from Sigma-Aldrich (St. Louis, MO, USA). All the primers for RT-qPCR were purchased from Bio Basic Inc., (Markham, ON, Canada). Anti-COX-2, anti-NF-κB, and anti-phospho-

NF-κB p65 antibodies were obtained from Cell Signaling Technology (Danvers, MA, USA). Anti-iNOS and anti-β-actin antibodies were from Sigma-Aldrich (St. Louis, MO, USA). Clarity Western ECL Substrate was purchased from Bio-Rad Laboratories (Hercules, CA, USA).

4.2. Preparation of Plant Extracts

Ficus lindsayana collection was conducted following the guidelines and regulations of the legislation and deposited at Thailand Natural History Museum (THNHM, Bangkok, Thailand), Thailand Science Park, under a code of Chantarasuwan 040117-1. The dried samples of *Ficus lindsayana* root and latex were ground. The powder of *Ficus lindsayana* latex (FLL) was soaked with deionized water at room temperature in the ratio of 1:10 *w/v*. Then, the aqueous fraction was filtrated and freeze-dried by lyophilizer to obtain FLL extract (FLLE). The powder of *Ficus lindsayana* root (FLR) was soaked with 80% ethanol overnight at room temperature in the ratio of 1:10 *w/v* and this was repeated twice. The ethanolic extract was concentrated by a rotary evaporator and freeze-dried by lyophilizer, obtaining FLR extract (FLRE). The extracts were kept at −30 °C until use.

4.3. Phytochemical Analysis

The total flavonoid and total phenolic contents were determined by the colorimetric method using the aluminum chloride and the Folin–Ciocalteu reagent, respectively, published in the previous publications [72,73], with slight modifications. The catechin and apigenin equivalents in each extract were estimated as mg CE and APE/g extract, respectively, using a standard curve to represent total flavonoid content. Total phenolic content was presented as mg gallic acid (GAE) or chlorogenic acid (CGAE)/g extract, equivalent to the standard curves of gallic acid and chlorogenic acid, respectively.

HPLC was performed to analyze known phenolics [31] and chlorogenic acids (CGAs), including neochlorogenic acid (3-CQA), cryptochlorogenic acid (4-CQA), and chlorogenic acid (5-CQA) (IUPAC name) [74] existing in the FL extracts as previously described, with slight modification. The C18 column (250 mm × 4.6 mm, 5 µm) was used. Gradient elution was performed using two solvents: A (0.1% trifluoroacetic acid (TFA) in water) and B (100% methanol) for detection and determining phenolic compounds with a flow rate of 1.0 mL/min and detection at 280 and 325 nm. The CGA chromatographic separation was carried out using gradient mode with mobile phase A (0.3% TFA in water) and mobile phase B (100% acetonitrile) with a flow rate of 1 mL/min and detection at 280. The phytochemical contents were determined by using a gradient system of mobile phase A (1% acetic acid in water) and mobile phase B (100% acetonitrile) with a flow rate of 0.7 mL/min and detection at 280. The peak area and retention time of the extracted sample used in the present HPLC method were determined to compare with standard curves of various concentrations of standard apigenin, catechin, chlorogenic acid, coumaric acid, ferulic acid, gallic acid, hydroxybenzoic acid, protocatechuic acid, vanillic acid, 3-CQA,4-CQA, and 5-CQA.

Moreover, identification and quantification of phenolics were performed utilizing liquid chromatography–electrospray ionization tandem mass spectrometry (LC-ESI-MS/MS), with a well-established procedure and validation as previously reported [75,76].

4.4. Determination of Antioxidant Activities

The 2,2′-azinobis-(3-ethylbenzothiazoline-6-sulfonic acid) (ABTS) and the 2,2-diphenyl-1-picrylhydrazyl (DPPH) assays were performed according to the previous studies [77,78] with slight modifications to assess radical scavenging ability of the extracts. Using the following equation, both antioxidant activities were estimated as a % inhibition.

$$\text{ABTS}^{\bullet+} \text{ or DPPH}^{\bullet} \text{ scavenging effect (\%)} = (\text{Abs}_{\text{control}} - \text{Abs}_{\text{extract}}) \times 100/\text{Abs}_{\text{control}}$$

The radical scavenging activity of ABTS or DPPH was expressed as SC50, which represents the concentration of the extract (mg/mL) required to scavenge 50% of the radicals.

4.5. Cell Culture

Macrophage-like cells, RAW 264.7, were purchased from CLS-Cell Lines Service, Germany, and cultured in Dulbecco's Modified Eagle Medium (DMEM, Sigma, St. Louis, MO, USA) supplemented with L-glutamine, 10% heat-inactivated fetal bovine serum (FBS, Sigma, St. Louis, MO, USA) and 1% penicillin/streptomycin solution (FBS, Sigma, St. Louis, MO, USA). The cells were maintained in a Corning® 60 mm Ultra-low attachment culture dish at 37 °C in a 5% CO_2 humidified atmosphere (CO_2 incubator, Thermo Scientific, Waltham, MA, USA) and sub-cultured every three days.

Human blood samples from healthy individuals (five samples) anonymized by the laboratory were taken from Maharaj Hospital, Chiang Mai, Thailand, and kept in a heparinized tube. Human peripheral blood mononuclear cells (PBMCs) were isolated using Ficoll–Hypaque separation, as directed in the manufacturer's instructions [79]. The remained red blood cells (RBCs) were employed in a hemolysis test. This study was granted a certificate of exemption by the Research Ethics Committee of the Faculty of Medicine, Chiang Mai University (No. EXEMPTION 4744/2017). Consent to participate was not applicable because of anonymous data collection. All methods were carried out in accordance with relevant guidelines and regulations.

3T3-L1 adipocyte cells from ATCC (American Type Culture Collection) were cultured in DMEM with L-glutamine supplemented with 10% FBS and 1% penicillin/streptomycin solution and maintained at 37 °C in a 5% CO_2 humidified atmosphere CO_2 incubator. After reaching confluence on day 2, 3T3-L1 preadipocytes were differentiated by adding 0.5 mM 3-isobutyl-1-methylxanthine (IBMX), 0.5 µg/mL dexamethasone, 5 µg/mL insulin and 10% FBS for 72 h, followed by another 72 h in the same medium without IBMX and dexamethasone. Complete cell differentiation was obtained by incubating the cells in DMEM containing 10% FBS for six days.

4.6. Cytotoxicity

Cytotoxicity of FLLE and FLRE was examined in RAW 264.7 macrophages. The cells (25,000 cells/well) were plated into a 96-well cell culture plate and incubated for 24 h. The cells were then treated with different concentrations of FLLE or FLRE (0–800 µg/mL) for 48 h. Next, the cytotoxicity of the extract was determined by MTT assay as described elsewhere [80,81]. Briefly, MTT (0.5 mg/mL) in DMEM was added to each well. Then, the plates were further incubated for four hours and the medium was removed. Formazan crystals were dissolved with 100 µL of dimethyl sulfoxide (DMSO). The absorbance was measured at 560 nm and percentages of cell viability were calculated.

Human peripheral blood mononuclear cells (PBMCs) were used to investigate the biosafety and cytotoxicity of the extracts for human immune cells. The isolated PBMCs were plated into a 96-well plate at the proper density (8×10^4 cells/well) and incubated for 24 h. Next, the cells were treated with various concentrations of FLLE or FLRE (0–800 µg/mL) for 48 h.

In 3T3-L1 adipocytes, the cells were plated in a 96-well plate (3000 cells/well) and incubated for two days. Then, the cells were differentiated by induction media, differentiation media, and maturation media. Until the cells became mature adipocytes, the cells were treated with various concentrations of FLLE or FLRE (0–200 µg/mL).

The cytotoxicity of the extracts was determined in the PBMCs and mature adipocytes by SRB assay, as described previously [82]. The percent cell survival was calculated as follows.

$$\% \text{ Cellular Viability} = ((\text{Abs of treatment group})/(\text{Abs of control group})) \times 100$$

The inhibitory concentration of 20% (IC20) or a non-toxic concentration was used for further experiments.

4.7. Hemolysis Assay

A hemolysis assay was used to determine the hemolytic effect of the FLLE and FLRE. In brief, human RBCs were collected after the separation of PBMCs from whole blood. The 5% RBCs suspension was then mixed with several concentrations of the extracts and incubated at 37 °C for 3 h. The hemolysis induction was measured as described previously [83]. The hemolysis guideline indicates that when <10%, hemolysis is non-hemolysis, and >25% hemolysis is a high hemolysis induction.

4.8. Adipogenesis

To determine the effect of FLLE and FLRE on adipogenesis, the extracts at 50, 100, and 200 μg/mL were added during the adipocyte transformation process (days 1–12). Cells cultured with the vehicle (DMSO) in all three types of transformation medium were set as the untreated control.

After the treatment, the cells were then fixed in fresh 4% paraformaldehyde and the lipid droplets were stained with a 60% Oil Red O diluted in 100% 2-isopropanol, as previously described. The stained-intracellular lipid droplets were dissolved in 100% 2-isopropanol and the absorbance was measured by spectrometry at 520 nm (Gen5, BioTek). The experiment was performed in triplicate and repeated three times, independently.

4.9. Glucose Uptake Assay

Insulin resistance was induced in mature adipocytes by 50 ng/mL TNF-α and they were treated with or without the extract for 24 h. Then, the cells were washed with PBS and starved with low-glucose DMEM for 3 h. After washing, 1 mg/mL bovine serum albumin containing 100 mmol/L 2-NBDG-glucose and 50 nmol/L insulin was added to the cells and they were incubated at 37 °C for 1 h. The fluorescence intensity of intracellular 2-NBDG-glucose was measured by lysis of the cells with 90% DMSO and by placing the lysate in a dark place for fluorescence measurement (excitation at 485 nm and emission at 535 nm).

4.10. Lipolysis Assay

Adipocyte lipolysis was determined by measurement of released glycerol in a culture medium. The glycerol assay kit (Sigma Aldrich, St. Louis, MO, USA) was used following the instruction of the manufacturer. Afterward, insulin resistance was induced in mature adipocytes by 50 ng/mL TNF-α and they were treated with or without the extracts for 24 h; the culture supernatant was collected to determine free glycerol content. A total of 25 μL of each supernatant was added to 100 μL of Free Glycerol Reagent in a 96-well plate. The mixture was incubated for 15 min at room temperature. The absorbance was measured at 540 nm. The amount of glycerol was calculated using the equation of the standard curve in the formula below.

$$\text{Free glycerol } (\mu g/mL) = (\text{Abs}_{540} - (\text{y-interception}))/\text{Slope}$$

4.11. Measurement of Inflammatory Mediator and Adipogenic mRNA Expressions by Reverse Transcription–Quantitative Polymerase Chain Reaction (RT-qPCR)

After the treatment, total RNA was extracted from the cells and quantified by nanodrop spectrophotometer. Then, total RNA was reverse-transcribed into cDNA. mRNA level was measured by reverse transcription-quantitative polymerase chain reaction (RT-qPCR) using specific primers for TNF-α (sense, 5′-TCTCATGCACCACCATCAAGGACT-3′; antisense,5′-CCACTCTCCCTTTGCAGAACTCA-3′), iNOS (sense, 5′-TCTTTGACGCTCGGAACTGTAG CA-3′; antisense, 5′-ACCTGATGTTGCCATTGTTGGTGG-3′), COX-2 (sense, 5′-TACTACAC CAGGGCCCTTCC-3′; antisense, 5′- CATATTTGAGCCTTGGGGGT-3′), IL-1β (sense, 5′-AAGGGCTGCTTCCCAACCTTTGAC-3′; antisense, 5′-ATACTGCCTGCCTGAAGCTCTTG T-3′), IL-6 (sense, 5′-ATCCAGTTGCCTTCTTGGGACTGA-3′; antisense, 5′-TAAGCCTCCG ACTTGTGAAGTGGT-3′), MCP-1 (sense, 5′-CACTCACCTGCTGCTACTCA-3′; antisense, 5′-AGGGCCGGGGTATGTAACT-3′), CEBPα (sense, 5′-GCAAAGCCAAGAAGTCGGTG-

3′; antisense, 5′- TCACTGGTCAACTCCAGCAC-3′), PPARγ (sense, 5′-TCCGCTGATGCACT GCCTAT-3′; antisense, 5′-GGAATGCGAGTGGTCTTCCA-3′), β-actin (sense, 5′-ACACCCC AGCCATGTACG-3′; antisense, 5′-TGGTGGTGAAGCTGTAGCC-3′), and GAPDH (sense, 5′-ACCACAGTCCATGCCATCAC-3′; antisense, 5′-TCCACCACCCTGTTGCTGTA-3′). The results of the target mRNA were relative to the housekeeping gene mRNA level, and the values obtained in the presence or absence of the extracts were expressed in relation to the values obtained in the control group.

4.12. Determination of Nitric Oxide Production

RAW 264.7 macrophages were plated in a 96-well plate and cultured for 24 h. The cells were then pretreated for 1 h with a non-toxic concentration of FLLE or FLRE (0–200 g/mL). After that, 1 μg/mL LPS was added to each well and incubated for 24 h. The culture supernatant was then collected to investigate NO generation using Griess reagent assay. Griess reagent and supernatant were mixed and incubated for 15 min at room temperature, in the dark. The absorbance was measured at 540 nm. In addition, the treated cells were subjected to MTT assay for the determination of the cell viability.

4.13. Enzyme-Linked Immunosorbent (ELISA) Assay

TNF-α or IL-6 levels secreted from the treated cells to the culture media were assessed using a sandwich Enzyme Link Immuno-Sorbent Assay performed according to manufacturers' guidelines (BioLegend's ELISA MAXTM Deluxe Set, San Diego, CA, USA).

4.14. Western Blotting

The treated cells were collected to prepare protein samples. The samples were subjected to 10% SDS-PAGE, and the proteins were electrically transferred to a nitrocellulose membrane. The target proteins were probed with specific antibodies (anti-COX-2 antibody (1:2000), anti-iNOS antibody (1:2000), anti- β-actin antibody (1:10,000), anti-NF-κB antibody (1:1000), and anti-phospho-NF-κB p65 (1:1000)). The enhanced chemiluminescence (ECL) method was used for the protein detection. The iNOS, COX-2, and β-actin visible bands were 131, 74, and 42 kDa, respectively.

4.15. Statistical Analysis

All values are reported as mean $\pm$ standard derivation (X $\pm$ SD) of three independent tests using triplicate samples. The one-way analysis of variance (ANOVA), followed by Tukey's multiple comparison tests was employed using Prism 9.4.1 software to determine overall differences among the treatment groups. Statistical significance is noted when the p values < 0.05.

5. Conclusions

In conclusion, FLLE and FLRE showed adipogenesis induction ability by increasing lipid accumulation, suggesting that the extracts might prevent hypertrophic adipocytes, leading to the reduction in inflammation, dysfunction, and insulin resistance of the cells. Moreover, FLLE and FLRE could improve insulin sensitivity in TNF-α-induced adipocytes via the decrease in MCP-1 expression, which may reduce inflammatory cascades and improve adipocyte function. Furthermore, FLRE exhibited anti-inflammation activity via the suppression of inflammation-related molecule expression. The extracts were less toxic, as determined by in vitro cytotoxic assays. Finally, the knowledge from the present study provides scientific data and useful information on the biological potential of *Ficus lindsayana*. However, identification of bioactive compounds and in vivo safety assessment must be performed for further development and use as either a herbal medicine or a functional ingredient.

Author Contributions: Conceptualization, J.K., P.B., A.I., A.W., P.T. and P.P.; methodology, U.S. and P.P.; validation, J.K., P.B. and P.P.; formal analysis, J.K., P.B., D.R., T.Y., A.I., A.W., P.T. and P.P.; investigation, J.K., P.B., D.R., T.Y., B.C. and U.S., and P.P.; resources, B.C.; data curation, J.K., P.B. and P.P.; writing—original draft preparation, J.K., P.B. and P.P.; writing—review and editing, J.K., P.B., A.I., A.W., P.T. and P.P.; visualization, J.K. and P.B.; supervision, A.I., A.W., P.T. and P.P.; project administration, P.P.; funding acquisition, B.C. and P.P. All authors have read and agreed to the published version of the manuscript.

Funding: This research was funded by The Agricultural Research Development Agency (Public Organization), Thailand, funding number CRP6105022130 and The Faculty of Medicine Research Fund, Chiang Mai University, funding number 016-2560.

Institutional Review Board Statement: This study was granted a certificate of exemption by the Research Ethics Committee of the Faculty of Medicine, Chiang Mai University (No. EXEMPTION 4744/2017).

Informed Consent Statement: Consent to participate was not applicable because of anonymous data collection.

Data Availability Statement: The datasets used and/or analyzed during the current study are available from the corresponding author on reasonable request.

Acknowledgments: This manuscript was proofread by Ruth Leatherman, RN, native English Proofreader, Research Administration Section, Faculty of Medicine, Chiang Mai University, Chiang Mai, 50200 Thailand.

Conflicts of Interest: The authors declare no conflicts of interest.

References

1. McArdle, M.A.; Finucane, O.M.; Connaughton, R.M.; McMorrow, A.M.; Roche, H.M. Mechanisms of obesity-induced inflammation and insulin resistance: Insights into the emerging role of nutritional strategies. *Front. Endocrinol.* **2013**, *4*, 52. [CrossRef]
2. Weisberg, S.P.; McCann, D.; Desai, M.; Rosenbaum, M.; Leibel, R.L.; Ferrante, A.W. Obesity is associated with macrophage accumulation in adipose tissue. *J. Clin. Investig.* **2003**, *112*, 1796–1808. [CrossRef]
3. Esser, N.; Legrand-Poels, S.; Piette, J.; Scheen, A.J.; Paquot, N. Inflammation as a link between obesity, metabolic syndrome and type 2 diabetes. *Diabetes Res. Clin. Pract.* **2014**, *105*, 141–150. [CrossRef]
4. Hajer, G.R.; van Haeften, T.W.; Visseren, F.L.J. Adipose tissue dysfunction in obesity, diabetes, and vascular diseases. *Eur. Heart J.* **2008**, *29*, 2959–2971. [CrossRef]
5. Zhang, Q.; Zhu, B.; Li, Y. Resolution of Cancer-Promoting Inflammation: A New Approach for Anticancer Therapy. *Front. Immunol.* **2017**, *8*, 71. [CrossRef]
6. Khanna, R.D.; Karki, K.; Pande, D.; Negi, R.; Khanna, R.S. Inflammation, Free Radical Damage, Oxidative Stress and Cancer. *Interdiscip. J. Microinflamm.* **2014**, *1*. [CrossRef]
7. Hunter, P. The inflammation theory of disease. The growing realization that chronic inflammation is crucial in many diseases opens new avenues for treatment. *EMBO Rep.* **2012**, *13*, 968–970. [CrossRef]
8. Goldfine, A.B.; Silver, R.; Aldhahi, W.; Cai, D.; Tatro, E.; Lee, J.; Shoelson, S.E. Use of salsalate to target inflammation in the treatment of insulin resistance and type 2 diabetes. *Clin. Transl. Sci.* **2008**, *1*, 36–43. [CrossRef] [PubMed]
9. Ramos-Zavala, M.G.; González-Ortiz, M.; Martínez-Abundis, E.; Robles-Cervantes, J.A.; González-López, R.; Santiago-Hernández, N.J. Effect of Diacerein on Insulin Secretion and Metabolic Control in Drug-Naïve Patients with Type 2 Diabetes: A randomized clinical trial. *Diabetes Care* **2011**, *34*, 1591–1594. [CrossRef] [PubMed]
10. Osafo, N.; CAgyare; Obiri, D.D.; Antwi, A.O. Nonsteroidal Anti-Inflammatory Drugs (NSAIDs); Updated on 1 May 2023. 2023. Available online: https://www.ncbi.nlm.nih.gov/books/NBK547742/ (accessed on 30 November 2023).
11. Wongrakpanich, S.; Wongrakpanich, A.; Melhado, K.; Rangaswami, J. A Comprehensive Review of Non-Steroidal Anti-Inflammatory Drug Use in the Elderly. *Aging Dis.* **2018**, *9*, 143–150. [CrossRef] [PubMed]
12. Vinayagam, R.; Xu, B. Antidiabetic properties of dietary flavonoids: A cellular mechanism review. *Nutr. Metab.* **2015**, *12*, 60. [CrossRef]
13. Batra, P.; Sharma, A.K. Anti-cancer potential of flavonoids: Recent trends and future perspectives. *3 Biotech.* **2013**, *3*, 439–459. [CrossRef] [PubMed]
14. Elisha, I.L.; Dzoyem, J.-P.; McGaw, L.J.; Botha, F.S.; Eloff, J.N. The anti-arthritic, anti-inflammatory, antioxidant activity and relationships with total phenolics and total flavonoids of nine South African plants used traditionally to treat arthritis. *BMC Complement. Altern. Med.* **2016**, *16*, 307. [CrossRef]
15. Ramchoun, M.; Harnafi, H.; Alem, C.; Benlyas, M.; Elrhaffari, L.; Amrani, S. Study on antioxidant and hypolipidemic effects of polyphenol-rich extracts from Thymus vulgaris and Lavendula multifida. *Pharmacogn. Res.* **2009**, *1*, 106–112.

16. Ahmed, F.; Urooj, A. Traditional uses, medicinal properties, and phytopharmacology of *Ficus racemosa*: A review. *Pharm. Biol.* **2010**, *48*, 672–681. [CrossRef]
17. Cheng, J.-X.; Zhang, B.-D.; Zhu, W.-F.; Zhang, C.-F.; Qin, Y.-M.; Abe, M.; Akihisa, T.; Liu, W.-Y.; Feng, F.; Zhang, J. Traditional uses, phytochemistry, and pharmacology of *Ficus hispida* L.f.: A review. *J. Ethnopharmacol.* **2020**, *248*, 112204. [CrossRef] [PubMed]
18. Shi, Y.; Mon, A.M.; Fu, Y.; Zhang, Y.; Wang, C.; Yang, X.; Wang, Y. The genus *Ficus* (Moraceae) used in diet: Its plant diversity, distribution, traditional uses and ethnopharmacological importance. *J. Ethnopharmacol.* **2018**, *226*, 185–196. [CrossRef]
19. Lansky, E.P.; Paavilainen, H.M.; Pawlus, A.D.; Newman, R.A. *Ficus* spp. (fig): Ethnobotany and potential as anticancer and anti-inflammatory agents. *J. Ethnopharmacol.* **2008**, *119*, 195–213. [CrossRef]
20. Deepa, P.; Sowndhararajan, K.; Kim, S.; Park, S.J. A role of *Ficus* species in the management of diabetes mellitus: A review. *J. Ethnopharmacol.* **2018**, *215*, 210–232. [CrossRef]
21. Mahmoudi, S.; Khali, M.; Benkhaled, A.; Benamirouche, K.; Baiti, I. Phenolic and flavonoid contents, antioxidant and antimicrobial activities of leaf extracts from ten Algerian *Ficus carica* L. *varieties*. *Asian Pac. J. Trop. Biomed.* **2016**, *6*, 239–245. [CrossRef]
22. Keshari, A.K.; Kumar, G.; Kushwaha, P.S.; Bhardwaj, M.; Kumar, P.; Rawat, A.; Kumar, D.; Prakash, A.; Ghosh, B.; Saha, S. Isolated flavonoids from *Ficus racemosa* stem bark possess antidiabetic, hypolipidemic and protective effects in albino Wistar rats. *J. Ethnopharmacol.* **2016**, *181*, 252–262. [CrossRef]
23. Olaokun, O.O.; McGaw, L.J.; van Rensburg, I.J.; Eloff, J.N.; Naidoo, V. Antidiabetic activity of the ethyl acetate fraction of *Ficus lutea* (Moraceae) leaf extract: Comparison of an in vitro assay with an in vivo obese mouse model. *BMC Complement. Altern. Med.* **2016**, *16*, 110. [CrossRef] [PubMed]
24. Misbah, H.; Abdul Aziz, A.; Aminudin, N. Antidiabetic and antioxidant properties of *Ficus deltoidea* fruit extracts and fractions. *BMC Complement. Altern. Med.* **2013**, *13*, 118. [CrossRef] [PubMed]
25. Jasmine, R.; Manikandan, K.; Karthikeyan, K. Evaluating the antioxidant and anticancer property of *Ficus carica* fruits. *Afr. J. Biotechnol.* **2015**, *14*, 634–641. [CrossRef]
26. Chandrashekhar, C.; Latha, K.; Vagdevi, H.; Vaidya, V. Anthelmintic activity of the crude extracts of *Ficus racemosa*. *Int. J. Green. Pharm.* **2008**, *2*, 100. [CrossRef]
27. Beentje, H. Flora of Singapore precursors, 29: A new name for *Ficus dubia* Wall. ex King (Moraceae). *Gard. Bull. Singap.* **2021**, *73*, 307–308. [CrossRef]
28. Chantarasuwan, B.; Thongaree, S. Five species of Ficus (Moraceae) new for Thailand. *Thai For. Bull.* **2006**, *34*, 25–37.
29. Gupta, D.; Bleakley, B.; Gupta, R.K. Dragon's blood: Botany, chemistry and therapeutic uses. *J. Ethnopharmacol.* **2008**, *115*, 361–380. [CrossRef]
30. Pompimon, W.; Udomputtimekakul, P.; Chaisena, A.; Wattananon, S.; Arsa, A.; Konsantha, K.; Nuntasaen, N. Anti-Syncytium (MC99+ 1A2) and Anti-Bacterial Activities from Twigs and Stems of *Ficus dubia*. *J. Pharm. Res. Int.* **2021**, *32*, 84–91. [CrossRef]
31. Suttisansanee, U.; Pitchakarn, P.; Ting, P.; Inthachat, W.; Thiyajai, P.; Rodthayoy, D.; Karinchai, J.; Chantarasuwan, B.; Nuchuchua, O.; Temviriyanukul, P. Health-promoting bioactivity and in vivo genotoxicity evaluation of a hemiepiphyte fig, *Ficus dubia*. *Food Sci. Nutr.* **2021**, *9*, 2269–2279. [CrossRef]
32. Chansriniyom, C.; Nooin, R.; Nuengchamnong, N.; Wongwanakul, R.; Petpiroon, N.; Srinuanchai, W.; Chantarasuwan, B.; Pitchakarn, P.; Temviriyanukul, P.; Nuchuchua, O. Tandem mass spectrometry of aqueous extract from *Ficus dubia* sap and its cell-based assessments for use as a skin antioxidant. *Sci. Rep.* **2021**, *11*, 16899. [CrossRef]
33. Hu, R.; Chantana, W.; Pitchakarn, P.; Subhawa, S.; Chantarasuwan, B.; Temviriyanukul, P.; Chewonarin, T. *Ficus dubia* latex extract prevent DMH-induced rat early colorectal carcinogenesis through the regulation of xenobiotic metabolism, inflammation, cell proliferation and apoptosis. *Sci. Rep.* **2022**, *12*, 15472. [CrossRef] [PubMed]
34. Hu, R.; Chantana, W.; Pitchakarn, P.; Subhawa, S.; Chantarasuwan, B.; Temviriyanukul, P.; Chewonarin, T. *Ficus dubia* latex extract induces cell cycle arrest and apoptosis by regulating the NF-κB pathway in inflammatory human colorectal cancer cell lines. *Cancers* **2022**, *14*, 2665. [CrossRef]
35. Kim, J.-Y.; van de Wall, E.; Laplante, M.; Azzara, A.; Trujillo, M.E.; Hofmann, S.M.; Schraw, T.; Durand, J.L.; Li, H.; Li, G.; et al. Obesity-associated improvements in metabolic profile through expansion of adipose tissue. *J. Clin. Investig.* **2007**, *117*, 2621–2637. [CrossRef]
36. Lu, Q.; Li, M.; Zou, Y.; Cao, T. Induction of adipocyte hyperplasia in subcutaneous fat depot alleviated type 2 diabetes symptoms in obese mice. *Obesity* **2014**, *22*, 1623–1631. [CrossRef] [PubMed]
37. Panday, D.R.; Rauniar, G.P. Effect of root-extracts of *Ficus benghalensis* (Banyan) in memory, anxiety, muscle co-ordination and seizure in animal models. *BMC Complement. Altern. Med.* **2016**, *16*, 429. [CrossRef] [PubMed]
38. Aziz, F.M. Protective Effects of latex of *Ficus carica* L. against lead acetate-induced hepatotoxicity in rats. *Jordan. J. Biol. Sci.* **2012**, *5*, 175–182.
39. Ibraheim, Z.Z.; Nafady, A.M.; Mostafa, M.A.; Amin, F.M. Antioxidant activity and total flavonoids content of aerial parts of *Ficus pyriformis* Hook. & Arn. (Moraceae) Cultivated in Egypt. *Am. J. Chem.* **2015**, *5*, 23–27.
40. Ali, B.; Mujeeb, M.; Aeri, V.; Mir, S.; Faiyazuddin, M.; Shakeel, F. Anti-inflammatory and antioxidant activity of *Ficus carica* Linn. leaves. *Nat. Prod. Res.* **2012**, *26*, 460–465. [CrossRef]
41. Naveed, M.; Hejazi, V.; Abbas, M.; Kamboh, A.A.; Khan, G.J.; Shumzaid, M.; Ahmad, F.; Babazadeh, D.; FangFang, X.; Modarresi-Ghazani, F.; et al. Chlorogenic acid (CGA): A pharmacological review and call for further research. *Biomed. Pharmacother.* **2018**, *97*, 67–74. [CrossRef]

42. Chen, L.; Teng, H.; Cao, H. Chlorogenic acid and caffeic acid from *Sonchus oleraceus* Linn synergistically attenuate insulin resistance and modulate glucose uptake in HepG2 cells. *Food Chem. Toxicol.* **2019**, *127*, 182–187. [CrossRef]
43. Liao, C.-C.; Ou, T.-T.; Wu, C.-H.; Wang, C.-J. Prevention of diet-induced hyperlipidemia and obesity by caffeic acid in C57BL/6 Mice through regulation of hepatic lipogenesis gene expression. *J. Agric. Food Chem.* **2013**, *61*, 11082–11088. [CrossRef]
44. Hwang, S.J.; Kim, Y.-W.; Park, Y.; Lee, H.-J.; Kim, K.-W. Anti-inflammatory effects of chlorogenic acid in lipopolysaccharide-stimulated RAW 264.7 cells. *Inflamm. Res.* **2013**, *63*, 81–90. [CrossRef] [PubMed]
45. Schröter, D.; Neugart, S.; Schreiner, M.; Grune, T.; Rohn, S.; Ott, C. Amaranth's 2-caffeoylisocitric acid—An anti-inflammatory caffeic acid derivative that impairs NF-κB signaling in LPS-challenged RAW 264.7 macrophages. *Nutrients* **2019**, *11*, 571. [CrossRef] [PubMed]
46. Huang, D.-W.; Shen, S.-C.; Wu, J.S.-B. Effects of caffeic acid and cinnamic acid on glucose uptake in insulin-resistant mouse hepatocytes. *J. Agric. Food Chem.* **2009**, *57*, 7687–7692. [CrossRef] [PubMed]
47. Park, C.-H.; Min, S.-Y.; Yu, H.-W.; Kim, K.; Kim, S.; Lee, H.-J.; Kim, J.-H.; Park, Y.-J. Effects of apigenin on RBL-2H3, RAW264.7, and HaCaT cells: Anti-Allergic, anti-inflammatory, and skin-protective activities. *Int. J. Mol. Sci.* **2020**, *21*, 4620. [CrossRef]
48. Tian, C.; Liu, X.; Chang, Y.; Wang, R.; Lv, T.; Cui, C.; Liu, M. Investigation of the anti-inflammatory and antioxidant activities of luteolin, kaempferol, apigenin and quercetin. *S. Afr. J. Bot.* **2020**, *137*, 257–264. [CrossRef]
49. Ji, G.; Zhang, Y.; Yang, Q.; Cheng, S.; Hao, J.; Zhao, X.; Jiang, Z. Genistein suppresses LPS-induced inflammatory response through inhibiting NF-κB following AMP kinase activation in RAW 264.7 macrophages. *PLoS ONE* **2012**, *7*, e53101. [CrossRef]
50. Shin, H.-K.; Seo, C.-S.; Jeong, S.-J.; Yoo, S.-R.; Lee, N.-R. Quantitative analysis and in vitro Anti-inflammatory effects of gallic acid, ellagic acid, and quercetin from *Radix Sanguisorbae*. *Pharmacogn. Mag.* **2016**, *12*, 104–108. [CrossRef]
51. Jung, U.J.; Cho, Y.-Y.; Choi, M.-S. Apigenin ameliorates dyslipidemia, hepatic steatosis and insulin resistance by modulating metabolic and transcriptional profiles in the liver of high-fat diet-induced obese mice. *Nutrients* **2016**, *8*, 305. [CrossRef]
52. Feng, X.; Weng, D.; Zhou, F.; Owen, Y.D.; Qin, H.; Zhao, J.; Yu, W.; Huang, Y.; Chen, J.; Fu, H.; et al. Activation of PPARγ by a natural flavonoid modulator, apigenin ameliorates obesity-related inflammation via regulation of macrophage polarization. *EBioMedicine* **2016**, *9*, 61–76. [CrossRef]
53. Zhang, Q.; de Mejia, E.G. Protocatechuic acid attenuates adipogenesis-induced inflammation and mitochondrial dysfunction in 3T3-L1 adipocytes by regulation of AMPK pathway. *J. Funct. Foods* **2020**, *69*, 103972. [CrossRef]
54. Kong, L.; Xu, M.; Qiu, Y.; Liao, M.; Zhang, Q.; Yang, L.; Zheng, G. Chlorogenic acid and caffeine combination attenuates adipogenesis by regulating fat metabolism and inhibiting adipocyte differentiation in 3T3-L1 cells. *J. Food Biochem.* **2021**, *45*, e13795. [CrossRef]
55. Adam, Z.; Khamis, S.; Ismail, A.; Hamid, M. *Ficus deltoidea*: A potential alternative medicine for diabetes mellitus. *Evid.-Based Complement. Altern. Med.* **2012**, *2012*, 632763. [CrossRef]
56. Sartipy, P.; Loskutoff, D.J. Monocyte chemoattractant protein 1 in obesity and insulin resistance. *Proc. Natl. Acad. Sci. USA* **2003**, *100*, 7265–7270. [CrossRef] [PubMed]
57. Kern, L.; Mittenbühler, M.J.; Vesting, A.J.; Ostermann, A.L.; Wunderlich, C.M.; Wunderlich, F.T. Obesity-induced TNFα and IL-6 signaling: The missing link between obesity and inflammation—Driven liver and colorectal cancers. *Cancers* **2018**, *11*, 24. [CrossRef] [PubMed]
58. Han, M.S.; White, A.; Perry, R.J.; Camporez, J.-P.; Hidalgo, J.; Shulman, G.I.; Davis, R.J. Regulation of adipose tissue inflammation by interleukin 6. *Proc. Natl. Acad. Sci. USA* **2020**, *117*, 2751–2760. [CrossRef] [PubMed]
59. Ji, C.; Chen, X.; Gao, C.; Jiao, L.; Wang, J.; Xu, G.; Fu, H.; Guo, X.; Zhao, Y. IL-6 induces lipolysis and mitochondrial dysfunction, but does not affect insulin-mediated glucose transport in 3T3-L1 adipocytes. *J. Bioenerg. Biomembr.* **2011**, *43*, 367–375. [CrossRef] [PubMed]
60. Rebollo-Hernanz, M.; Zhang, Q.; Aguilera, Y.; Martín-Cabrejas, M.A.; de Mejia, E.G. Phenolic compounds from coffee by-products modulate adipogenesis-related inflammation, mitochondrial dysfunction, and insulin resistance in adipocytes, via insulin/PI3K/AKT signaling pathways. *Food Chem. Toxicol.* **2019**, *132*, 110672. [CrossRef] [PubMed]
61. Zhang, B.; Berger, J.; Hu, E.-D.; Szalkowski, D.; White-Carrington, S.; Spiegelman, B.M.; Moller, D.E. Negative regulation proliferator-activated gene expression of peroxisome receptor-y contributes to the antiadipogenic effects of tumor. *Mol. Endocrinol.* **1996**, *10*, 1457–1466. [PubMed]
62. Wu, Z.; Xie, Y.; Morrison, R.F.; Bucher, N.L.R.; Farmer, S.R. PPAR induces the insulin-dependent glucose transproter GLUT4 in the absence of C/EBP during the conversion of 3T3 fibroblast into adipocytes. *Am. Soc. Clin. Investig.* **1998**, *101*, 22–32. [CrossRef]
63. Wu, Z.; Rosen, E.D.; Brun, R.; Hauser, S.; Adelmant, G.; Troy, A.E.; McKeon, C.; Darlington, G.J.; Spiegelman, B.M. Cross-regulation of C/EBP and PPAR controls the transcriptional pathway of adipogenesis and insulin sensitivity. *Mol. Cell* **1999**, *3*, 151–158. [CrossRef]
64. Santiago, L.A.; Saguinsin, S.G.C.; Reyes, A.M.L.; Guerrero, R.P.; Nuguid, A.M.N.; Santos, A.C.N. Total phenolic and flavonoid contents and free radical scavenging components of *Ficus nota* Merr. (Moraceae) ethanolic leaf extract. *Int. Food Res. J.* **2017**, *24*, 2050–2058.
65. Mollace, V.; Muscoli, C.; Masini, E.; Cuzzocrea, S.; Salvemini, D. Modulation of prostaglandin biosynthesis by nitric oxide and nitric oxide donors. *Pharmacol. Rev.* **2005**, *57*, 217–252. [CrossRef] [PubMed]
66. Jeong, J.B.; Jeong, H.J. Rheosmin, a naturally occurring phenolic compound inhibits LPS-induced iNOS and COX-2 expression in RAW264.7 cells by blocking NF-κB activation pathway. *Food Chem. Toxicol.* **2010**, *48*, 2148–2153. [CrossRef] [PubMed]

67. De Luca, C.; Olefsky, J.M. Inflammation and insulin resistance. *FEBS Lett.* **2008**, *582*, 97–105. [CrossRef] [PubMed]
68. Nworu, C.S.; Nwuke, H.C.; Akah, P.A.; Okoye, F.B.C.; Esimone, C.O. Extracts of *Ficus exasperata* leaf inhibit topical and systemic inflammation in rodents and suppress LPS-induced expression of mediators of inflammation in macrophages. *J. Immunotoxicol.* **2012**, *10*, 302–310. [CrossRef] [PubMed]
69. Jung, H.W.; Son, H.Y.; Van Minh, C.; Kim, Y.H.; Park, Y. Methanol extract of Ficus leaf inhibits the production of nitric oxide and proinflammatory cytokines in LPS-stimulated microglia via the MAPK pathway. *Phytother. Res.* **2008**, *22*, 1064–1069. [CrossRef] [PubMed]
70. Swantek, J.L.; Cobb, M.H.; Geppert, T.D. Jun N-Terminal Kinase/Stress-Activated Protein Kinase (JNK/SAPK) is required for lipopolysaccharide stimulation of tumor necrosis factor alpha (TNF-alpha) translation by blocking JNK/SAPK. *Mol. Cell. Biol.* **1997**, *17*, 6274–6282. [CrossRef]
71. Huang, F.; Cao, J.; Liu, Q.; Zou, Y.; Li, H.; Yin, T. MAPK/ERK signal pathway involved expression of COX-2 and VEGF by IL-1β induced in human endometriosis stromal cells in vitro. *Int. J. Clin. Exp. Pathol.* **2013**, *6*, 2129–2136.
72. Baba, S.A.; Malik, S.A. Determination of total phenolic and flavonoid content, antimicrobial and antioxidant activity of a root extract of *Arisaema jacquemontii* Blume. *J. Taibah Univ. Sci.* **2015**, *9*, 449–454. [CrossRef]
73. Budluang, P.; Pitchakarn, P.; Ting, P.; Temviriyanukul, P.; Wongnoppawich, A.; Imsumran, A. Anti-inflammatory and anti-insulin resistance activities of aqueous extract from *Anoectochilus burmannicus*. *Food Sci. Nutr.* **2017**, *5*, 486–496. [CrossRef]
74. Craig, A.P.; Fields, C.; Liang, N.; Kitts, D.; Erickson, A. Performance review of a fast HPLC-UV method for the quantification of chlorogenic acids in green coffee bean extracts. *Talanta* **2016**, *154*, 481–485. [CrossRef] [PubMed]
75. Chupeerach, C.; Temviriyanukul, P.; Thangsiri, S.; Inthachat, W.; Sahasakul, Y.; Aursalung, A.; Wongchang, P.; Sangkasa-Ad, P.; Wongpia, A.; Polpanit, A.; et al. Phenolic profiles and bioactivities of ten original lineage beans in thailand. *Foods* **2022**, *11*, 3905. [CrossRef] [PubMed]
76. Sirichai, P.; Kittibunchakul, S.; Thangsiri, S.; On-Nom, N.; Chupeerach, C.; Temviriyanukul, P.; Inthachat, W.; Nuchuchua, O.; Aursalung, A.; Sahasakul, Y.; et al. Impact of drying processes on phenolics and in vitro health-related activities of indigenous plants in Thailand. *Plants* **2022**, *11*, 294. [CrossRef] [PubMed]
77. Chatthongpisut, R.; Schwartz, S.J.; Yongsawatdigul, J. Antioxidant activities and antiproliferative activity of Thai purple rice cooked by various methods on human colon cancer cells. *Food Chem.* **2015**, *188*, 99–105. [CrossRef] [PubMed]
78. Wang, H.-F.; Wang, Y.-K.; Yih, K.-H. DPPH free-radical scavenging ability, total phenolic content, and chemical composition analysis of forty-five kinds of essential oils. *J. Cosmet. Sci.* **2008**, *59*, 509–522. [CrossRef] [PubMed]
79. Bittersohl, H.; Steimer, W. Chapter 9—Intracellular concentrations of immunosuppressants. In *Personalized Immunosuppression in Transplantation*; Oellerich, M., Dasgupta, A., Eds.; Elsevier: San Diego, CA, USA, 2016; pp. 199–226.
80. Buacheen, P.; Karinchai, J.; Inthachat, W.; Butkinaree, C.; Jankam, C.; Wongnoppavich, A.; Imsumran, A.; Chewonarin, T.; Pimpha, N.; Temviriyanukul, P.; et al. The Toxicological Assessment of *Anoectochilus burmannicus* Ethanolic-Extract-Synthesized Selenium Nanoparticles Using Cell Culture, Bacteria, and *Drosophila melanogaster* as Suitable Models. *Nanomaterials* **2023**, *13*, 2804. [CrossRef]
81. Tolosa, L.; Donato, M.T.; Gómez-Lechón, M.J. General Cytotoxicity Assessment by Means of the MTT Assay. In *Protocols in In Vitro Hepatocyte Research*; Vinken, M., Rogiers, V., Eds.; Springer: New York, NY, USA, 2015; pp. 333–348.
82. Vichai, V.; Kirtikara, K. Sulforhodamine B colorimetric assay for cytotoxicity screening. *Nat. Protoc.* **2006**, *1*, 1112–1116. [CrossRef]
83. Suganthy, N.; Muniasamy, S.; Archunan, G. Safety assessment of methanolic extract of *Terminalia chebula* fruit, *Terminalia arjuna* bark and its bioactive constituent 7-methyl gallic acid: In vitro and in vivo studies. *Regul. Toxicol. Pharmacol.* **2017**, *92*, 347–357. [CrossRef]

pharmaceuticals

MDPI

Article

Chemical Composition, Antioxidant, Anticancer, and Antibacterial Activities of Roots and Seeds of *Ammi visnaga* L. Methanol Extract

Ibrahim M. Aziz [1,*], Rawan M. Alshalan [1], Humaira Rizwana [1], Fetoon Alkhelaiwi [1], Abdulaziz M. Almuqrin [2], Reem M. Aljowaie [1] and Noorah A. Alkubaisi [1]

1 Department of Botany and Microbiology, College of Science, King Saud University, Riyadh 11451, Saudi Arabia; ralshalaan@ksu.edu.sa (R.M.A.); hrizwana@ksu.edu.sa (H.R.); falklewiy@ksu.edu.sa (F.A.); raljowaie@ksu.edu.sa (R.M.A.); nalkubaisi@ksu.edu.sa (N.A.A.)

2 Department of Clinical Laboratory Sciences, College of Applied Medical Sciences, King Saud University, Riyadh 12372, Saudi Arabia; aalmuqrin@ksu.edu.sa

* Correspondence: iaziz@ksu.edu.sa

Abstract: For centuries, plants and their components have been harnessed for therapeutic purposes, with *Ammi visnaga* L. (Khella) being no exception to this rich tradition. While existing studies have shed light on the cytotoxic and antimicrobial properties of seed extracts, there remains a noticeable gap in research about the antimicrobial, antioxidant, and anticancer potential of root extracts. This study seeks to address this gap by systematically examining methanol extracts derived from the roots of *A. visnaga* L. and comparing their effects with those of seed extracts specifically against breast cancer cells. Notably, absent from previous investigations, this study focuses on the comparative analysis of the antimicrobial, antioxidant, and anticancer activities of both root and seed extracts. The methanol extract obtained from *A. visnaga* L. seeds demonstrated a notably higher level of total phenolic content (TPC) than its root counterpart, measuring 366.57 ± 2.86 and 270.78 ± 2.86 mg GAE/g dry weight of the dry extract, respectively. In the evaluation of antioxidant activities using the DPPH method, the IC_{50} values for root and seed extracts were determined to be 193.46 ± 17.13 µg/mL and 227.19 ± 1.48 µg/mL, respectively. Turning our attention to cytotoxicity against breast cancer cells (MCF-7 and MDA-MB-231), both root and seed extracts displayed similar cytotoxic activities, with IC_{50} values of 92.45 ± 2.14 µg/mL and 75.43 ± 2.32 µg/mL, respectively. Furthermore, both root and seed extracts exhibited a noteworthy modulation of gene expression, upregulating the expression of caspase and Bax mRNA levels while concurrently suppressing the expression of anti-apoptotic genes (Bcl-xL and Bcl-2), thereby reinforcing their potential as anticancer agents. *A. visnaga* L. seed extract outperforms the root extract in antimicrobial activities, exhibiting lower minimum inhibitory concentrations (MICs) of 3.81 ± 0.24 to 125 ± 7.63 µg/mL. This highlights the seeds' potential as potent antibacterial agents, expanding their role in disease prevention. Overall, this study underscores the diverse therapeutic potentials of *A. visnaga* L. roots and seeds, contributing to the understanding of plant-derived extracts in mitigating disease risks.

Keywords: natural products; medicinal plants; anticancer potential; herbal treatment; lung disease

1. Introduction

Medicinal plant-based compounds provide an extensive array of chemical diversity, which plays a vital role in the exploration and advancement of contemporary medicinal therapies [1–3]. Over the past few decades, numerous natural plant-derived compounds have been identified, exhibiting antioxidative, anticancer, anti-inflammatory, and antibacterial properties explained by their ability to activate a variety of signaling transduction pathways [4–8]. Approximately 25% of current medicines are derived from plants, underscoring the profound impact of botanical sources in pharmaceuticals. Moreover, globally, up to 200 species are recognized as therapeutic plants, emphasizing the rich diversity and potential within the plant kingdom for medicinal applications [9].

Ammi visnaga, commonly known as Khella and Bishop's Weed, is an annual aromatic herb belonging to the *Apiaceae* family. Originating from the Mediterranean region, this herb has proliferated globally, extending its presence to Europe, Asia, and North America. The widespread distribution of *A. visnaga* underscores its adaptability and its integration into diverse ecosystems beyond its native habitat [10,11]. For centuries, the utilization of plants and plant components in the treatment of diseases has been a pervasive practice, and *A. visnaga* L. stands as no exception to this historical trend [12]. Moreover, *A. visnaga* L. has earned recognition in the literature and works of diverse Arab chemists and physicians, attesting to its well-documented medicinal and therapeutic characteristics [12,13]. The therapeutic efficacy of *A. visnaga* L. is intricately linked to its rich phytochemical composition, encompassing diverse bioactive constituents such as furanochromones and pyranocoumarins. Recent years have witnessed a discernible surge in scholarly interest directed toward elucidating the pharmacological properties inherent to *A. visnaga* L. [14–17]. Furthermore, notable chemical constituents found in substantial concentrations in this botanical specimen encompass butanoic acid, 2-methyl-, pentyl ester, (Z)-β-ocimene, D-limonene, linalool, pulegone, lavandulyl-butyrate, marmesin, isoimperatorin, heraclenin, isopimpinellin, nonhydroxylic coumarins, ammirin, alloimperatorin, khellin, visnagin, and acetylated flavonoids, in addition to the essential oil [18,19]. The essential oil derived from *A. visnaga* L. has been demonstrated to possess notable antiviral, antibacterial, and larvicidal properties. Furthermore, the antioxidant activity of the plant can be attributed to its flavonoid content. These beneficial properties of *A. visnaga* have been recognized and utilized for therapeutic purposes for over 7000 years [12,20,21]. The odorant volatile compounds responsible for the aroma of *A. visnaga* are found in flowers, leaves, stems, peels, and roots [22]. Aqueous extracts of *A. visnaga* seeds have shown significant improvement in conditions such as uremia, nephrolithiasis, and hyperbilirubinemia. These beneficial effects have been reported in various studies [23–25]. In addition, it has been observed that the aqueous extract of *A. visnaga* exhibits potential benefits in reducing blood sugar levels and is believed to possess hypoglycemic effects in rats [26]. Previous research has provided evidence of the significant inhibitory effects of *A. visnaga* L. extracts on the growth of bacteria and fungi [27,28].

A. visnaga L. extracts have been reported to possess therapeutic potential in the treatment of stomach pains and moderate anginal symptoms. It is also used as a supportive therapy for minor respiratory tract obstruction in asthma or spastic bronchitis, as well as postoperative treatment for disorders related to the presence of urinary calculi. The plant and its extracts are also utilized as a lithotriptic drug in the treatment of kidney stones. It is also used internally as an emmenagogue to control menstruation, as a diuretic, and to treat vertigo and diabetes. Aerial parts infusions have also been used to cure headaches [12,29,30]. Additionally, these extracts have demonstrated the ability to reduce blood pressure and to alleviate bronchial spasms [31,32]. A recent study has provided evidence of the cytotoxic effects of *A. visnaga* seed extract on a human liver cancer cell line (HuH-7) [33].

Cytotoxic agents cause apoptosis in susceptible target cells by activating death signaling pathways. Chemotherapeutic agents induce apoptosis by activating death receptor systems simultaneously or sequentially, disrupting mitochondrial function and proteolytic processing of caspases [4]. Thus, the cell death pathway may occur in several sites; however, the precise molecular pathways for each medication and unique target cell have not been completely elucidated. In the present study, changes in caspase-3, -8, -9, and Bax (pro-apoptotic) genes and anti-apoptotic genes (Bcl-xL and Bcl-2) following apoptosis stimulation by methanol extracts of *A. visnaga* L. in MCF-7 and MDA-MB-231 cells was revealed. Apoptosis, or programmed cell death, is a critical component of many processes that occur in response to environmental stimuli. According to research, there are two primary apoptotic routes in mammalian cells: the extrinsic or death receptor pathway and the intrinsic or mitochondrial system. The activation of caspases is connected with the induction of cell death in both extrinsic and intrinsic apoptotic pathways [34]. Aspase-8 is mostly active in the extrinsic apoptotic route, while caspase-9 activation is associated with the mitochondrial or intrinsic pathway [35]. Caspases may be activated in anticancer treatment by stimulating the extrinsic route or by activating the intrinsic pathway at the mitochondria [36]. Increased Bax expression in breast cancer cells enhances sensitivity to apoptotic stimuli and reduces tumor growth [37]. Another anti-apoptotic protein that inhibits apoptosis is Bcl-xL [38]. Bcl-xL expression has been correlated to the progression of breast cancer [39]. While Bcl-xL suppresses apoptosis, it is regarded as a critical molecule in the induction of chemoresistance [40]. On the other hand, past research has extensively explored the cytotoxic and antibacterial effects of seed extracts; a comparative analysis with root extracts regarding antimicrobial, antioxidant, and anticancer properties remains unexplored. The chemical mechanisms underlying the biological effects of *A. visnaga* roots and seed extracts remain enigmatic. This study aims to fill this gap by evaluating the phytochemical composition and antioxidant properties of *A. visnaga* L. root extracts compared to seed extracts, utilizing the 1,1-diphenyl-2-picryl hydrazyl (DPPH) scavenging assay and 2,2′-azino-bis (3-ethylbenzothiazoline-6-sulfonic acid) (ABTS) assay. Additionally, it seeks to assess the potential effects of *A. visnaga* L. roots compared to seed extracts against breast cancer (MCF-7) and MDA-MB-231 cells. This study further aims to elucidate the underlying mechanisms through qPCR-based mRNA expression profiling of selected pro- and anti-apoptosis marker genes. Moreover, antibacterial activity against Gram-positive and Gram-negative bacteria will be explored using the minimum inhibitory concentration (MIC) and minimum bactericidal concentration (MBC) methods.

2. Results

2.1. Chemical Composition of Methanol Roots and Seeds Extracts of A. visnaga L.

GC-MS/FID analysis was conducted to analyze the methanol extract of *A. visnaga* L. roots and seeds for phytochemical components. The identified compounds are presented in Table 1 and Figure 1A. In the root methanol extract, the predominant phytochemical compound identified was Docosanolide (73.39%), followed by Angecin (10.75%) and 2,5-Dimethyl-5-Nitrohexanal (10.70%). On the other hand, the major phytochemical compound in the methanol extract of the seeds was 2-Benzoyl-3-Methyl-2,3-Diaza (54.60%), followed by 2-Methoxy-4-Propyl-Phenol (24.96%) and 6-Octadecenoic Acid (10.68%) (Table 2 and Figure 1B).

Table 1. GC-MS identified volatile components from the methanol roots extract of *A. visnaga* L.

Peak	Compound Name	Retention Time (min)	Peak Area %	Area
1	1-Butoxy-2-Propanol Acetate	5.04	5.36	14,009
2	5-Methyl-2-Heptanamine	6.97	8.22	21,484
3	(-)-Curcuhydroquinone	9.39	9.03	31,466
4	Di-Isodecyl Phthalate	9.76	3.66	9559
5	2,5-Dimethyl-5-Nitrohexanal	12.56	10.70	27,988
6	3-Methyl-2h-Cyclohepta[B]Furan	14.98	2.85	59,272
7	Angecin	19.24	10.75	223,303
8	9-Octadecenoic Acid	20.52	8.11	168,542
9	6-Methoxy-2-Oxo-(2h)-Furo[2,3-H]-1-Benzopyran	21.60	1.54	32,007
10	Docosanolide	22.32	73.39	1,524,375

2.2. Antioxidant Activity

2.2.1. Total Phenolic Content (TPC) and Total Flavonoid Content (TFC)

The methanol extract derived from the seeds of *A. visnaga* L. displayed a higher TPC level, measuring 366.57 ± 2.86 ± 4.09 mg GAE/g dry weight of the dry extract than the roots extract measured value of 270.78 ± 2.86 mg GAE/g dry weight of the dry extract, according to the correlation coefficient (R^2 = 0.977). Regarding the TFC, the seeds of *A. visnaga* L. contained an amount of 242.10 ± 3.07 mg QE/g dry weight of the dry extract, while the roots exhibited a slightly lower TFC value of 214.46 ± 2.86 mg QE/g dry weight of the dry extract, according to the correlation coefficient ($R^2 = 0.965$), indicating a highly significant correlation between the TFC and the extract from both roots and seeds of *A. visnaga* L.

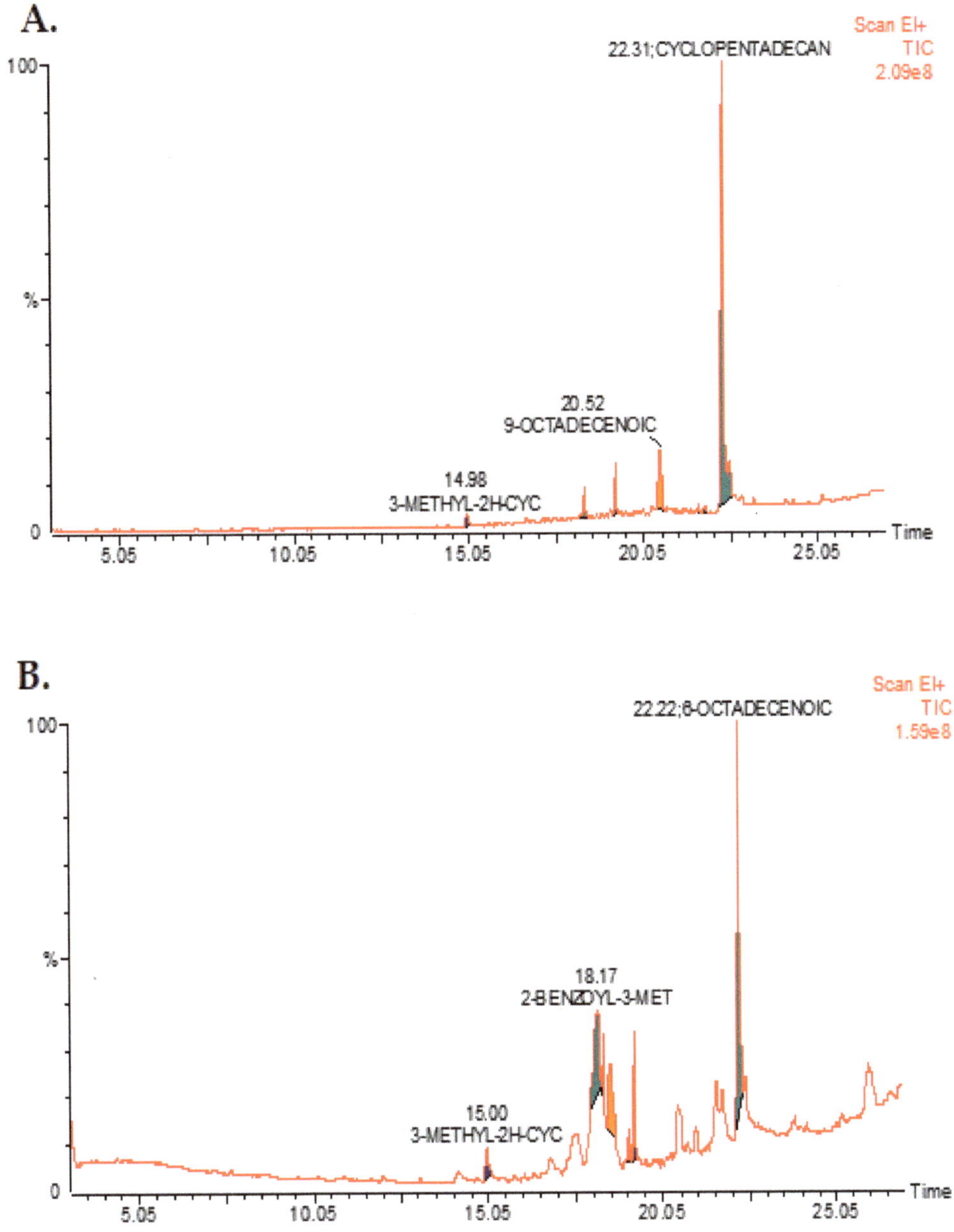

Figure 1. The GC-MS spectrum of the compounds extracted from *A. visnaga* L., specifically from the roots (**A**) and seeds (**B**), is shown in Figures 1A and 1B, respectively. For the analysis, a methanol extract was used, and the GC-MS instrument was programmed for 30 min. Each peak observed in the spectrum represents an identified compound, and the presence of a large peak indicates the major compound in the extract.

Table 2. GC-MS identified volatile components from the methanol seeds extract of *A. visnaga* L.

Peak	Compound Name	Retention Time (min)	Peak Area %	Area
1	Camphor	9.59	0.68	151,747
2	4-Methyl-1-Methyl 3-Cyclohexen-1-Ol	10.12	0.75	167,952
3	3-Cyclohexene-1-Methanol	10.35	4.04	908,773
4	4-Phenyl2-Butanone	11.00	3.34	750,682
5	Isocaryophyllen	13.76	0.51	114,170
6	Trans-α-Bergamotene	13.87	1.14	256,370
7	3-Methyl-2h-Cyclohepta[B]Furan	14.98	2.85	59,272
8	2-Benzoyl-3-Methyl-2,3-Diaza	18.17	54.60	450,1224
9	1-Methyl-5-Phenyltetrazole	18.34	1.92	158,385
10	2-Methoxy-4-Propyl-Phenol	18.54	24.96	2,057,664
11	Neophytadiene	19.09	0.510	42,337
12	Angecin	19.24	5.66	466,675
13	6-Octadecenoic Acid	22.22	10.68	880,313

2.2.2. DPPH and ABTS Radical Scavenging Activity

The antioxidant capacity of the phytochemicals extracted from the roots and seeds of *A. visnaga* L. was assessed using two methods: DPPH and ABTS radical scavenging activity. The results, presented in Figure 2, were compared with vitamin C (IC_{50} of 83.45 ± 1.24 μg/mL). Higher concentrations of the extract led to enhanced DPPH and ABTS radical activities. In the DPPH assay, the root extract exhibited an IC50 value of 193.46 ± 17.13, while the ABTS assay showed a value of 188.74 ± 2.69 μg/mL (Figure 2A). Similarly, the seed extract demonstrated improved DPPH and ABTS radical scavenging abilities with increasing concentration, yielding IC_{50} values of 227.19 ± 1.48 and 221.94 + 1.32 μg/mL, respectively (Figure 2B).

2.3. *Cytotoxic Activity*

Root and seed extracts of *A. visnaga* L. exhibited a dose-dependent inhibition of proliferation, as illustrated in (Figure 3). Remarkably, compared to the positive control (doxorubicin), the methanol extracts from both *A. visnaga* L. roots and seeds demonstrated robust cytotoxic activity against MCF-7 and MDA-MB-231 cells. The results indicated a significant ($p < 0.05$) difference between untreated and treated cells at varied doses. While 50 μg/mL of roots and seeds extracts showed limited inhibition of MCF-7 and MDA-MB-231 cell growth, higher concentrations of roots extract exhibited a gradient cytotoxic effect, with significant viability reduction ($p < 0.05$) at 100–400 μg/mL. The IC_{50} values of MCF-7 and MDA-MB-231 cells were 92.45 ± 2.14 and 75.43 ± 2.32 μg/mL, respectively (Figure 3A). Similar trends were observed with the seed extract, displaying IC_{50} values of 87.35 ± 2.44 and 72.49 ± 1.36 μg/mL for MCF-7 and MDA-MB-231 cells, respectively (Figure 3B). Notably, the seed extract demonstrated a more potent cytotoxic effect than the root extract against both cell lines.

2.4. *Effects of A. visnaga L., Root and Seeds Extracts on MCF-7 and MDA-MB-231 Induced Apoptosis Signaling*

The effect of *A. visnaga* L. roots and seeds extract on apoptosis signaling in MCF-7 and MDA-MB-231 cells was assessed after 48 h using qPCR. As shown in Figure 4A,B, there was a significant increase in caspase-3, -8, and -9 mRNA levels in MCF-7 and MDA-MB-231 cells treated with roots and seeds extracts of *A. visnaga* L. compared to the control untreated cells. Furthermore, the extracts significantly upregulated Bax mRNA expression while significantly downregulating the anti-apoptotic genes *Bcl-2* and *Bcl-xL* in treated MCF-7 and MDA-MB-231 cells, relative to the control untreated cells ($p < 0.05$). It is noteworthy that MDA-MB-231 cells treated with *A. visnaga* L. roots and seeds extracts exhibited greater sensitivity than MCF-7 cells.

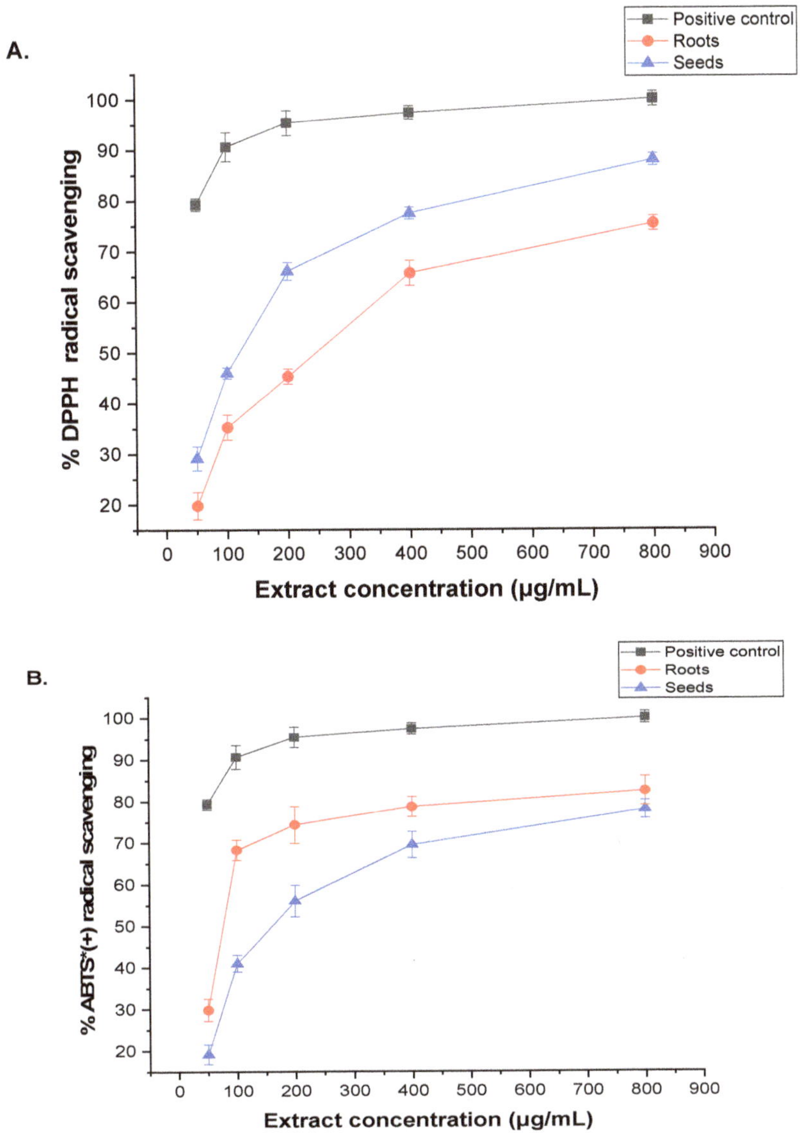

Figure 2. DPPH and ABTS estimation of (**A**) roots and (**B**) seeds of *A. visnaga* L. extracts. The presented statistics are mean values based on three replicates ± SD. * = radical cation.

2.5. Antibacterial Activity of Roots and Seeds of A. visnaga L. Extracts

The antibacterial efficacy of methanol extracts derived from both roots and seeds of *A. visnaga* L. was systematically investigated against six selected bacterial strains, with results compared to Chloramphenicol (Tables 3 and 4). Remarkably, the seeds of *A. visnaga* L exhibited superior antibacterial activity, demonstrating MIC values ranging from 3.81 ± 0.24 to 125 ± 7.63 µg/mL, outperforming the root extract (MIC, 7.81 ± 1.74 to 62.5 ± 3.53 µg/mL). Among the strains, S. *epidermidis* (MTCC 12228) and *S. aureus* were the most sensitive to seed extract with MIC (3.81 ± 0.28 and 3.81 ± 0.24 µg/mL, respectively). Weaker antibacterial effects were observed against *P. aeruginosa* (MTCC 27853) with MIC values of (62.5 ± 3.53 μg/mL) and MBC of (125 ± 5.69 μg/mL) when tested with seeds of *A. visnaga* L. extract. Interestingly, Gram-negative bacteria, including *P. aeruginosa* (MTCC 27853), *K. pneumoniae* (MTCC 13883), and *E. coli* (ATCC 25922), displayed lower sensitivity compared to Gram-positive bacteria, suggesting varied susceptibility to *A. visnaga* L. extracts.

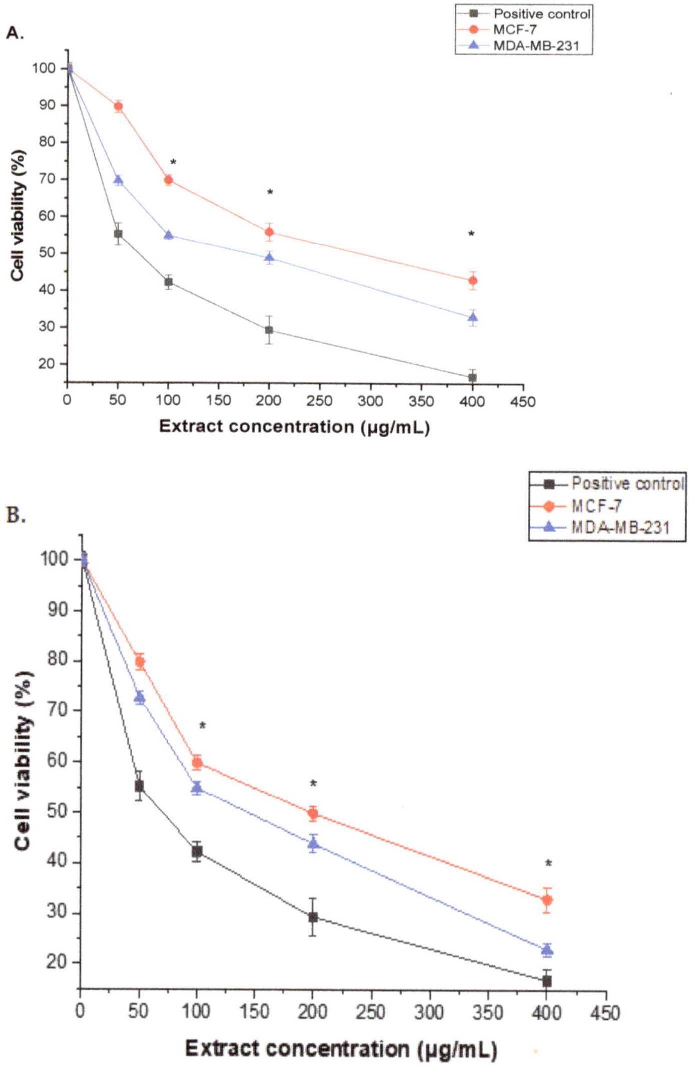

Figure 3. The cytotoxicity of *A. visnaga* L. extracts derived from roots (**A**) and seeds (**B**) was examined using the MTT assay for 24 h, with concentrations ranging from 0 to 400 μg/mL. The results, represented as the mean ± SD of three independent experiments, demonstrated a statistically significant difference from the control (* = $p < 0.05$). In particular, the cytotoxic effects of the extracts on MCF-7 and MDA-MB-231 cells were assessed.

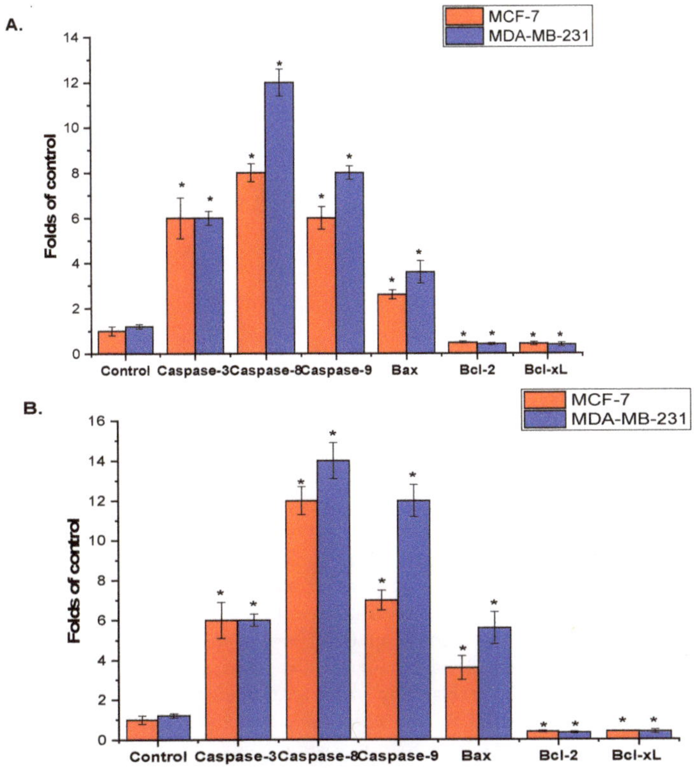

Figure 4. Illustration of the qPCR-based mRNA expression analysis of selected pro- and anti-apoptosis marker genes in MCF-7 and MDA-MB-231 cells treated with extracts derived from *A. visnaga* L. roots (**A**) and seeds (**B**). The results demonstrate a statistically significant difference from the control, indicated by (* = $p < 0.05$).

Table 3. The inhibitory zone, MIC, and MBC of roots of *A. visnaga* L. extracts.

Bacterium/Dilution	Positive Control	500 µg/mL	250 µg/mL	125 µg/mL	62.5 µg/mL	MIC (µg/mL)	MBC (µg/mL)
S. aureus (MTCC 29213)	25 ± 1.24	21 ± 1.62	18 ± 0.64	14 ± 1.38	12 ± 1.36	7.81 ± 1.74	15.62 ± 3.84
S. epidermidis (MTCC 12228)	26 ± 1.14	22 ± 2.34	19 ± 2.36	14 ± 0.98	12 ± 1.39	7.81 ± 0.54	15.62 ± 1.83
B. subtilis (MTCC 10400)	24 ± 0.42	21 ± 3.93	19 ± 1.44	13 ± 1.65	11 ± 1.69	15.62 ± 1.43	31.25 ± 1.23
E. coli (ATCC 25922)	25 ± 2.15	20 ± 1.64	15 ± 1.66	12 ± 2.37	6 ± 0.39	31.25 ± 1.23	62.5 ± 3.76
K. pneumoniae (MTCC 13883)	22 ± 1.35	17 ± 132	13 ± 1.25	8 ± 1.45	6 ± 0.93	31.25 ± 1.45	62.5 ± 3.53
P. aeruginosa (MTCC 27853)	28 ± 2.27	19 ± 0.64	14 ± 0.44	11 ± 1.27	5 ± 0.83	62.5 ± 3.53	125 ± 5.69

Table 4. The inhibitory zone, MIC, and MBC of seeds of *A. visnaga* L. extracts against selected bacteria strains.

Bacterium/Dilution	Positive Control	500 µg/mL	250 µg/mL	125 µg/mL	62.5 µg/mL	MIC (µg/mL)	MBC (µg/mL)
S. aureus (MTCC 29213)	25 ± 1.24	18 ± 2.65	16 ± 1.33	12 ± 2.36	8 ± 0.69	3.81 ± 0.24	7.81 ± 2.43
S. epidermidis (MTCC 12228)	26 ± 1.14	23 ± 0.98	18 ± 1.36	12 ± 1.93	8 ± 0.76	3.81 ± 0.28	7.81 ± 1.34
B. subtilis (MTCC 10400)	24 ± 0.42	20 ± 1.35	12 ± 1.95	10 ± 0.64	9 ± 0.36	15.63 ± 1.63	31.25 ± 2.65
E. coli (ATCC 25922)	25 ± 2.15	18 ± 0.59	14 ± 1.25	10 ± 1.44	8 ± 0.35	50 ± 5.73	100 ± 3.57
K. pneumoniae (MTCC 13883)	22 ± 1.35	18 ± 0.92	11 ± 0.84	9 ± 0.39	5 ± 0.23	125 ± 7.63	250 ± 5.66
P. aeruginosa (MTCC 27853)	28 ± 2.27	17 ± 0.85	12 ± 0.37	9 ± 0.33	6 ± 0.25	31.25 ± 5.27	62.5 ± 4.65

3. Discussion

For centuries, pharmaceutical compounds derived from plants, including alkaloids, polyphenols, terpenoids, flavonoids, ursolic acid, paclitaxel, camptothecin, podophyllotoxin, and combretastatin, have been utilized for various purposes [41]. These natural products possess diverse properties, such as anticancer, antioxidant, anti-inflammatory, and antibacterial effects [42,43]. Despite previous studies emphasizing the cytotoxic and antibacterial effects of *A. visnaga* L. seed extracts, an unexplored avenue involves comparing the potential of root extracts as antimicrobial, antioxidant, and anticancer agents as against seed extracts. Therefore, the objective of this study was to analyze the chemical composition of methanol extracts obtained from both the roots and seeds of *A. visnaga* L. using GC/MS. Additionally, we aimed to assess the anticancer, antioxidant, and antibacterial activities of the methanol extracts derived from the roots and compare them with the seed extracts. Furthermore, we employed qPCR-based mRNA expression profiling of selected pro- and anti-apoptosis marker genes to explore the potential of apoptosis induction.

The chemical constituents of *A. visnaga* are well known and have been reported by many researchers in numerous studies throughout the years. Numerous chemical components of *A. visnaga*, notably γ-pyrones (Furanochromone Derivatives), have been the subject of previous research. The two principal ones are visnagin and khellin [44,45], together with 4-norvisnagin, khellinol, visamminol, ammiol, and khellol [46]. In addition to khellinin, khellinone, and visnaginone [10], other significant γ-pyrones are 5,7-dihydroxy-2-methyl-γ-pyrone-7-O-glucoside [12]. The most prevalent components of *A. visnaga* essential oils were also discovered to be isoamyl 2-methylbutyrate, isoamyl isobutyrate, iso-butyl-2-methylbutyrate, 2-methylbutyl 2-methylbutyrate, 2-methylbutyl isobutyrate, and isoamyl isovalerate [45,47]. Our study involved the analysis of various phytochemical compounds using GC-MS. Docosanolide (73.39%) was identified as the main photochemical component in the obtained methanol extract of roots. According to a preliminary investigation, docosanol administration had distinct effects on human melanoma and CHO-K1 cells, considerably affecting their rates of proliferation but not their viability. The composition of *A. visnaga* L. has been the subject of numerous investigations. *A. visnaga* L. was shown to contain important phytochemical substances, including (Z)-β-ocimen and oxygenated monoterpenes such D-limonene, linalool, pulegone, and lavandulyl-butyrate, in a recent study. According to [44], the major components of the essential oil derived from ripe fruits of *A. visnaga* L. were reported as nerol (29.98%), α-bisabolol (20.86%), and butylated hydroxytoluene (18.55%). The differences in chemical composition observed among *A. visnaga* L. plants may be attributed to various ecological and genetic factors. Factors such as soil type and properties, soil management practices, and environmental stress can influence the modulation of specific enzyme groups responsible for regulating biosynthetic pathways. These factors can ultimately impact the production and abundance of phytochemical compounds in the plant [10,48,49].

Significant secondary metabolites, such as quercetin, kaempferol, rhamnocitrin, and rhamnetin, are known to be present in *A. visnaga* L., predominantly in its aerial parts. Extensive research has been conducted by multiple investigators, including [12,50], to identify and study these compounds. The presence of phenolic compounds in *A. visnaga* L. contributes to its potential pharmacological activities and associated health benefits. However, the yield of these phenolic compounds in the extract solvent can be influenced by various factors. These factors include the type of solvent used, the extraction method employed, the extraction time, and temperature, as well as the composition and physical properties of the sample [51–53]. In the conducted study, the methanol extracts of *A. visnaga* L. roots and seeds were analyzed for their TPC. The TPC values were determined to be 270.78 ± 2.86 and 366.57 ± 2.86 ± 4.09 mg GAE dry weight of the dry extract, respectively. Additionally, the investigation included the assessment of TFC, which plays a vital role as a major plant pigment with radical scavenging activity and contributes to plant coloration. The TFC levels in *A. visnaga* L. seeds and roots were found to be 242.10 ± 3.07 and 214.46 ± 2.86 mg QE per dry weight of the dry extract, respectively. It is worth noting that the TPC and TFC values obtained in our study were found to be higher than those reported in previous studies. For instance, a recent investigation reported TPC and TFC values of 76.75 ± 2.31 mg GA per gram dry weight of the dry extract and 11.75± 0.02 mg QE per gram dry weight of the dry extract, respectively, in an ethanolic extract derived from the aerial portion of *A. visnaga* L. [54]. In contrast to the findings in this research, another recent study conducted by [55] reported different results regarding the TPC and TFC in an ethanolic extract of the aerial part of *A. visnaga* L. Specifically, their study indicated that a 70% methanolic extract exhibited the highest TPC value of 176 mg GAE per gram dry weight of the dry extract and TFC value of 22 mg QE per dry weight of the dry extract. These values differ from the TPC and TFC values obtained in our study for the roots and seeds of *A. visnaga* L. It is important to acknowledge the variability that can arise in the composition and content of phenolic compounds and flavonoids due to different extraction methods and plant sources. The analysis of the essential oil derived from *A. visnaga* L. revealed a range of TPC values from 7.26 ± 1.68 mg GA per gram. Furthermore, these ranged between 5.82 ± 0.79 mg QE per gram [19]. According to a recent study conducted by El Karkouri et al. in 2020, the crude extract of *A. visnaga* L. polyphenols obtained from Morocco's Middle Atlas using Soxhlet extraction with 70% methanol yielded a content of 7.16 mg GAE per gram of phenolic components. This finding provides specific information on the phenolic content of the crude extract derived from *A. visnaga* L. in the mentioned geographical region, highlighting its potential phenolic composition and content [56]. The findings suggest the efficacy of alcoholic solvents for phenolic compound extraction, promoting safe human consumption [57,58]. Phenolic compounds have been investigated for their efficacy as robust hydrogen donors in the context of scavenging the DPPH radicalTop of Form [59].

Very few studies have examined the antioxidant properties of *A. visnaga* [12]. The investigation conducted in this research concerning the biological activities of extracts derived from the roots and seeds of *A. visnaga* L. revealed noteworthy antioxidant capabilities, as assessed through the scavenging of DPPH and ABTS radicals. The IC_{50} values for DPPH and ABTS scavenging activities were determined to be 193.46 ± 17.13 µg/mL and 227.19 ± 1.48 µg/mL, respectively. Moreover, the ABTS assay indicated IC_{50} values of 188.74 ± 2.69 µg/mL for the roots extract and 221.94 ± 1.32 µg/mL for the seeds extract, juxtaposed against the established reference standard, ascorbic acid (IC_{50} of 83.45 ± 1.24 µg/mL). Consistent with antecedent research, the findings presented herein align with a previous investigation wherein an ethanolic extract derived from the aerial component of *A. visnaga* L. demonstrated the utmost efficacy in scavenging DPPH radicals, registering a prominent activity level of 89.21% at a concentration of 3 mg/mL. This observation notably diverged from the outcomes associated with ethanol and acetone extracts at the corresponding concentration [55]. In a recent investigation, the essential oil exhibited a diminished capacity to attenuate the concentration of the DPPH free radicals, as evidenced by an obtained IC_{50} value of 4.13 ± 0.22 mg/mL. This potency stands in notable contrast to the reference antioxidant, butylated hydroxytoluene, which demonstrated a significantly superior IC_{50} value of 0.17 ± 0.01 mg/mL [19].

Flavonoids, renowned for their antioxidant and anticancer properties, play a role in inducing apoptosis, autophagy, and reducing cancer cell proliferation and invasiveness [60]. The current study aimed to assess the cytotoxic and apoptotic effects of *A. visnaga* L. roots and seeds extracts on MCF-7 and MDA-MB-231 cells. Earlier research highlighted the anticancer potential of flavonoids in *A. visnaga* leaf extract against human breast cancer BT-20 cells [61]. In a separate study, the antineoplastic efficacy of naphthoquinone was elucidated through its isolation from the leaves of the plant, specifically in the context of its impact on laryngeal cancer cells [62]. The anticancer impact of *A. visnaga* L. seeds extract was more prominent at higher concentrations, with an IC_{50} of 87.35 ± 2.44 and 72.49 ± 1.36 µg/mL for MCF-7 and MDA-MB-231 cells, respectively. In comparison, the root extract had a lower cytotoxic effect than the seed extract, with IC_{50} of 92.45 ± 2.14 and 75.43 ± 2.32 µg/mL against MCF-7 and MDA-MB-231 cells.

In a recent study, methanolic crude extracts from *A. marina*'s L. leaves exhibited potent anticancer activity against MDA-MB 231, with an IC_{50} of 480 µg/mL, showcasing superior effects compared to other extracts. The methanolic extract induced a time-dependent reduction in cell growth, suppressing it by 40%, 44%, and 59% after 24, 48, and 72 h, respectively [63]. Another study found that *A. visnaga* L. seed extract significantly decreased the viability of human hepatic carcinoma (HuH-7 cells) at concentrations of 1000 µg/mL and higher after 48 h [33].

Apoptosis, or programmed cell death, is intricately connected to various disorders, including cancer [64]. This fundamental biological process involves three primary pathways: the intrinsic pathway, regulated by mitochondria; the extrinsic pathway, mediated by death receptors; and endoplasmic reticulum stress-dependent signaling transduction. Caspase-8 serves as a mediator in the extrinsic pathway, activating executioner caspases -6 and -7 to initiate apoptosis. Simultaneously, caspase-9 acts as an important upstream mediator in the intrinsic route, initiating apoptosis by activating caspases -3 and -7 [65]. Caspase-3 engages in interactions with both caspase-8 and caspase-9, thereby showcasing its involvement in both exogenous and endogenous apoptotic properties [66]. Our RT-qPCR results showed that methanol extracts from *A. visnaga* L. root and seed, when applied to MCF-7 and MDA-MB-231 cells, increased the expression of caspase-3, -8, -9, and Bax mRNA levels while decreasing the expression of anti-apoptotic genes Bcl-2 and Bcl-xL. An early investigation demonstrated mitochondrial membrane potential dysfunction induced by *A. visnaga* L. extract, influencing the transcriptional overexpression of Bax and Bcl-2 [67]. In line with this, a recent study suggested that *A. visnaga* L. seed extract was found to upregulate caspase-3 mRNA expression in treated HuH-7 cells while downregulating Bcl-2 gene expression [33].

The rise of multidrug-resistant bacteria poses a significant challenge in treating infections and pathogenic diseases, emphasizing the urgent need to explore novel antimicrobial compounds for combatting these pathogens. Antimicrobial resistance (AMR) stands as a growing global public health threat, impacting individuals worldwide. It denotes an upsurge in the prevalence of hazardous microorganisms, including bacteria and fungi, that have developed resistance to one or more antimicrobial treatments, often referred to as multi-resistant organisms. Antibiotic resistance can manifest through various mechanisms, such as gene mutations, the production of antibiotic hydrolytic enzymes, or the horizontal gene transfer (HGT) of resistance-conferring genes. HGT, predominantly occurring between bacteria of the same species, is recognized as a major contributor to the current AMR crisis [68].

Despite significant efforts made over the past decade, natural plant-derived compounds persist as crucial and effective sources of antibacterial and anticancer agents [4].

Globally, approximately 200 plant species are recognized as medicinal plants, and they play a substantial role in the production of modern medications. These plants contribute to the synthesis of an impressive 25% to 50% of the medicines available today [9]. This study explored the antibacterial potential of methanol extracts from both roots and seeds of *A. visnaga* L., revealing potent antibacterial activity against tested bacteria. Notably, *A. visnaga* L. seeds exhibited remarkable antibacterial activity, with a MIC range from 3.81 ± 0.24 to 125 ± 7.63 μg/mL, compared to the root extract (MIC, 7.81 ± 1.74 to 62.5 ± 3.53 μg/mL). *S. epidermidis* (MTCC 12228) and *S. aureus* were notably more susceptible to the seeds with MIC (3.81 ± 0.28 and 3.81 ± 0.24 μg/mL, respectively) and roots extracts of *A. visnaga* L. with MIC (7.81 ± 0.54 and 7.81 ± 1.74 μg/mL, respectively), compared to other bacteria. Conversely, the lowest activity was observed against *P. aeruginosa* (MTCC 27853), *K. pneumoniae* (MTCC 13883), and *E. coli* (ATCC 25922), suggesting Gram-negative bacteria's greater resistance to *A. visnaga* L. for both extracts, a phenomenon linked to the structural characteristics of the Gram-negative cell wall [69]. Numerous studies have been conducted to explore the antibacterial properties of *A. visnaga* L. extracts. In one particular investigation, the ethanolic extract derived from the fruit of *A. visnaga* L. demonstrated remarkable efficacy against the Gram-positive bacterium *Enterococcus faecalis*, with a MIC value of 5 mg/mL. Additionally, this extract exhibited antibacterial activity against Gram-negative bacteria, including *E. coli* and *K. pneumoniae*, with a MIC value of 12.5 mg/mL [27]. Earlier research also indicated antibacterial potential in the aerial sections of *A. visnaga* L. extracts, particularly the methanolic extract at 10 mg/mL, which demonstrated efficiency against B. cereus strains for swarming motility and biofilm formation [55]. Numerous researchers have conducted investigations on the antibacterial activities of *A. visnaga* L. essential oils, and their effectiveness against various pathogens has been demonstrated. These studies have shown that *A. visnaga* L. essential oils exhibit notable efficacy against pathogens such as *E. coli*, *P. aeruginosa*, and *K. pneumoniae* strains [20,47,70].

In the field of in vivo research, an early study assessed the toxicity of plant extracts, which is a critical step in guaranteeing their safety for ingestion. This entails finding safe levels that do not injure cells, tissues, or organisms [71]. In a recent study involving female Wistar rats, the administration of a 1 g/kg dosage of hydroalcoholic *A. visnaga* L. extract orally for 90 days did not show any significant impact on the liver, kidneys, or spleen. Additionally, the hematological examination revealed no noteworthy changes except for an increase in white blood cell count [72]. Furthermore, a previous investigation on Albino rats was also demonstrated that *A. visnaga* L. seed ethanolic extract, administered at doses of 150, 300, and 600 mg/kg bw/d for 14 days, did not induce organ toxicity (liver, kidney, brain, spleen, heart, testis, and ovary) or mortality [73].

One limitation of this study is the absence of in vivo experiments, as they were not the primary focus of our research. Further investigations, encompassing both in vitro and in vivo trials, are essential to comprehensively explore the putative bioactivity of *A. visnaga* L. against infectious diseases.

4. Materials and Methods

4.1. *A. visnaga L. Root and Seeds Extract Preparation*

The dried plant material, comprising roots and seeds of *A. visnaga* L., was procured from a supermarket located in Riyadh, Saudi Arabia. Using a mortar and pestle, a regular blender, and an electric sieve system, the plant material was meticulously crushed into a fine powder. The preparation followed a previously established protocol [74]. In summary, approximately 300 g of *A. visnaga* L. seed and root powder were separately placed in glass jars and soaked in 1000 mL of 95% methanol. These mixtures were then subjected to agitation on a rotary shaker for 72 h. After the designated time, the mixtures were filtered through a Whatman filter paper, and the filtrates were dried at 80 °C until complete evaporation of the methanol, resulting in the crude extract of *A. visnaga*. The extracts were subsequently weighed and dissolved in methanol to achieve the desired concentration. The extracts were then diluted with dimethylsulfoxide (DMSO) (Sigma-Aldrich, Ayrshire, UK) at a concentration of 0.1% and used as a negative control. Finally, the prepared extracts were stored in sealed vials, protected from light, at a temperature of 4 °C, until further utilization.

4.2. Determination of Phytochemicals from the Methanol Roots and Seeds Extracts of A. visnaga L.

The methanol extracts of *A. visnaga* L. roots and seeds were subjected to analysis using a Chromatography-mass spectrometry (GC–MS) system manufactured by Agilent Technologies Inc. Stevens Creek Blvd, Santa Clara, CA, USA. The GC–MS system was equipped with an Agilent 5977A MSD system. The volatile compounds present in the methanol extract were purified using a capillary column with dimensions of 30 m × 0.25 mm and a 0.25 μm film thickness. Helium gas was employed as the carrier gas, with a flow rate of 0.5 mL/min. During the analysis, the injector temperature was maintained at 250 °C. The oven temperature was programmed as follows: initially, it was held at 70 °C for 3 min, then increased by 3 °C/min to reach 100 °C, and held for 3 min. Subsequently, the temperature was further increased to 120 °C at a rate of 10 °C/min and maintained for 3 min. Finally, the temperature was raised to 220 °C at a rate of 10 °C/min. The mass spectrum settings included an electron impact (EI) source, with the ionization temperature set at 230 °C and the electron energy at 70 eV. The quadrupole temperature was maintained at 150 °C, and the interface temperature was set to 280 °C. The quantity scanning range for the mass spectrum analysis ranged from 20 amu to 500 amu.

4.3. Antioxidant Activity

4.3.1. Analysis of TPC

The TPC of *A. visnaga* L. roots and seeds was determined using the Folin-Ciocalteu method, as described in a previous study conducted by [75]. In brief, approximately 0.05 mL of the *A. visnaga* L. root and seed extracts were separately mixed with 0.25 mL of Folin-Ciocalteau reagent (0.5 N), and the mixture was incubated for 10 min. Next, 2.5 mL of 0.5 M sodium carbonate solution was added, followed by an additional 30-min incubation. The optical density (OD) of the samples was measured at 765 nm against a reagent blank with a VR-2000.0 spectrophotometer (JP Selecta, Barcelona, Spain). Gallic acid was used as a standard at concentrations ranging from 10 to 100 mg/mL. The TPC was calculated as mg GAE per gram of extract at various concentrations, as mentioned in that study.

4.3.2. Analysis of TFC

The method described by Ordonez et al. was employed to assess the TFC in the extracts of *A. visnaga* L. roots and seeds [76]. In this method, approximately 0.1 mL of the *A. visnaga* L. root and seed extracts were separately incubated with 2.0 mL of a 2% AlCl3 solution for 30 min. Following incubation, the absorbance of the extract was measured using an ELX-808 microplate reader (BioTek Laboratories, LL, Shoreline, WA, USA) at a wavelength of 420 nm. A standard curve was generated using various concentrations (10–100 mg/mL) of quercetin as the reference standard. The TFC was determined by comparing the absorbance of the extracts to the standard quercetin curve. The results were expressed as mg QE/g per gram of extract.

4.3.3. DPPH Scavenging Assay

The antioxidative activity of *A. visnaga* L. roots and seeds was assessed through the utilization of the DPPH (1,1-diphenyl-2-picrylhydrazyl) scavenging assay, as outlined in a study conducted by [77]. The extracts of *A. visnaga* L. roots and seeds were prepared at four different concentrations (100, 200, 400, and 800 μg/mL). For each concentration, approximately 0.5 mL of the extract was mixed with 0.375 mL of methanol and a DPPH solution (2 mL, 0.08 mM). The reaction mixture was then placed in a dark environment and incubated for 30 min. After incubation, the OD of the mixture was measured at 517 nm using a spectrophotometer. Ascorbic acid was used as a positive control at known concentrations (μg/mL). The results were reported as IC_{50} values, which were calculated using Graph Pad Prism software (version 5.0, La Jolla, CA, USA), and the percentage of DPPH scavenging activity was determined.

4.3.4. ABTS Assay

The ABTS assay was performed by following the experimental procedure outlined by [78]. The assay was carried out by first mixing the ABTS solution (192 mg/50 mL) with the K2S2O8 solution (140 mM). Consequently, the reaction mixture was placed in the dark at room temperature for about 12 h. In addition, the ABTS solution was mixed with methanol to achieve an OD of 0.70 ± 0.02 at 734 nm. Furthermore, fifty microliters of each concentration of the extract (both roots and seeds) were thoroughly mixed with 3 mL of diluted ABTS. Moreover, the mixture was incubated for 6 min in dark conditions. Subsequently, the OD was measured at 734 nm using a VR-2000.0 spectrophotometer (JP Selecta, Barcelona, Spain). It is worth mentioning that the positive control utilized in this study was ascorbic acid (μg/mL). Lastly, the results were represented as percentages of DPPH and IC50 values.

4.4. *Cell Culture and Cytotoxicity Assays*

The two types of breast cancer cells, namely, MCF-7 (ATCC HTB-22) and MDA-MB-231 (ATCC HTB-26), were cultured in DMEM (Qiagen, Germantown, MD, USA). Moreover, the culture media were supplemented with 1% penicillin/streptomycin and 10% fetal bovine serum (FBS). Additionally, the cells were maintained at a temperature of 37 °C in a humidified atmosphere with 5% CO_2. Furthermore, the media were changed every 2–3 days to ensure optimal cell growth, as outlined in a study conducted by [79]. To assess the cytotoxicity of *A. visnaga* L. root and seed extracts, the MTT assay was conducted on MCF-7 and MDA-MB-231 cells. This method relies on mitochondrial dehydrogenases in living cells to convert MTT into formazan crystals [80,81]. First, the cells were seeded in 96-well microtiter plates at a density of 1×10^4 cells per well. Subsequently, after 24 h of incubation at 37 °C in a 5% CO_2 atmosphere, fresh media were added to the wells. In addition, a range of different concentrations of *A. visnaga* L. root and seed extracts (ranging from 50 μg/mL to 400 μg/mL) were carefully added to the wells. The plates were then incubated at 37 °C for 24 h under the same aforementioned conditions. After the 24-h incubation period, approximately 10 μL of MTT reagent (5 mg/mL) was meticulously added to each well. Moreover, a further incubation of 30 min was conducted. Consequently, 100 μL of DMSO was added to the wells and incubated for an additional 10 min. The absorbance of the samples was measured using a microtiter plate reader at a wavelength of 590 nm using an ELX-808 microplate reader (BioTek Laboratories, LL, Shoreline, WA, USA), with positive and negative controls used for comparison. The cell viability (%) was then calculated. Notably, the experiment was performed in triplicate to ensure reliable results. The mean value was considered for data analysis, and the IC_{50} value was subsequently determined using the GraphPad Prism software.

4.5. *Apoptosis Coding Genes Assay*

The evaluation of apoptosis coding genes was carried out as originally described by [34], with minor modifications. Precisely 2×10^5 MCF-7 and MDA-MB-231 cells were seeded into six-well plates containing 3 mL of culture medium. The culture medium was then mixed with roots or seeds extracts of *A. visnaga L* (100 μg/mL), respectively. After a 48-h incubation at 37 °C, the wells were washed with phosphate-buffered saline (PBS) and trypsinized using 0.25% trypsin prepared in 0.53 mM EDTA. The cells were centrifuged at 500× *g* for 5 min at 4 °C, and the upper liquid phase was discarded. The resulting pellet was used for rRT-PCR analysis to assess the expressions of apoptosis-coding genes.

To extract cellular RNA from the cancer cells, an RNeasy Micro Kit (Qiagen, Hilden, Germany) was used following the manufacturer's instructions. The extracted RNA was then subjected to qPCR using the one-step RT^2 SYBR® Green/ROX™ qPCR Master Mix. For each sample, a master mix was prepared by combining the following components: Go

Taq Qpcr master mix (2×) (10μL), one-step RT mix (0.4 μL), CXL (0.33 μL), F primer (0.4 μL), R primer (0.4 μL), RNase-free water (8.5 μL), and RNA template (4 μL). The mixture was thoroughly mixed, centrifuged, and transferred to the RT^2 PCR Array Loading Reservoir. The RT^2 Profiler PCR Array was tightly sealed with optical thin Wall Cap Strips and placed in a pre-programmed real-time instrument (7500 Applied Biosystems).

The rRT-PCR reactions were carried out in a 7500 Fast real-time PCR (7500 Fast; Applied Biosystems, Foster City, CA, USA) using the following cycling conditions: reverse transcription at 37 °C for 15 min, and initial PCR denaturation at 95 °C for 10 min. Each PCR cycle consisted of denaturation at 95 °C for 10 s, annealing at 60 °C for 30 s, and extension at 72 °C for 30 s. A total of forty cycles were performed. Melting curve analysis was performed to confirm the specificity of amplification and to ensure there were no primer dimers present. The results were analyzed using the $2^{-\Delta\Delta Cq}$ method, as described by [82]. Furthermore, Delta Cq (ΔCq) values were obtained for the different genes and, to normalize the data, these values were based on the expression of GAPDH amplified from the same samples. The fold change in expression was then calculated by comparing it to the expression of the untreated control cells. The specific oligo sequences used for the PCR amplification can be found in Table 5.

Table 5. The primer sequences of various genes involved in apoptosis and anti-apoptotic genes.

Gene Name	Primers Sequence	Reference
Caspase-3	F: 5′-GCTGGATGCCGTCTAGAGTC-3′ R: 5′-ATGTGTGGATGATGCTGCCA-3′	[83]
Caspase-8	F: 5′-AGAAGAGGGTCATCCTGGGAGA-3′ R: 5′-TCAGGACTTCCTTCAAGGCTGC-3′	[84]
Caspase-9	F: 5′-ATTGCACAGCACGTTCACAC-3′ R: 5′-TATCCCATCCCAGGAAGGCA-3′	[83]
Bax	F: 5′-GAGCTAGGGTCAGAGGGTCA-3′ R: 5′-CCCCGATTCATCTACCCTGC-3′	[83]
Bcl-2	F: 5′-ACCTACCCAGCCTCCGTTAT-3′ R: 5′-GAACTGGGGGAGGATTGTGG-3′	[83]
Bcl-XL	F: 5′-CAGAGCTTTGAACAGGTAG-3′ R: 5′-GCTCTCGGGTGCTGTATTG-3′ R: 5′-GGGCGGATTAGGGCTTCC-3′	[85]
GAPDH	F: 5′-CGGAGTCAACGGATTTGGTC-3′ R: 5′-AGCCTTCTCCATGGTCGTGA-3′	[86]

4.6. *Antibacterial Activity*

4.6.1. Microbial Strain

The antibacterial activity of the root and seed methanol extracts of *A. visnaga* was evaluated against several bacterial pathogens that included both Gram-positive and Gram-negative strains. In addition, the selected Gram-positive strains, such as *Bacillus subtilis* (MTCC-10400), Staphylococcus aureus (MTCC-29213), and *Staphylococcus epidermidis* (MTCC-12228), were included in this study. Additionally, three Gram-negative strains, namely *Klebsiella pneumoniae* (MTCC-13883), *Escherichia coli* (ATCC-25922), and *Pseudomonas aeruginosa* (MTCC-27853), were utilized. It is important to note that all of these bacterial strains were obtained from the King Khalid University Hospital in Riyadh, Saudi Arabia.

4.6.2. Disc Diffusion Method

The agar disc diffusion method, widely recognized as the gold standard, was employed in this study, following previously established procedures [87] with minor adaptations. Specifically, we utilized methanol extracts derived from *A. visnaga* L. root and seed for our analysis. Our investigation into the antimicrobial activity was conducted on nutrient agar. To cultivate the tested bacteria, they were initially incubated in nutrient agar for 24 h at 37 °C. Subsequently, a bacterial inoculum of 1×10^6 CFU/mL saline was incubated on nutrient agar for another 24 h. For the application of the bacterial inoculum, approximately 0.1 mL was evenly spread on nutrient agar plates using an "L" rod. To assess the impact of the methanol extract of *A. visnaga* L. root and seed, 20 μg of each extract was placed on separate filter paper discs (6 mm in diameter) and then incubated for 24 h. It's important to note that Chloramphenicol (20 μg/mL) served as our positive control, while a 0.1% DMSO solution in nutrient broth was used as the negative control. The resulting zones of inhibition surrounding each well-containing methanol extract of *A. visnaga* L. root and seed were measured in diameter following an overnight incubation [88].

4.6.3. Determination of MIC and MBC

The antibacterial activity of methanol extracts obtained from the roots and seeds of *A. visnaga* L. was investigated concerning both Gram-positive and Gram-negative bacteria. The evaluation was carried out using the MIC and MBC methods of broth dilution, as originally described by [89]. However, minor modifications were implemented in the assay procedure for this study. The assay was carried out employing microtiter plates. Firstly, approximately 300 μL of nutrient broth medium was added to each well. Subsequently, a series of dilutions of the root and seed extracts (ranging from 1.56 to 800 μg/mL) were separately added to different plates. Following this, 20 μL of inoculum containing 1×10^5 CFU/mL was added to all the wells. The microtiter plates were then incubated at 37 °C for 18 h. The presence or absence of bacterial growth was determined by visually observing changes in turbidity. Hence, meticulous examination of all the wells in the microtiter plate was conducted to discern any discernible alterations in turbidity, which would indicate bacterial growth. It is noteworthy that Chloramphenicol (20 μg/mL) and 0.1% DMSO served as the positive and negative controls, respectively. MBC determinations were confirmed by spreading the culture from wells that showed no growth onto nutrient agar plates, following the methodology described by [90].

4.7. Statistical Analysis

To analyze the data, a One-Way ANOVA was conducted, and a significant level was observed. It is important to note that all experiments were performed in triplicates, and the mean standard deviation (SD) was utilized for the analysis. To determine statistical significance, a threshold of "p" value > 0.05 was adopted.

5. Conclusions

In this study, the primary objective was to evaluate the antioxidant, anticancer, and antibacterial properties of a methanol extract obtained from the roots and seeds of *A. visnaga* L. To this end, the phenolic compounds and flavonoids present in *A. visnaga* L. were analyzed, suggesting its potential as an antioxidant agent. Comparing the roots and seeds of *A. visnaga* L. to the positive control, we observed significant antioxidant, cytotoxic, and antibacterial activities in both samples. The methanolic extracts from both roots and seeds exhibited heightened antioxidant activity, with the seeds extract displaying superior antioxidant, anticancer, and antibacterial effects compared to the root extract. These findings collectively suggest that *A. visnaga* extracts harbor antioxidant, cytotoxic, and antibacterial properties, indicating their potential clinical use as therapeutic agents for reducing disease risk.

Author Contributions: Conceptualization, I.M.A.; methodology, I.M.A.; software, I.M.A.; validation, H.R. and N.A.A.; formal analysis, I.M.A.; investigation, F.A.; resources, I.M.A. data curation, F.A.; writing—original draft preparation, R.M.A. (Rawan M. Alshalan) and I.M.A.; writing—review and editing, R.M.A. (Rawan M. Alshalan), F.A. and H.R.; visualization, R.M.A. (Rawan M. Alshalan) and N.A.A.; supervision, N.A.A., A.M.A. and R.M.A. (Reem M. Aljowaie); project administration, N.A.A.; funding acquisition, N.A.A., A.M.A. and R.M.A. (Reem M. Aljowaie). All authors have read and agreed to the published version of the manuscript.

Funding: This research received no external funding.

Institutional Review Board Statement: Not applicable.

Informed Consent Statement: Informed consent was obtained from all subjects involved in this study.

Data Availability Statement: Data is contained within the article.

Acknowledgments: The authors thank the Researchers Supporting Project number (RSP2024R418), King Saud University, Riyadh, Saudi Arabia.

Conflicts of Interest: The authors declare no conflicts of interest.

References

1. Panche, A.N.; Diwan, A.D.; Chandra, S.R. Flavonoids: An overview. *J. Nutr. Sci.* **2016**, *5*, e47. [CrossRef]
2. Paz, J.E.W.; Contreras, C.R.; Munguía, A.R.; Aguilar, C.N.; Inungaray, M.L.C. Phenolic content and antibacterial activity of extracts of Hamelia patens obtained by different extraction methods. *Braz. J. Microbiol.* **2018**, *49*, 656–661. [CrossRef]
3. Bourais, I.; Elmarrkechy, S.; Taha, D.; Mourabit, Y.; Bouyahya, A.; El Yadini, M.; Machich, O.; El Hajjaji, S.; El Boury, H.; Dakka, N. A Review on Medicinal Uses, Nutritional Value, and Antimicrobial, Antioxidant, Anti-Inflammatory, Antidiabetic, and Anticancer Potential Related to Bioactive Compounds of J. regia. *Food Rev. Int.* **2022**, *39*, 6199–6249. [CrossRef]
4. Hashem, S.; Ta, A.; Akhtar, S.; Nisar, S.; Sageena, G.; Ali, S.; Al-Mannai, S.; Therachiyil, L.; Mir, R.; Elfaki, I. Targeting cancer signaling pathways by natural products: Exploring promising anti-cancer agents. *Biomed. Pharmacother.* **2022**, *150*, 113054. [CrossRef] [PubMed]
5. Bhilkar, P.; Bodhne, A.; Yerpude, S.; Madankar, R.; Somkuwar, S.; Chaudhary, A.; Lambat, A.; Desimone, M.; Sharma, R.; Chaudhary, R. Phyto-derived metal nanoparticles: Prominent tool for biomedical applications. *OpenNano* **2023**, *14*, 100192. [CrossRef]
6. Gahtori, R.; Tripathi, A.H.; Kumari, A.; Negi, N.; Paliwal, A.; Tripathi, P.; Joshi, P.; Rai, R.C.; Upadhyay, S.K. Anticancer plant-derivatives: Deciphering their oncopreventive and therapeutic potential in molecular terms. *Future J. Pharm. Sci.* **2023**, *9*, 14. [CrossRef]
7. Goel, H.; Kumar, R.; Tanwar, P.; Upadhyay, T.K.; Khan, F.; Pandey, P.; Kang, S.; Moon, M.; Choi, J.; Choi, M. Unraveling the therapeutic potential of natural products in the prevention and treatment of leukemia. *Biomed. Pharmacother.* **2023**, *160*, 114351. [CrossRef]
8. Nirmala, N.S.; Krishnan, N.B.; Vivekanandan, V.; Thirugnanasambantham, K. Anti-inflammatory Potential of Lead Compounds and Their Derivatives from Medicinal Plants. In *Bioprospecting of Tropical Medicinal Plants*; Springer: Berlin/Heidelberg, Germany, 2023; pp. 1199–1232.
9. Adedokun, K.A.; Imodoye, S.O.; Bello, I.O.; Lanihun, A.-A. Therapeutic potentials of medicinal plants and significance of computational tools in anti-cancer drug discovery. In *Phytochemistry, Computational Tools and Databases in Drug Discovery*; Elsevier: Amsterdam, The Netherlands, 2023; pp. 393–455.
10. Hashim, S.; Jan, A.; Marwat, K.B.; Khan, M.A. Phytochemistry and medicinal properties of *Ammi visnaga* (Apiacae). *Pak. J. Bot.* **2014**, *46*, 861–867.
11. Oakeley, H. *Modern Medicines from Plants: Botanical Histories of Some of Modern Medicine's Most Important Drugs*; CRC Press: Boca Raton, FL, USA, 2023.
12. Khalil, N.; Bishr, M.; Desouky, S.; Salama, O. *Ammi visnaga*, L. a potential medicinal plant: A review. *Molecules* **2020**, *25*, 301. [CrossRef] [PubMed]
13. Saad, B.; Azaizeh, H.; Said, O. Tradition and perspectives of Arab herbal medicine: A review. *Evid.-Based Complement. Altern. Med.* **2005**, *2*, 475–479. [CrossRef]
14. Patel, K.; Rahman, M.; Kumar, V.; Verma, A.; Patel, D.K. Visnagin: A New Perspective of Medicinal Importance, Physiological Functions, Phytochemistry, Pharmacology and Analytical Aspects of Active Phytoconstituents of *Ammi visnaga*. *Nat. Prod. J.* **2019**, *9*, 197–206. [CrossRef]
15. Golkar, P.; Akbari, R.; Bazarganipour, M.; Javed, R. Biochemical and phytochemical responses of *Ammi visnaga* L. (Apiaceae) callus culture elicited by SiO_2 and graphene Oxide-SiO_2 nanoparticles. *Plant Physiol. Biochem.* **2023**, *200*, 107741. [CrossRef] [PubMed]
16. Bahmanpoor, N.; Hamdi, S.M.M.; Ataee, R. Real-Time-RT PCR Study of Extract of *Ammi visnaga* on Pseudomonas aeruginosa Exo A and Exo S Genes Expression. *Iran. J. Med. Microbiol.* **2023**, *17*, 186–193. [CrossRef]
17. Mohamed, Z.; Abdel-Motaal, F.F. Antioxidant and Antifungal Activities of *Ammi visnaga* Aqueous Extract Prevent Oxidative Stress Biomarkers and DNA Damage in Experimental Rats Infected with *Aspergillus glaucus*. *Biol. Bull.* **2023**, *50*, 1125–1142. [CrossRef]
18. Elgamal, M.H.A.; Shalaby, N.M.; Duddeck, H.; Hiegemann, M. Coumarins and coumarin glucosides from the fruits of *Ammi majus*. *Phytochemistry* **1993**, *34*, 819–823. [CrossRef]
19. Kamal, F.Z.; Stanciu, G.D.; Lefter, R.; Cotea, V.V.; Niculaua, M.; Ababei, D.C.; Ciobica, A.; Ech-Chahad, A. Chemical composition and antioxidant activity of *Ammi visnaga* L. essential oil. *Antioxidants* **2022**, *11*, 347. [CrossRef]
20. Feirouz, B.; Salima, K.-G. Antibacterial activity and chemical composition of *Ammi visnaga* L. essential oil collected from Boumerdes (Algeria) during three periods of the plant growth. *J. Essent. Oil Bear. Plants* **2014**, *17*, 1317–1328. [CrossRef]

21. El Hachlafi, N.; Benkhaira, N.; Al-Mijalli, S.H.; Mrabti, H.N.; Abdnim, R.; Abdallah, E.M.; Jeddi, M.; Bnouham, M.; Lee, L.-H.; Ardianto, C. Phytochemical analysis and evaluation of antimicrobial, antioxidant, and antidiabetic activities of essential oils from Moroccan medicinal plants: *Mentha suaveolens*, *Lavandula stoechas*, and *Ammi visnaga*. *Biomed. Pharmacother.* **2023**, *164*, 114937. [CrossRef]
22. Bakkali, F.; Averbeck, S.; Averbeck, D.; Idaomar, M. Biological effects of essential oils—A review. *Food Chem. Toxicol.* **2008**, *46*, 446–475. [CrossRef]
23. Khan, Z.A.; Assiri, A.M.; Al-Afghani, H.M.; Maghrabi, T.M. Inhibition of oxalate nephrolithiasis with *Ammi visnaga* (AI-Khillah). *Int. Urol. Nephrol.* **2001**, *33*, 605–608. [CrossRef]
24. Yadav, R.D.; Jain, S.; Alok, S.; Mahor, A.; Bharti, J.P.; Jaiswal, M. Herbal plants used in the treatment of urolithiasis: A review. *IJPSR* **2011**, *2*, 1412–1420.
25. Kilicaslan, I.; Coskun, S. Spontaneous stone passage: Is it *Ammi visnaga* effect? *Urol. Res.* **2012**, *40*, 799–800. [CrossRef]
26. Jouad, H.; Maghrani, M.; Eddouks, M. Hypoglycemic effect of aqueous extract of *Ammi visnaga* in normal and streptozotocin-induced diabetic rats. *J. Herb. Pharmacother.* **2002**, *2*, 19–29. [CrossRef] [PubMed]
27. Ghareeb, A.M.; Zedan, T.H.; Gharb, L. Antibacterial and antifungal activities of *Ammi visnaga* extracts against pathogenic microorganisms. *Iraqi J. Sci.* **2011**, *52*, 30–36.
28. Amin, J.N.; Murad, A.; Motasem, A.-M.; Ibrahem, S.R.; Ass'ad, J.M.; Ayed, A.M. Phytochemical screening and in-vitro evaluation of antioxidant and antimicrobial activities of the entire Khella plant (*Ammi visnaga.* L.) a member of palestinian flora. *Int. J. Pharmacogn. Phytochem. Res.* **2015**, *7*, 137–143.
29. Batanouny, K.; Abou Tabl, S.; Shabana, M.S. Wild Medicinal Plants in Egypt (An Inventory to Support Onservation and Sustainable Use). *Cairo Egypt Palm Press C* **1999**, *154*, 1–48.
30. Farnsworth, N.R.; Krause, E.C.; Bolton, J.L.; Pauli, G.F.; van Breemen, R.B.; Graham, J.G. The university of Illinois at Chicago/National institutes of health center for botanical dietary supplements research for women's health: From plant to clinical use. *Am. J. Clin. Nutr.* **2008**, *87*, 504S–508S. [CrossRef]
31. Lee, J.-K.; Jung, J.-S.; Park, S.-H.; Park, S.-H.; Sim, Y.-B.; Kim, S.-M.; Ha, T.-S.; Suh, H.-W. Anti-inflammatory effect of visnagin in lipopolysaccharide-stimulated BV-2 microglial cells. *Arch. Pharmacal Res.* **2010**, *33*, 1843–1850. [CrossRef]
32. Kwon, M.-S.; Lee, J.-K.; Park, S.-H.; Sim, Y.-B.; Jung, J.-S.; Won, M.-H.; Kim, S.-M.; Suh, H.-W. Neuroprotective effect of visnagin on kainic acid-induced neuronal cell death in the mice hippocampus. *Korean J. Physiol. Pharmacol.* **2010**, *14*, 257–263. [CrossRef]
33. Arafah, M.W.; Almutairi, B.; Al-Zharani, M.; Alkahtane, A.A.; Al-Otibi, F.O.; Ali, D.; Alghamdi, W.M.; Alanazi, I.S.; Aljarba, N.H.; Alhoshani, N.M. The protective effect of Ammi visnaga extract against human hepatic cancer. *J. King Saud Univ.-Sci.* **2021**, *33*, 101540. [CrossRef]
34. Ferreira, E.; Cronjé, M.J. Selection of suitable reference genes for quantitative real-time PCR in apoptosis-induced MCF-7 breast cancer cells. *Mol. Biotechnol.* **2012**, *50*, 121–128. [CrossRef] [PubMed]
35. Yapasert, R.; Banjerdpongchai, R. Gambogic Acid and Piperine Synergistically Induce Apoptosis in Human Cholangiocarcinoma Cell via Caspase and Mitochondria-Mediated Pathway. *Evid.-Based Complement. Altern. Med.* **2022**, *2022*, 6288742. [CrossRef]
36. Bhadra, K. A Mini Review on Molecules Inducing Caspase-Independent Cell Death: A New Route to Cancer Therapy. *Molecules* **2022**, *27*, 6401. [CrossRef] [PubMed]
37. Hussain, M.S.; Gupta, G.; Afzal, M.; Alqahtani, S.M.; Samuel, V.P.; Kazmi, I.; Alzarea, S.I.; Saleem, S.; Dureja, H.; Singh, S.K. Exploring the role of lncrna neat1 knockdown in regulating apoptosis across multiple cancer types: A review. *Pathol.-Res. Pract.* **2023**, *252*, 154908. [CrossRef] [PubMed]
38. Hashem, R.; Al-Obaidi, Z.F.; Samawi, F.T.; Baher, H. Analysis of anti-apoptotic protein (Bcl-xl) levels and mRNA expression in infertile patients. *Afr. J. Reprod. Health* **2022**, *26*, 63–71. [PubMed]
39. Bernal, C.; Otalora, A.; Cañas, A.; Barreto, A.; Prieto, K.; Montecino, M.; Rojas, A. Regulatory Role of the RUNX2 Transcription Factor in Lung Cancer Apoptosis. *Int. J. Cell Biol.* **2022**, *2022*, 5198203. [CrossRef]
40. Lopez, A.; Reyna, D.E.; Gitego, N.; Kopp, F.; Zhou, H.; Miranda-Roman, M.A.; Nordstrøm, L.U.; Narayanagari, S.-R.; Chi, P.; Vilar, E. Co-targeting of BAX and BCL-XL proteins broadly overcomes resistance to apoptosis in cancer. *Nat. Commun.* **2022**, *13*, 1199. [CrossRef] [PubMed]
41. Salmerón-Manzano, E.; Garrido-Cardenas, J.A.; Manzano-Agugliaro, F. Worldwide research trends on medicinal plants. *Int. J. Environ. Res. Public Health* **2020**, *17*, 3376. [CrossRef] [PubMed]
42. Réthy, B.; Csupor-Löffler, B.; Zupkó, I.; Hajdú, Z.; Máthé, I.; Hohmann, J.; Rédei, T.; Falkay, G. Antiproliferative activity of Hungarian Asteraceae species against human cancer cell lines. Part I. *Phytother. Res. Int. J. Devoted Pharmacol. Toxicol. Eval. Nat. Prod. Deriv.* **2007**, *21*, 1200–1208. [CrossRef] [PubMed]
43. Ramakrishna, W.; Kumari, A.; Rahman, N.; Mandave, P. Anticancer activities of plant secondary metabolites: Rice callus suspension culture as a new paradigm. *Rice Sci.* **2021**, *28*, 13–30. [CrossRef]
44. Günaydin, K.; Beyazit, N. The chemical investigations on the ripe fruits of *Ammi visnaga* (Lam.) Lamarck growing in Turkey. *Nat. Prod. Res.* **2004**, *18*, 169–175. [CrossRef]
45. Zrira, S.; Elamrani, A.; Pellerin, P.; Bessière, J.-M.; Menut, C.; Benjilali, B. Isolation of Moroccan *Ammi visnaga* oil: Comparison between hydrodistillation, steam distillation and supercritical fluid extraction. *J. Essent. Oil Bear. Plants* **2008**, *11*, 30–35. [CrossRef]

46. Jabboury, Z.E.; Ousaaid, D.; Gašić, U.; Janaćković, P.; Stevanovic, Z.D.; Kolašinac, S.; Benjelloun, M.; Ghadraoui, L.E. Unraveling the Phytochemical Profile Variability and Antioxidant Activities of Different Parts of *Ammi visnaga* (L) Collected from Taounate Region. *Chem. Afr.* **2023**, 1–7. [CrossRef]
47. Soro, K.; Sabri, L.; Amalich, S.; Khabbal, Y.; Zair, T. Chemical composition of Moroccan *Ammi visnaga* L. (Lam.) and antibacterial activity of its essential oil against extended-spectrum beta-lactamase-producing and not producing bacteria. *Phytotherapie* **2015**, *13*, 168–175. [CrossRef]
48. Samuel, A.D.; Tit, D.M.; Melinte, C.E.; Iovan, C.; Purza, L.; Gitea, M.; Bungau, S. Enzymological and physicochemical evaluation of the effects of soil management practices. *Rev. Chim.* **2017**, *68*, 2243–2247. [CrossRef]
49. Samuel, A.D.; Bungau, S.; Tit, D.M.; Melinte, C.E.; Purza, L.; Badea, G.E. Effects of long term application of organic and mineral fertilizers on soil enzymes. *Rev. Chim.* **2018**, *69*, 2608–2612. [CrossRef]
50. Osama, S.; El Sherei, M.; Al-Mahdy, D.A.; Bishr, M.; Salama, O. Effect of salicylic acid foliar spraying on growth parameters, γ-pyrones, phenolic content and radical scavenging activity of drought stressed *Ammi visnaga* L. plant. *Ind. Crops Prod.* **2019**, *134*, 1–10. [CrossRef]
51. Tan, K.W.; Kassim, M.J. A correlation study on the phenolic profiles and corrosion inhibition properties of mangrove tannins (*Rhizophora apiculata*) as affected by extraction solvents. *Corros. Sci.* **2011**, *53*, 569–574. [CrossRef]
52. Aourabi, S.; Driouch, M.; Sfaira, M.; Mahjoubi, F.; Hammouti, B.; Emran, K. Influence of phenolic compounds on antioxidant and anticorrosion activities of *Ammi visnaga* extracts obtained ultrasonically in three solvent systems. *Int. J. Electrochem. Sci.* **2019**, *14*, 6376–6393. [CrossRef]
53. Isleroglu, H.; Turker, I. Ultrasonic-assisted extraction and thermal stability of phytochemicals from fenugreek leaves. *J. Appl. Res. Med. Aromat. Plants* **2022**, *30*, 100390. [CrossRef]
54. Aourabi, S.; Driouch, M.; Ammor, K.; Sfaira, M.; Touhami, M.E.; Mahjoubi, F. Evaluation of anticorrosion and antioxidant activities of ethanolic extract of *Ammi visnaga*. *Anal Bioanal Electrochem.* **2018**, *10*, 912–929.
55. Imane, B.; Ouafa, R.; Rachid, D. Antimicrobial and antioxidant activity of *Ammi visnaga* (L) phenolic extracts and their effects on planktonic and biofilm growth of food spoilage *Bacillus cereus*. *Int. J. Biosci.* **2016**, *9*, 32–47.
56. El Karkouri, J.; Drioiche, A.; Soro, A.; Ailli, A.; Benhlima, N.; Bouzoubaa, A.; El Makhoukhi, F.; Oulhaj, H.; Elombo, F.K.; Zair, T. Identification and antioxidant activity of *Ammi Visnaga* L. Polyphenols from the Middle Atlas in Morocco. *Mediterr. J. Chem.* **2020**, *10*, 649. [CrossRef]
57. Shi, J.; Nawaz, H.; Pohorly, J.; Mittal, G.; Kakuda, Y.; Jiang, Y. Extraction of polyphenolics from plant material for functional foods—Engineering and technology. *Food Rev. Int.* **2005**, *21*, 139–166. [CrossRef]
58. Alara, O.R.; Abdurahman, N.H.; Ukaegbu, C.I. Extraction of phenolic compounds: A review. *Curr. Res. Food Sci.* **2021**, *4*, 200–214. [CrossRef] [PubMed]
59. Babbar, N.; Oberoi, H.S.; Sandhu, S.K.; Bhargav, V.K. Influence of different solvents in extraction of phenolic compounds from vegetable residues and their evaluation as natural sources of antioxidants. *J. Food Sci. Technol.* **2014**, *51*, 2568–2575. [CrossRef] [PubMed]
60. Kopustinskiene, D.M.; Jakstas, V.; Savickas, A.; Bernatoniene, J. Flavonoids as anticancer agents. *Nutrients* **2020**, *12*, 457. [CrossRef]
61. Kooti, W.; Servatyari, K.; Behzadifar, M.; Asadi-Samani, M.; Sadeghi, F.; Nouri, B.; Zare Marzouni, H. Effective medicinal plant in cancer treatment, part 2: Review study. *J. Evid.-Based Complement. Altern. Med.* **2017**, *22*, 982–995. [CrossRef]
62. Sharaf, M.; El-Ansari, M.; Saleh, N. New flavonoids from Avicennia marina. *Fitoterapia* **2000**, *71*, 274–277. [CrossRef]
63. Behbahani, M.; Sadeghi-aliabadi, H. Evalution of cytotoxic effect of some extracts of *Avicennia marina* against MDA-MB 231 human breast cancer cell line. *Pharm. Sci.* **2010**, *16*, 229–238.
64. Park, W.; Wei, S.; Kim, B.-S.; Kim, B.; Bae, S.-J.; Chae, Y.C.; Ryu, D.; Ha, K.-T. Diversity and complexity of cell death: A historical review. *Exp. Mol. Med.* **2023**, *55*, 1573–1594. [CrossRef]
65. Lossi, L. The concept of intrinsic versus extrinsic apoptosis. *Biochem. J.* **2022**, *479*, 357–384. [CrossRef] [PubMed]
66. Jiang, M.; Qi, L.; Li, L.; Li, Y. The caspase-3/GSDME signal pathway as a switch between apoptosis and pyroptosis in cancer. *Cell Death Discov.* **2020**, *6*, 112. [CrossRef]
67. Wang, X.; Peng, P.; Pan, Z.; Fang, Z.; Lu, W.; Liu, X. Psoralen inhibits malignant proliferation and induces apoptosis through triggering endoplasmic reticulum stress in human SMMC7721 hepatoma cells. *Biol. Res.* **2019**, *52*, 34. [CrossRef] [PubMed]
68. Roberts, M.; Burgess, S.; Toombs-Ruane, L.; Benschop, J.; Marshall, J.; French, N. Combining mutation and horizontal gene transfer in a within-host model of antibiotic resistance. *Math. Biosci.* **2021**, *339*, 108656. [CrossRef]
69. Singh, G.; Kapoor, I.; Singh, P.; de Heluani, C.S.; de Lampasona, M.P.; Catalan, C.A. Chemistry, antioxidant and antimicrobial investigations on essential oil and oleoresins of Zingiber officinale. *Food Chem. Toxicol.* **2008**, *46*, 3295–3302. [CrossRef] [PubMed]
70. Satrani, B.; Farah, A.; Fechtal, M.; Talbi, M.; Boumari, M. Chemical composition and antimicrobial and antifungal activities of the essential oil of *Ammi visnaga* (L.) Lam. *Acta. Bot. Gal* **2004**, *151*, 65–71. [CrossRef]
71. Abebe, M.S.; Asres, K.; Bekuretsion, Y.; Abebe, A.; Bikila, D.; Seyoum, G. Sub-chronic toxicity of ethanol leaf extract of *Syzygium guineense* on the biochemical parameters and histopathology of liver and kidney in the rats. *Toxicol. Rep.* **2021**, *8*, 822–828. [CrossRef]
72. Ndayambaje, M.; Wahnou, H.; Sow, M.; Chgari, O.; Habyarimana, T.; Karkouri, M.; Limami, Y.; Naya, A.; Oudghiri, M. Exploring the multifaceted effects of *Ammi visnaga*: Subchronic toxicity, antioxidant capacity, immunomodulatory, and anti-inflammatory activities. *J. Toxicol. Environ. Health Part A* **2023**, *87*, 150–165. [CrossRef]

73. Koriem, K.M.; Arbid, M.S.; El-Attar, M.A. Acute and subacute toxicity of *Ammi visnaga* on rats. *Interdiscip. Toxicol.* **2019**, *12*, 26–35. [CrossRef]
74. Al-Hadhrami, R.M.S.; Hossain, M.A. Evaluation of antioxidant, antimicrobial and cytotoxic activities of seed crude extracts of *Ammi majus* grown in Oman. *Egypt. J. Basic Appl. Sci.* **2016**, *3*, 329–334. [CrossRef]
75. Wolfe, K.L.; Liu, R.H. Apple peels as a value-added food ingredient. *J. Agric. Food Chem.* **2003**, *51*, 1676–1683. [CrossRef] [PubMed]
76. Ordonez, A.; Gomez, J.; Vattuone, M. Antioxidant activities of *Sechium edule* (Jacq.) Swartz extracts. *Food Chem.* **2006**, *97*, 452–458. [CrossRef]
77. Tian, M.; Wu, X.; Lu, T.; Zhao, X.; Wei, F.; Deng, G.; Zhou, Y. Phytochemical analysis, antioxidant, antibacterial, cytotoxic, and enzyme inhibitory activities of *Hedychium flavum* rhizome. *Front. Pharmacol.* **2020**, *11*, 572659. [CrossRef] [PubMed]
78. Yu, X.; Zhao, M.; Liu, F.; Zeng, S.; Hu, J. Antioxidants in volatile Maillard reaction products: Identification and interaction. *LWT-Food Sci. Technol.* **2013**, *53*, 22–28. [CrossRef]
79. Kis, B.; Pavel, I.Z.; Avram, S.; Moaca, E.A.; Herrero San Juan, M.; Schwiebs, A.; Radeke, H.H.; Muntean, D.; Diaconeasa, Z.; Minda, D. Antimicrobial activity, in vitro anticancer effect (MCF-7 breast cancer cell line), antiangiogenic and immunomodulatory potentials of *Populus nigra* L. buds extract. *BMC Complement. Med. Ther.* **2022**, *22*, 74. [CrossRef]
80. Riss, T.L.; Moravec, R.A.; Niles, A.L.; Duellman, S.; Benink, H.A.; Worzella, T.J.; Minor, L. Cell viability assays. In *Assay Guidance Manual [Internet]*; Eli Lilly & Company: Indianapolis, IN, USA; National Center for Advancing Translational Sciences: Bethesda, MD, USA, 2016; pp. 1–31.
81. Sukumaran, A.; Sweety, V.K.; Vikas, B.; Joseph, B. Cytotoxicity and Cell Viability Assessment of Biomaterials. In *Cytotoxicity-Understanding Cellular Damage and Response*; Intechopen: London, UK, 2023. [CrossRef]
82. Schmittgen, T.D.; Livak, K.J. Analyzing real-time PCR data by the comparative CT method. *Nat. Protoc.* **2008**, *3*, 1101–1108. [CrossRef]
83. Alotaibi, M.R.; Hassan, Z.K.; Al-Rejaie, S.S.; Alshammari, M.A.; Almutairi, M.M.; Alhoshani, A.R.; Alanazi, W.A.; Hafez, M.M.; Al-Shabanah, O.A. Characterization of apoptosis in a breast cancer cell line after IL-10 silencing. *Asian Pac. J. Cancer Prev. APJCP* **2018**, *19*, 777.
84. Honarpisheh, M.; Desai, J.; Marschner, J.A.; Weidenbusch, M.; Lech, M.; Vielhauer, V.; Anders, H.-J.; Mulay, S.R. Regulated necrosis-related molecule mRNA expression in humans and mice and in murine acute tissue injury and systemic autoimmunity leading to progressive organ damage, and progressive fibrosis. *Biosci. Rep.* **2016**, *36*, e00425. [CrossRef]
85. Buskaran, K.; Bullo, S.; Hussein, M.Z.; Masarudin, M.J.; Mohd Moklas, M.A.; Fakurazi, S. Anticancer Molecular Mechanism of Protocatechuic Acid Loaded on Folate Coated Functionalized Graphene Oxide Nanocomposite Delivery System in Human Hepatocellular Carcinoma. *Materials* **2021**, *14*, 817. [CrossRef]
86. Jiang, Q.; Yang, M.; Qu, Z.; Zhou, J.; Zhang, Q. Resveratrol enhances anticancer effects of paclitaxel in HepG2 human liver cancer cells. *BMC Complement. Altern. Med.* **2017**, *17*, 477. [CrossRef]
87. Salem, N.; Kefi, S.; Tabben, O.; Ayed, A.; Jallouli, S.; Feres, N.; Hammami, M.; Khammassi, S.; Hrigua, I.; Nefisi, S. Variation in chemical composition of *Eucalyptus globulus* essential oil under phenological stages and evidence synergism with antimicrobial standards. *Ind. Crops Prod.* **2018**, *124*, 115–125. [CrossRef]
88. Al-Dhabi, N.A.; Valan Arasu, M.; Vijayaraghavan, P.; Esmail, G.A.; Duraipandiyan, V.; Kim, Y.O.; Kim, H.; Kim, H.-J. Probiotic and antioxidant potential of Lactobacillus reuteri LR12 and Lactobacillus lactis LL10 isolated from pineapple puree and quality analysis of pineapple-flavored goat milk yoghurt during storage. *Microorganisms* **2020**, *8*, 1461. [CrossRef]
89. Basri, D.F.; Sandra, V. Synergistic interaction of methanol extract from *Canarium odontophyllum* Miq. Leaf in combination with oxacillin against methicillin-resistant *Staphylococcus aureus* (MRSA) ATCC 33591. *Int. J. Microbiol.* **2016**, *2016*, 5249534. [CrossRef]
90. Aljeldah, M.M.; Yassin, M.T.; Mostafa, A.A.-F.; Aboul-Soud, M.A. Synergistic Antibacterial Potential of Greenly Synthesized Silver Nanoparticles with Fosfomycin against Some Nosocomial Bacterial Pathogens. *Infect. Drug Resist.* **2022**, *16*, 125–142. [CrossRef] [PubMed]

pharmaceuticals

MDPI

Review

Anticancer Potential and Molecular Targets of Pristimerin in Human Malignancies

Kirti S. Prabhu [1,*,†], Serah Jessy [1,†], Shilpa Kuttikrishnan [1,†], Farina Mujeeb [2], Zahwa Mariyam [1], Ummu Habeeba [1], Nuha Ahmad [1], Ajaz A. Bhat [3] and Shahab Uddin [1,2,4,5,*]

1 Translational Research Institute, Academic Health System, Hamad Medical Corporation, Doha 3050, Qatar; serahjessym@gmail.com (S.J.); skuttikrishnan@hamad.qa (S.K.); v-zpurayil@hamad.qa (Z.M.); v-uhabeeba@hamad.qa (U.H.); nuha001ahmad@gmail.com (N.A.)

2 Department of Biosciences, Integral University, Lucknow 226026, Uttar Pradesh, India; farinam@iul.ac.in

3 Department of Human Genetics-Precision Medicine in Diabetes, Obesity, and Cancer Program, Sidra Medicine, Doha 26999, Qatar; abhat@sidra.org

4 Dermatology Institute, Academic Health System, Hamad Medical Corporation, Doha 3050, Qatar

5 Laboratory of Animal Research Center, Qatar University, Doha 2713, Qatar

* Correspondence: kprabhu@hamad.qa (K.S.P.); skhan34@hamad.qa (S.U.); Tel.: +974-443-90966 (K.S.P.); +974-402-53220 (S.U.); Fax: +974-443-98792 (S.U.)

† These authors contributed equally to this work.

Abstract: The growing global burden of malignant tumors with increasing incidence and mortality rates underscores the urgent need for more effective and less toxic therapeutic options. Herbal compounds are being increasingly studied for their potential to meet these needs due to their reduced side effects and significant efficacy. Pristimerin (PS), a triterpenoid from the quinone formamide class derived from the Celastraceae and Hippocrateaceae families, has emerged as a potent anticancer agent. It exhibits broad-spectrum anti-tumor activity across various cancers such as breast, pancreatic, prostate, glioblastoma, colorectal, cervical, and lung cancers. PS modulates several key cellular processes, including apoptosis, autophagy, cell migration and invasion, angiogenesis, and resistance to chemotherapy, targeting crucial signaling pathways such as those involving NF-κB, p53, and STAT3, among others. The main objective of this review is to provide a comprehensive synthesis of the current literature on PS, emphasizing its mechanisms of action and molecular targets with the utmost clarity. It discusses the comparative advantages of PS over current cancer therapies and explores the implications for future research and clinical applications. By delineating the specific pathways and targets affected by PS, this review seeks to offer valuable insights and directions for future research in this field. The information gathered in this review could pave the way for the successful development of PS into a clinically applicable anticancer therapy.

Keywords: Pristimerin; apoptosis; autophagy; reactive oxygen species; signaling pathways

1. Introduction

Cancer is a significant global health issue that has attracted attention due to its devastating impact on humans worldwide. Chemotherapy, radiotherapy, immunotherapy, genetic and targeted treatment, hormone therapy, and surgery represent subsets of the multifaceted approaches that have been employed in the pursuit of cancer treatment. Among the myriad therapeutic alternatives at our disposal, chemotherapy stands out as a widely recognized modality that exhibits remarkable efficacy in the management of neoplastic growths [1]. Nevertheless, it is crucial to recognize the possible drawbacks linked to chemotherapy, including the development of multidrug resistance (MDR) in cancer cells and the occurrence of severe drug-induced adverse effects. Henceforth, it is imperative to foster the development of more efficacious treatment modalities [2,3].

For centuries, traditional Chinese medicine (TCM) has been seen as a potential remedy for the challenges that cancer poses [4]. This choice is primarily driven by the remarkably diminished likelihood of encountering adverse effects and an elevated probability of achieving triumphant outcomes. Numerous naturally occurring compounds discovered within the realm of TCM have been scientifically validated for their remarkable anticancer attributes. Among these compounds are resveratrol, dioscin, berberine, curcumin, baicalein, wogonin, silibinin, quercetin, celastrol, and PS [1,4–9].

Triterpenoids are a class of essential compounds found in plants as specialized metabolites. Quinone methide triterpenoids, a specific group of compounds containing a quinone ring, have been of particular interest due to their cytotoxic and anti-tumoral activities [10]. Pristimerin (PS), 20α-3-hydroxy-2-oxo-24-nor-friedela-1-10,3,5,7-tetraen-carboxylicacid-29-methylester, with the molecular formula $C_{30}H_{40}O_4$ (Figure 1), a quinonemethide triterpenoid compound of indigenous origin, is taxonomically categorized within the families Celastraceae and Hippocrateaceae. In 1951, Bhatnagar and Divekar achieved the commendable feat of isolating PS from botanical specimens of *Pristimerae indica* and *P. grahami*. Consequently, in 1954, diligent efforts were made by Kulkarni and Shah to successfully ascertain its precise molecular structure, thus solidifying its scientific identity [11]. Pristimerin has various pharmacological properties including anticancer, antioxidant, anti-inflammatory, antibacterial, antimalarial, and insecticidal actions [11]. Recent pharmacokinetic prediction studies employing molecular docking and simulation methodologies indicate that PS exhibited a substantial binding energy of −10.9 kcal/mol when interacting with pri-miR-378a [12]. The molecular dynamics simulation provided evidence of a stable connection between the PS and miRNA complex [12]. PS has the potential to regulate cancer-causing miRNAs, making it a promising candidate for cancer prevention and treatment due to its precise control of miRNA activity. PS's therapeutic value has drawn the interest of an increasing number of researchers who have made important contributions to the field. These characteristics have been extensively reported in various scientific studies [1,11].

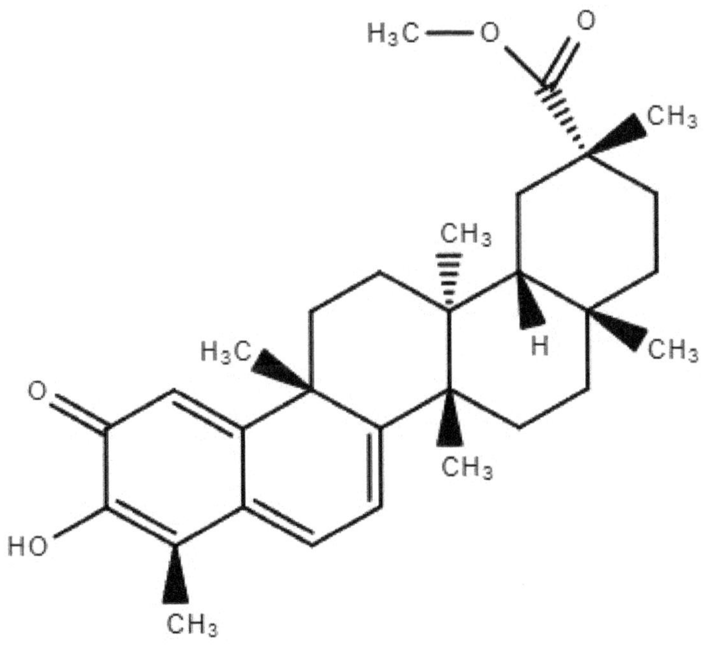

Figure 1. Chemical structure of Pristimerin.

PS demonstrates remarkable pharmacological efficacy in combating tumors through its capacity to selectively target and modulate a wide array of signal transduction pathways and molecular targets. These pathways encompass a myriad of intricate molecular interactions, such as the phosphatidylinositol 3-kinase (PI3K)/AKT pathway, the nuclear factor-kappaB (NF-kB) pathway, the reactive oxygen species (ROS)/mitogen-activated protein kinase (MAPK) pathway, the sonic hedgehog (Shh)/glioma-associated oncogene homolog 1 (Gli1) pathway, and the hypoxia-inducible factor 1a (HIF-1a)/sphingosine kinase 1 (SPHK1) pathway. Moreover, it significantly impacts the complex interaction between proteasome functioning and telomerase activity. PS exerts its anticancer effects via the induction of G1 phase arrest, apoptosis initiation, and autophagy facilitation in cancer cells. Furthermore, it induces inhibitory effects on the tumor cells through the modulation of cellular adhesion, reduction in cancer stem cell (CSC) activity, inhibition of the epithelial–mesenchymal transition (EMT), and inhibition of angiogenesis [11,13].

Several investigations have demonstrated that treating cancer cells with PS can reverse chemoresistance. Multiple studies have also shown that PS can increase the therapeutic effectiveness of various chemotherapeutic agents [14–16]. The primary aim of this review is to systematically consolidate the existing knowledge on the anticancer potential of PS, detailing how it interacts with and influences various molecular pathways to inhibit cancer progression. This review aims to provide a comprehensive resource for both researchers and clinicians, offering a clearer understanding of the multifunctional roles of PS in cancer therapy. By highlighting well-established and newly discovered mechanisms of PS, this synthesis encourages further research into its clinical applications and the development of novel therapeutic strategies that may incorporate or enhance the efficacy of PS.

This paper introduces several new scientific aspects of PS research. It examines the less explored molecular interactions of PS, particularly its ability to modulate proteasome functionality and telomerase activity. These areas are seldom the primary focus of cancer therapy studies but have shown promise in preliminary investigations. Additionally, this review discusses how PS has the potential to overcome chemoresistance, which is a major hurdle in current cancer treatment patterns. By elucidating the molecular basis for PS's ability to reverse resistance mechanisms, this work contributes to the frontier of cancer research. It suggests innovative approaches for integrating PS into existing treatment regimens, which not only deepens our understanding of PS's therapeutic scope but also establishes a foundational framework for future translational and clinical research in oncology.

2. Induction of Apoptosis

Apoptosis is a genetically regulated form of programmed cell death essential for eliminating unnecessary, damaged, or infected cells, thus maintaining cellular homeostasis [17]. The two main categories of apoptosis are the extrinsic death receptor system and the intrinsic mitochondrial pathway [18].

The death receptor pathway involves the activation of death receptors, such as Fas and tumor necrosis factor (TNF) receptor-1. This process results in the formation of a death-inducing signaling complex composed of the adaptor protein, the Fas-associated death domain, and initiator caspases, specifically caspase-8. In the context of the mitochondrial pathway, increased mitochondrial permeability results in the release of cytochrome-c, Apaf-1, and other apoptotic components into the cytoplasm. This event is followed by caspase activation and subsequent cellular death [1,11].

Several reports have documented that PS induces cell death both in vitro and in vivo (Tables 1 and 2) via the activation of mitochondrial signaling, caspase activation (both extrinsic and intrinsic), and PARP cleavage [5,19–22]. In addition, PS has been shown to induce apoptosis via the production of reactive oxygen species (ROS), resulting in significant cytotoxic effects across a diverse range of cancers [5,13,23–26].

Table 1. Anticancer activity of Pristimerin (PS) in in vitro models.

Cancer	Cell Lines	Mechanism of Action/s	PS Alone or/in Combination with Other Drug	References
Breast cancer	MDA-MB-231	Increased expression of RGS4 that suppressed migration and invasion	PS (0–3 μM)	[27]
	ADR-resistant MCF-7/ADR	Induced apoptosis via suppression of AKT pathway	PS (0–10 μM)	[16]
	MDA-MB-231	Enhanced autophagy induction	PS (5 μM) and paclitaxel (24 μM)	[15]
	MDA-MB-231, MDA-MB-468	Decreased levels of phosphorylated ASK1 and JNK	PS (0–0.6 μM)	[28]
	MCF-7, MDA-MB-231,4T1	Induced apoptosis, upregulated expression of miR-542-5p while downregulating DUB3 levels	PS (0–4 μM)	[29]
	epidermal growth factor receptor 2 (HER2)-positive SKBR3	Reduced fatty acid synthase and altered AKT, MAPK, and mTOR pathways	PS (0–10 μM)	[30]
Cervical cancer	HeLa	Activated ROS-dependent JNK, Bax, and PARP-1	PS	[25]
	HeLa, CasKi, SiHa	Induced ROS-dependent cell death	PS	[25]
Colorectal cancer	HCT116, HT-29	Inhibited Wnt/β-catenin signaling pathway	PS	[31]
	AOM/DSS model of colitis-associated colorectal cancer	Suppression of AKT and FOXO3 signaling	PS	[32]
Leukemia	HL-60	Induced apoptosis	PS	[26]
	K562	ROS-JNK-induced autophagy.	PS (0–0.8 μM)	[33]
Lung cancer	NCI-H1299	Targeted Shh/Gli1 signaling pathway	PS (0–500 nM)	[34]
	NCI-H1299	Decreased the rate of migration and invasion	PS (0–500 nM)	[34]
Ovarian cancer	OVCAR-5, MDAH-2774, SK-OV-3	Inhibited AKT/NF-k B/mTOR pathway	PS (0–10 μM)	[19]
Pancreatic cancer	AsPC-1, BxPC-3, PANC-1	Abrogated Chk1/53BP1-mediated DNA repair, suppressed NF-κB activity	PS (200 nM) + gemcitabine (500 nM)	[14,35]
	MiaPaCa-2, Panc-1	Inhibited hTERT via suppressing transcription factors	PS (0–5 μM)	[36]
	MiaPaCa-2, Panc-1	Induced inhibition of AKT/NF-κB/mTOR pathway	PS (5 μM) + proteasome inhibitors	[20]
Prostate	LNCaP, PC-3	Decreased level of survivin and Bcl-2, and Inhibited hTERT mRNA expression levels.	PS (0–10 μM)	[24,37,38]
	PC-3, LNCaP, C4-2B	Induced apoptosis	PS (0–5 μM)	[39]
Oral squamous cell carcinoma	CAL-27, SCC-25	G1 arrest via inhibition of MAPK/Erk1/2 and AKT pathway	PS (0–1 μM)	[40]

Table 2. Anticancer activity of Pristimerin (PS) in in vivo models.

Cancer	Animal Models	Mechanism of Action/s	PS Alone or/in Combination with Other Drug	References
Breast cancer	Breast cancer xenograft model	The inhibition of proteasomal activity and inhibition of tumor migration and invasion	PS (1 mg/kg)	[41]
	MDA-MB-231 tumor xenografts in nude mice	The stimulation of ROS/ASK1/JNK-mediated apoptosis and autophagy. Suppression of tumor growth	PS (0.5 mg/kg)	[28]
	Human breast cancer xenograft model	Suppression of VEGF, tumor growth, and angiogenesis	PS (3 mg/kg)	[42]
Cervical cancer	Tumor xenografts on nude mice	Apoptosis via mitochondrial signaling and activation of pro-apoptotic protein Bax	PS + Taxol	[43]
Colorectal cancer	Human colorectal cancer xenograft model	Inhibited tumor growth via targeting PI3K/AKT/mTOR pathway	PS (1 mg/kg)	[23]
	Human colorectal cancer xenograft model	Inhibited NF-κB signaling pathway	PS (1 mg/kg)	[44]
	Tumor xenograft in nude mice	Apoptosis through activation of the ROS/ER stress/JNK pathway	PS	[45]
Leukemia	Imatinib-resistant Bcr-Abl-T315I xenografts in mice	Suppressed TNFα-induced NFKB, as well as inhibition of the Bcr-Abl expression	PS (1 mg/kg)	[46]
Lung cancer	Human lung tumors xenograft model	Anticancer activity via targeting miR−23a/AKT/GSK3b pathway	PS (0.8 mg/kg) + cisplatin (2 mg/kg)	[47]
	Lung tissue samples from patients	Exerted anticancer activities through EphB4/CDC42/N-WASP pathway.	PS (0–8 μM)	[48]
Prostate cancer	Intra-tibial injection mouse model	Suppressed stem cell activity and angiogenesis via VEGF inhibition	PS (1.6 μM)	[49]

3. Induction of Autophagy

Autophagy is a critical process involved in the destruction of impaired organelles and aged proteins, as well as in the preservation of cellular homeostasis [50]. Autophagy in cancer biology serves a dual function, encompassing both tumor promotion and inhibition. The induction of autophagy in response to diverse cellular stressors plays a crucial role in regulating cell death, therefore offering a promising avenue for developing novel anticancer therapeutics [11,50]. ATG proteins encoded by autophagy-related genes (ATGs) help build the autophagosome [51]. The LC3 conversion (from LC3-I to LC3-II), which is recognized as a hallmark of autophagy [52], occurs when ATG4B combines with ATG7 to produce LC3II, which is formed by the conjugation of LC3-I and phosphatidylethanolamine. In cancer related to esophageal and cholangiocarcinoma, PS enhanced the ratio of LC3-II/LC3-I and increased the accumulation of autophagosomes [53]. Multiple in vitro investigations have demonstrated an upregulation of Beclin-1, ATG7, LC3-II, and p62 expression levels in malignancies associated with breast cancer (BC) and chronic myeloid leukemia (CML) [28,33,54]. Furthermore, the concurrent administration of PS and paclitaxel enhanced extracellular signal-related kinase (ERK)-mediated autophagic cell death. This was evidenced by an increase in the degradation of p62 and the expression of beclin1 [15]. In contrast, the study conducted by Zhang et al. [47] showed that PS had inhibitory effects on autophagy in lung cancer A549 and NCI-H446 cells. This was achieved by downregulating LC3BII and beclin1, ultimately enhancing the apoptotic response induced by cisplatin.

4. Inhibition of Cell Migration, Invasion and Metastasis

The metastasis of cancer encompasses a range of intricate cellular and molecular events, including cancer cell invasion, migration, and the establishment of metastatic colonies in clinical settings [11,55].

4.1. *Epithelial–Mesenchymal Transition (EMT)*

The inhibition of the epithelial–mesenchymal transition (EMT) involves the transformation of epithelial cells into mesenchymal cells, thereby enhancing the migratory and invasive capabilities of tumor cells [56,57]. Previous studies have demonstrated that treatment with PS significantly reduces the expression of key EMT markers including N-cadherin, fibronectin, vimentin, ZEB1, and Snail in both prostate and lung cancer cells, confirming its role in modulating EMT pathways [58,59]. Furthermore, the research by Shu et al. revealed that PS inhibits EMT in trophoblast cells via the miR-542-5p/EGFR signaling axis [60]. This effect of PS extends to suppressing proliferation, migration, and the EMT in trophoblast cells, while simultaneously inducing apoptosis. Notably, the downregulation of miR-542-5p, AGO2, and EGFR expression in these cells contributes to this phenomenon. Moreover, the co-treatment of PS with miR-542-5p silencing exhibited a synergistic effect, highlighting the potential of PS as a therapeutic agent for preventing embryo implantation in cases of ectopic pregnancy. In studies involving MDA-MB-231 triple-negative breast cancer cells, PS was shown to inhibit cell proliferation and revert EMT by upregulating E-cadherin and downregulating N-cadherin [61]. Additionally, PS suppresses the expression of integrin β3 mRNA and protein, which are crucial components of the heterodimeric transmembrane receptor associated with the EMT. Experimental data indicate that silencing integrin β3 enhances the anti-EMT effects of PS, whereas overexpressing this receptor diminishes its efficacy. In xenograft models, PS treatment led to the notable suppression of tumor growth, underscoring its potential utility in cancer therapy.

4.2. *Cell Adhesion and Cytoskeleton Inhibition*

Matrix metalloproteinases (MMPs) play a pivotal role in carcinoma development by modulating the tumor microenvironment. Notably, the proteins MMP2 and MMP9, which are crucial for facilitating invasion and metastasis, are downregulated by PS in a dose-dependent manner. This effect was specifically observed in EC9706 and EC109 cell lines, which are models for esophageal cancer, indicating the targeted action of PS on these enzymes [62,63]. Furthermore, PS has demonstrated significant efficacy in reducing lung cancer cell viability, migration, invasion, and capillary formation. These effects are mediated through the downregulation of the EphB4/CDC42/N-WASP signaling pathway. This pathway is critical for orchestrating mitochondrial-mediated intrinsic apoptosis and endoplasmic reticulum (ER) stress, thereby impeding cancer cell survival and spread [48]. Additional research involving the NCI-H1299 lung cancer cell line has shown that PS not only suppresses cell proliferation but also induces apoptosis. Alongside these effects, there was a notable reduction in the migration and invasion capabilities of H1299 cells, further supporting the potential of PS as a multifaceted therapeutic agent in the treatment of lung cancer [58].

5. Cancer Stem Cells (CSCs)

The inhibition of cancer stem cells (CSCs) is pivotal in understanding and managing carcinogenesis, tumor metastasis, and resistance to chemotherapy. Specific CSC markers such as CD44, aldehyde dehydrogenase (ALDH), and CD133 are integral to the processes of carcinogenesis, self-renewal, and therapy resistance. Additionally, transcription factors like NANOG, SOX-2, and OCT-4 have been implicated in the processes of metastasis and invasion, highlighting their roles in tumor progression and cellular invasiveness [64,65]. However, a significant challenge in CSC research is the identification of a precise and specific panel of CSC markers, as current markers often lack the specificity required for effective targeting and analysis. The natural compound PS has shown promising results in reducing the proportion of ALDH+ cells and inhibiting tumorsphere formation, suggesting its potential in targeting cellular mechanisms essential for CSC maintenance. In the context of uveal melanoma (UM), treatment with PS was found to decrease the levels of stemness-associated proteins such as Slug and Sox2, although the levels of Nanog and KLF4 remained unchanged, indicating selective effects on stem cell-associated pathways [64]. In prostate cancer, using the PC-3 cell line as a model, PS administration resulted in a reduction in the levels of CD44, CD133, and other stemness factors including KLF4, OCT4, and AGO2. This indicates its broad-spectrum activity against various markers associated with stemness [64]. Additionally, the efficacy of PS in eradicating CSCs in esophageal squamous cell carcinoma (ESCC) has been linked to its modulation of the NF-κB signaling pathway, further underscoring its therapeutic potential [64]. PS also demonstrates a potent anticancer effect against breast cancer stem cells, inducing cell death through both apoptosis and incomplete autophagy. The underlying mechanisms involve the inhibition of thioredoxin-1, activation of the ASK1 and JNK signaling pathways, and generation of reactive oxygen species (ROS), all of which are crucial to the PS-induced cell death process [28,54]. These findings support the role of PS as a multifaceted agent capable of targeting and modifying the behavior of cancer stem cells across different cancer types.

6. Angiogenesis Inhibition

Angiogenesis, the process of new blood vessel formation, is critical for various physiological functions but can contribute detrimentally to cancer development when aberrantly activated. In parallel, the formation of new lymphatic vessels, known as lymphangiogenesis, also plays a significant role in cancer progression [66]. Consequently, therapies that target these processes, particularly anti-angiogenic treatments, are crucial in the fight against cancer. Recent research has highlighted the efficacy of PS in inhibiting angiogenesis triggered by vascular endothelial growth factor (VEGF) in human umbilical vascular endothelial cells (HUVECs). This inhibition has been observed both in vitro and in vivo, marking PS as a potent inhibitor of angiogenic signaling pathways [67]. Further studies have shown that in hypoxic conditions, PS effectively suppresses the expression and phosphorylation of key regulatory proteins such as HIF-1α, SPHK-1, and AKT/GSK-3β in PC-3 prostate cancer cells. This suppression leads to a consequential decrease in VEGF levels and angiogenesis, underlining the potential of PS in targeted cancer therapies [68]. Additionally, PS has demonstrated significant anticancer activity in uveal melanoma cells by inhibiting TNFα-induced p65 translocation, IκBα phosphorylation, and NF-κB-dependent gene expression. These molecular interventions contribute to the reduced cell viability and diminished clonogenic, migration, and invasion capabilities of uveal melanoma cells. Remarkably, when PS is combined with vinblastine, a primary therapeutic agent, a synergistic effect is observed, enhancing the therapeutic outcome. Moreover, PS induces apoptosis in these cells, providing a multi-faceted approach to combat uveal melanoma [69].

7. PS and Targeted Pathways

Over the past several decades, extensive research has revealed that many chronic health issues stem from the dysregulation of genes primarily involved in cell cycle control, particularly in oncology. This dysregulation often leads to unchecked cellular proliferation and subsequent metastasis. PS, a naturally occurring compound, has been shown to impact a wide array of biological processes by interacting with multiple signaling pathways. Comprehensive in vitro and in vivo studies have highlighted PS's effectiveness in inhibiting cell proliferation and promoting apoptotic mechanisms, and their detailed results are presented in Table 1 and illustrated in Figure 2.

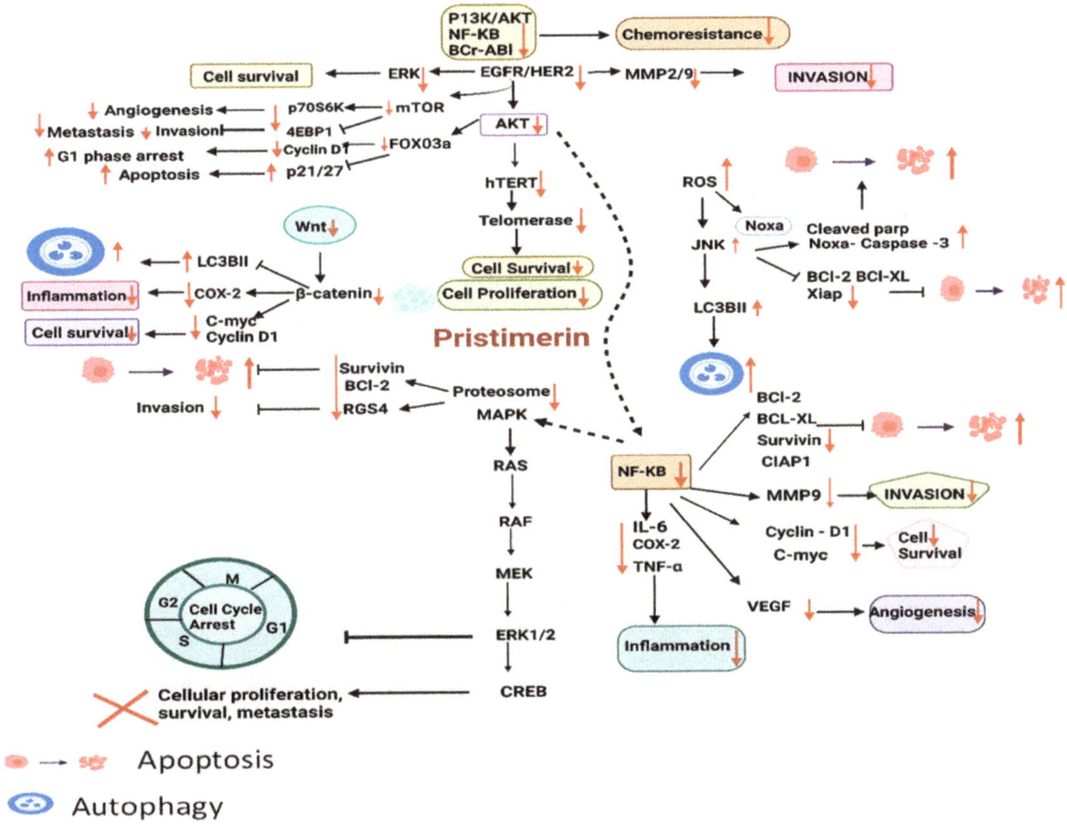

Figure 2. Schematic presentation of PS's anticancer mechanisms of action targeting various signaling cascades via upregulation and downregulation of different regulatory proteins.

The following sections provide a thorough overview of the anticancer activities attributed to PS, exploring its mechanisms of action and the specific signaling pathways it targets. These investigations have identified PS as a potent agent against a variety of cancer types, where it interrupts critical pathways involved in tumor growth and survival. Each cancer type responds differently, showcasing the adaptability and broad potential of PS as a key component in targeted cancer therapy.

7.1. PI3K/AKT Pathway

Phosphatidylinositol 3-kinase (PI3K/AKT/mTOR pathway cascade), or the PI3K/AKT pathway, is the most frequently altered pathway in humans for cancer development. This pathway plays a crucial role in several cellular processes, including cell cycle regulation, cell survival, metabolism, motility, angiogenesis, chemoresistance, and genomic stability [70]. The phosphorylation of Akt can trigger the subsequent phosphorylation of NF-kB, mTOR, and FoxO3a, which play a crucial role in cell growth, proliferation, survival, and angiogenesis [1]. Numerous research has yielded empirical data supporting the inhibitory efficacy of PS on the PI3K/AKT signaling pathway. In addition, PS treatment reduced the levels of mTOR-regulated phosphorylated S6K1 and phosphorylated 4E-BP1 [19,23,32,54].

Multiple biological processes are known to be linked to the PI3K/AKT pathway. Inhibiting AKT signaling reduces anti-apoptotic proteins while increasing pro-apoptotic molecules [71]. Previous studies have provided evidence indicating that PS can inhibit the transcription of FoxO3a-target genes, including cyclinD1 and Bcl-xL, while concurrently promoting the overexpression of the p21 and p27 genes [32]. PS also decreased angiogenesis by targeting many signaling pathways, including VEGF-induced AKT, ERK1/2, mTOR, and ribosomal protein S6 kinase [67]. These findings indicate that PS suppresses cell migration, invasion, and metastasis via affecting the PI3K/AKT pathway.

7.2. ROS Generation and MAPK Pathway

The three main subfamilies of mitogen-activated protein kinases (MAPKs) are extracellular signal-regulated kinases (ERKs), p38, and stress-activated protein kinases (JNK) [72]. According to published reports, PS increased phosphorylated JNK and p38 in K562 leukemic cells and BC while decreasing phosphorylated ERK [28,73]. Numerous research studies have shown that the activation of JNK is closely linked to the initiation of apoptosis in many cancers [25,28,33].

Reports were published that PS treatment leads to an increase in reactive oxygen species (ROS) generation, which in turn results in heightened mitochondrial permeability and a reduction in the mitochondrial membrane potential, which leads to cell death [21,23,24,28,71,74]. Moreover, it has been shown that increased levels of reactive oxygen species (ROS) have been associated with the buildup of unfolded proteins and endoplasmic reticulum (ER) stress, eventually resulting in cellular apoptosis [45]. ROS generated by PS triggers JNK activation. Numerous publications have shown that PS has the ability to trigger cellular apoptosis (Table 2) via the activation of the ROS/JNK signaling pathway [25,63,75,76]. According to recent research in colorectal cancer (CRC) cells, JNK inhibition [25,63,75,76] results in caspase suppression, which in turn causes apoptosis [45]. Furthermore, PS has been found to induce cell cycle arrest in the G1 phase, as well as apoptosis and autophagy [28]. These cellular responses were initiated by the ROS/ASK1/JNK signaling cascades.

7.3. NF-κB Pathway

The NF-kB transcription factors have been widely recognized for their role in the context of cancer [77]. The activation of NF-kB leads to the upregulation of NF-kB-dependent genes [78], and several other signaling pathways are thought to play important roles in this process. PS has been shown in multiple investigations to effectively suppress TNF-a or LPS-induced p-IKK, p-IkBα, and p65 translocation [35,44,46,63,69,79].

PS has significantly reduced the expression of NF-kB-dependent genes (those involved in apoptosis, invasion, and angiogenesis) and cytokines [19,20,32,35,44,46,63,69]. The inhibition of the AKT/mTOR pathway and NF-kB has also been shown to reduce tumor angiogenesis in osteosarcoma cells [80], which may improve the efficacy of anticancer medicines and radiation.

7.4. HIF-1a/SPHK-1 Pathway

Hypoxia, a common feature in advanced solid tumors, has been identified as a significant factor in the advancement of metastasis and the emergence of treatment resistance. The activation of hypoxia-inducible transcription factors facilitates the occurrence of this phenomenon [81,82]. The overexpression of the transcription factor known as hypoxia-inducible factor 1α (HIF-1α) in human cancers can be attributed to hypoxic conditions within the tumor. This event subsequently stimulates angiogenesis and augments the survival capabilities and proliferation of cancerous cells [83].

The inhibitory effects of PS have been seen in the context of hypoxia-induced sphere and colony growth. PS has been demonstrated to have an inhibitory effect on the activity of the cancer stem cell markers CD44, KLF4, OCT4, and AGO2. Similarly, other studies reported that PS had an inhibitory effect on many epithelial–mesenchymal transition (EMT) markers, including N-cadherin, fibronectin, vimentin, and ZEB1 [59,68].

SPHK1 stabilizes HIF-1a via a downstream pathway involving AKT and GSK-3b. The enzymatic activity of SPHK-1 increases in hypoxia, whereas ROS regulates its control. Several studies have shown that PS can potentially decrease the expression of HIF-1α via the inhibition of the SPHK-1 pathway. Further, sphingosine kinase-1 (SPHK-1) inhibition inhibited VEGF synthesis and cyclinD1 and CDK4 expression [1,68].

7.5. Ubiquitin–Proteosome Pathway

The ubiquitin–proteasome system coordinates physiological activities, including growth, death, cell cycle control, DNA repair, and antigen presentation [1]. The 26S eukaryotic proteasome comprises two 19S regulatory particles and one 20S catalytic particle. There are three catalytic sites on the 20S core particle: chymotrypsin-like (b5), trypsin-like (b2), and PGPH-like or caspase-like (b1) [84].

Different studies have shown that the conjugated ketone carbon (C6) of PS and the N-terminal threonine of the proteasomal b5 subunit have inhibitory effects on chymotrypsin-like activity. The inhibition results in polyubiquitination and subsequent modifications in the levels of Bax, p27, and IkBα, ultimately leading to the induction of cell death [39,43,85]. The suppression of Chk1 by PS has been found to cause a defect in DNA repair [86]. This could potentially broaden the use of olaparib in tumors that are proficient in BRCA but have TP53 mutations [86]. This suggests that PS can be used in combination with PARP inhibitor-based therapy.

Cancer cells exhibit increased expression of survivin, a protein that inhibits apoptosis and promotes cell survival by obstructing the mechanism of programmed cell death [1]. Several studies have shown that PS effectively decreases the levels of survivin by promoting its degradation via the ubiquitin–proteasome pathway, ultimately leading to apoptosis [37]. PS triggers apoptosis in prostate cancer cells via the generation of reactive oxygen species and the degradation of ubiquitin–proteasomes [24]. Additionally, PS decreases the invasiveness of breast cancer cells via enhancing RGS4 and suppressing proteasomal activity [41].

7.6. Wnt/β-Catenin Pathway

Wnt proteins function as critical mediators in a variety of important biological processes. The aberrant stimulation of the pathway mediated by Wnt/β-catenin can result in various illnesses, including cancers [1]. PS has shown the ability to modulate the Wnt/β-catenin pathway in MCF-7 breast cancer cells. This modulation is achieved by the targeting and downregulation of LRP6 expression and phosphorylation, resulting in a decrease in the total β-catenin levels. Additionally, PS treatment leads to an elevation in LC3-II levels, suggesting their potential involvement in the regulation of autophagy [54]. PS has also been seen to downregulate Wnt target genes, including cyclinD1, c-Myc, β-catenin, and cox-2, in HT-29 and HCT116 CRC cells [31].

Dishevelled (Dvl), a key component of Wnt/β-catenin signaling, increases β-catenin via phosphorylating/inactivating GSK3b and increasing AKT-Axin-GSK3b complex interaction [87]. Reports have shown that the degradation of β-catenin by GSK3b activation may cause PS-induced CRC cell death [31]. PS treatment decreased the p-AKT levels in MCF-7 breast cancer cells, suggesting that the PI3K/AKT pathway suppressed the Wnt/β-catenin pathway in breast cancer [54].

7.7. Shh/Gli1 Pathway

The sonic hedgehog (Shh)/glioma-associated oncogene homolog 1 (Gli1) signaling pathway is known to be aberrantly activated in various human neoplasms, playing a critical role in tumor development and progression. This pathway is divided into two branches: the canonical and the non-canonical pathways. In the canonical Shh pathway, tumor-produced Shh ligands negate the suppressive action of the Patched (PTCH) receptor on the Smoothened (SMO) protein. This de-repression of SMO initiates a cascade of molecular events that ultimately activates Gli1, a transcription factor responsible for modulating gene expression that affects numerous cellular processes critical to tumorigenesis [1]. A significant study by Lei et al. demonstrated that PS effectively disrupts this pathway. PS was shown to inhibit the nuclear localization of Gli1 in endothelial and pericyte cells within the tumor microenvironment. By preventing Gli1 from entering the nucleus, PS effectively shuts down the SHH/Gli1 signaling pathway, leading to a reduction in its ability to promote angiogenesis. This action results in the suppression of downstream signaling involved in the growth and maintenance of NCI-H1299 xenograft tumors, illustrating a potent anti-tumor mechanism of PS [34]. Through such targeted interference, PS holds promise as a therapeutic agent capable of mitigating the angiogenic and oncogenic potentials of the SHH/Gli1 pathway in cancer treatment.

7.8. Telomerase

Mammalian telomeres, which consist of a repetitive nucleotide sequence (TTAGGG), play a pivotal role in cellular aging and cancer biology. These sequences are capped and protected by a protein complex known as shelterin. This complex is critical for maintaining telomere integrity by preventing harmful end-to-end chromosomal fusions during the formation of the T-loop, a structure essential for telomere protection [1]. During cell division, these TTAGGG repeat sequences are progressively shortened, a process intrinsically linked to cellular aging known as senescence. This shortening mechanism serves as a natural limit to cell proliferation, thus acting as a barrier against the characteristic of uncontrolled cell growth in cancer. Notably, there is a strong correlation between the increased activity of the enzyme telomerase, which elongates telomeres, and the progression of cancer, underscoring the enzyme's role in tumorigenesis [88]. Recent studies have highlighted the efficacy of PS in combating cancer by targeting telomere dynamics. PS has been shown to inhibit the expression and activity of human telomerase reverse transcriptase (hTERT), the catalytic subunit of telomerase, in both pancreatic ductal adenocarcinoma and prostate cancer cells. This inhibition is mediated through the downregulation of several key transcription factors, including Sp1, c-Myc, NF-kB, and STAT-3, which are crucial for hTERT transcriptional activation. Furthermore, PS impacts the PI3K/AKT pathway, a significant regulator of cell survival and proliferation. It inhibits the phosphorylation of AKT and subsequently hTERT, leading to a reduction in telomerase activity. This effect contributes to telomere shortening and promotes the induction of senescence, thus impeding the proliferation of cancer cells [36,38]. By disrupting these critical cellular pathways, PS not only impedes cancer progression but also has potential as a therapeutic agent in oncology.

8. Role of PS in Overcoming Multidrug Resistance and Enhancing Chemotherapeutic Efficacy

Multidrug resistance (MDR) represents a significant challenge in cancer therapy, as cancer cells can develop resistance to a variety of chemotherapeutic agents, each with distinct molecular structures and mechanisms of action. One of the key players in MDR is the ATP-binding cassette (ABC) transporter family, particularly ABCB1 (P-glycoprotein, Pgp), which functions as a potent drug efflux pump. The elevation of ABCB1, along with the multidrug resistance-associated protein 1 (MRP1/ABCC1) and the breast cancer resistance protein [89–91]. PS has shown potential in overcoming ABCB1-mediated chemotherapeutic drug resistance. In human oral epidermoid carcinoma cells (KBv200), PS has been found to disrupt ABCB1 stability independently of its mRNA expression, highlighting a novel approach to mitigating MDR [92]. Additionally, PS has demonstrated efficacy against imatinib-resistant chronic myeloid leukemia (CML) cells both in vitro and in vivo by inhibiting NF-κB and Bcr-Abl, key factors in the development of resistance [46]. Moreover, PS has been linked to the reversal of MDR in multidrug-resistant MCF-7/ADR breast cancer cells through its association with the AKT signaling pathway, emphasizing its role in broader MDR contexts [16].

The integration of natural products with conventional chemotherapeutics has emerged as a promising strategy to enhance anticancer efficacy [1]. The integration of natural products with conventional chemotherapeutics has emerged as a promising strategy to enhance anticancer efficacy. For instance, PS has shown synergistic effects with 5-fluorouracil (5-FU) in ESCC [63], and when combined with paclitaxel (taxol), it has enhanced anti-tumor activities through ROS-mediated mitochondrial dysfunction in cervical cancer cells [43]. Together, they inhibit ERK1/2 [15], triggering autophagy in human BC cells. Additionally, the combination of PS and cisplatin in A549 and NCI-H446 lung cancer cells has been effective in inducing apoptosis by inhibiting the AKT/GSK3β and miRNA-23a signaling pathways [47]. In pancreatic cancer, PS augments the cytotoxic effects of gemcitabine by blocking the NF-κB activation that is typically induced by gemcitabine treatment [14,35]. Furthermore, the co-administration of PS and bortezomib has shown cytotoxic effects against myeloma, illustrating the broad potential of PS in enhancing the effectiveness of multiple chemotherapeutic regimens [85].

9. Conclusions and Future Perspectives

The potential of Chinese herbal therapy, particularly PS, in cancer treatment is being increasingly recognized. PS's effectiveness against cancer is mediated through several mechanisms, including the induction of autophagy, regulation of inflammation-related tumorigenesis, enhancement of chemosensitivity, and modulation of the tumor microenvironment and immune response. Its ability to inhibit cell proliferation, trigger apoptosis, prevent tumor metastasis and invasion, and suppress angiogenesis positions PS as a promising anticancer agent.

Despite the promising anticancer effects demonstrated by PS, significant research gaps remain that need to be addressed to advance PS from laboratory research to clinical applications. The extraction process of PS is inefficient, limiting its bioavailability and hindering further development. There is a critical need to understand the pharmacokinetics and pharmacodynamics of PS in diverse population groups. Detailed studies are required to explore how PS is metabolized and distributed in the human body, and how these processes vary by genetic makeup, age, and comorbid conditions. This understanding will be vital for optimizing dosages and minimizing potential side effects in clinical settings.

Furthermore, while PS has shown potential in modulating several cancer-related pathways, the exact molecular interactions and the potential for off-target effects remain underexplored. Future investigations should focus on the specificity of PS towards its molecular targets and its interaction with other cellular components in the tumor microenvironment. Such studies could elucidate the unintended impacts of PS, thereby refining its therapeutic profile. Additionally, comprehensive in vivo studies and clinical trials are needed to validate the efficacy and safety of PS observed in vitro. These studies should aim to establish robust clinical protocols and assess long-term outcomes to fully harness PS's potential as a part of integrated cancer therapy. The integration of advanced technologies like CRISPR gene editing and AI-driven predictive models could further delineate the role of PS in cancer therapy, providing deeper insights and accelerating its clinical translation.

Author Contributions: K.S.P. and S.K.: writing original draft, figure preparation; S.J.: writing, reviewing, figure preparation and editing F.M., Z.M., U.H. and N.A.: writing and reviewing; A.A.B.: writing, critical reviewing and editing; S.U.: conceptualization, supervision, critical reviewing and editing the manuscript. All authors have read and agreed to the published version of the manuscript.

Funding: The Medical Research Centre at Hamad Medical Corporation, Doha, Qatar supported this work under the approved project numbers MRC-01-21-472.

Institutional Review Board Statement: Not applicable.

Informed Consent Statement: Not applicable.

Data Availability Statement: Not applicable.

Acknowledgments: The authors are thankful to the Qatar National Library for supporting the partial funding of publication charges.

Conflicts of Interest: The authors declare no conflicts of interest.

List of Abbreviations

ABCB1	ATP-Binding Cassette Subfamily B member 1
AIF	Apoptosis-Inducing Factor
ATG	autophagy-related gene
BC	breast cancer
CAC	colitis-associated colorectal cancer
CML	chronic myeloid leukemia
CRC	colorectal cancer
CSCs	cancer stem cells
DVL	Dishevelled
EMT	epithelial–mesenchymal transition
ESCC	esophageal squamous cell carcinoma
HCC	hepatocellular carcinoma
HIF1-α	Hypoxia-Inducing Factor1—α
Htert	human telomerase reverse transcriptase
HUVEC	human umbilical vein endothelial cell
JNK	c-Jun NH(2)-terminal kinase
MDR	multidrug resistance
MMP	matrix metalloproteinase
NAC	N-Acetyl Cystine
NF-kB	nuclear factor-kB
PS	Pristimerin
ROS	reactive oxygen species
TCM	traditional Chinese medicine
TME	tumor microenvironment
TNF	tumor necrosis factor
UM	uveal melanoma
VEGF	vascular endothelial growth factor

References

1. Chen, R.Z.; Yang, F.; Zhang, M.; Sun, Z.G.; Zhang, N. Cellular and Molecular Mechanisms of Pristimerin in Cancer Therapy: Recent Advances. *Front. Oncol.* **2021**, *11*, 671548. [CrossRef] [PubMed]
2. Bukowski, K.; Kciuk, M.; Kontek, R. Mechanisms of Multidrug Resistance in Cancer Chemotherapy. *Int. J. Mol. Sci.* **2020**, *21*, 3233. [CrossRef]
3. Zhang, Q.Y.; Wang, F.X.; Jia, K.K.; Kong, L.D. Natural Product Interventions for Chemotherapy and Radiotherapy-Induced Side Effects. *Front. Pharmacol.* **2018**, *9*, 1253. [CrossRef]
4. Xiang, Y.; Guo, Z.; Zhu, P.; Chen, J.; Huang, Y. Traditional Chinese medicine as a cancer treatment: Modern perspectives of ancient but advanced science. *Cancer Med.* **2019**, *8*, 1958–1975. [CrossRef] [PubMed]
5. Al-Tamimi, M.; Khan, A.Q.; Anver, R.; Ahmad, F.; Mateo, J.M.; Raza, S.S.; Alam, M.; Buddenkotte, J.; Steinhoff, M.; Uddin, S. Pristimerin mediated anticancer effects and sensitization of human skin cancer cells through modulation of MAPK signaling pathways. *Biomed. Pharmacother.* **2022**, *156*, 113950. [CrossRef]
6. Rauf, A.; Abu-Izneid, T.; Khalil, A.A.; Imran, M.; Shah, Z.A.; Emran, T.B.; Mitra, S.; Khan, Z.; Alhumaydhi, F.A.; Aljohani, A.S.M.; et al. Berberine as a Potential Anticancer Agent: A Comprehensive Review. *Molecules* **2021**, *26*, 7368. [CrossRef]
7. Tomeh, M.A.; Hadianamrei, R.; Zhao, X. A Review of Curcumin and Its Derivatives as Anticancer Agents. *Int. J. Mol. Sci.* **2019**, *20*, 1033. [CrossRef]
8. Xiao, Q.; Zhu, W.; Feng, W.; Lee, S.S.; Leung, A.W.; Shen, J.; Gao, L.; Xu, C. A Review of Resveratrol as a Potent Chemoprotective and Synergistic Agent in Cancer Chemotherapy. *Front. Pharmacol.* **2018**, *9*, 1534. [CrossRef] [PubMed]
9. Rauf, A.; Imran, M.; Khan, I.A.; Ur-Rehman, M.; Gilani, S.A.; Mehmood, Z.; Mubarak, M.S. Anticancer potential of quercetin: A comprehensive review. *Phytother. Res.* **2018**, *32*, 2109–2130. [CrossRef]
10. Huong, D.T.L.; Son, N.T. Pristimerin: Natural Occurrence, Biosynthesis, Pharmacology, and Pharmacokinetics. *Rev. Bras. Farmacogn.* **2024**, *34*, 467–480. [CrossRef]
11. Li, J.J.; Yan, Y.Y.; Sun, H.M.; Liu, Y.; Su, C.Y.; Chen, H.B.; Zhang, J.Y. Anti-Cancer Effects of Pristimerin and the Mechanisms: A Critical Review. *Front. Pharmacol.* **2019**, *10*, 746. [CrossRef]
12. Mathur, A.; Singh, A.; Hussain, Y.; Mishra, A.; Meena, A.; Mishra, N.; Luqman, S. Regulating pri/pre-microRNA up/down expressed in cancer proliferation, angiogenesis and metastasis using selected potent triterpenoids. *Int. J. Biol. Macromol.* **2024**, *257 Pt 1*, 127945. [CrossRef]

13. Yousef, B.A.; Hassan, H.M.; Zhang, L.Y.; Jiang, Z.Z. Anticancer Potential and Molecular Targets of Pristimerin: A Mini- Review. *Curr. Cancer Drug Targets* **2017**, *17*, 100–108. [CrossRef]
14. Jiang, Z.; Zhao, Y.; Zhao, Y.; Liu, Y.; Tao, L. Pristimerin synergizes with gemcitabine through abrogating Chk1/53BP1-mediated DNA repair in pancreatic cancer cells. *Food Chem. Toxicol.* **2021**, *147*, 111919. [CrossRef]
15. Lee, Y.; Na, J.; Lee, M.S.; Cha, E.Y.; Sul, J.Y.; Park, J.B.; Lee, J.S. Combination of pristimerin and paclitaxel additively induces autophagy in human breast cancer cells via ERK1/2 regulation. *Mol. Med. Rep.* **2018**, *18*, 4281–4288. [CrossRef] [PubMed]
16. Xie, G.; Yu, X.; Liang, H.; Chen, J.; Tang, X.; Wu, S.; Liao, C. Pristimerin overcomes adriamycin resistance in breast cancer cells through suppressing Akt signaling. *Oncol. Lett.* **2016**, *11*, 3111–3116. [CrossRef]
17. Ke, B.; Tian, M.; Li, J.; Liu, B.; He, G. Targeting Programmed Cell Death Using Small-Molecule Compounds to Improve Potential Cancer Therapy. *Med. Res. Rev.* **2016**, *36*, 983–1035. [CrossRef] [PubMed]
18. Elmore, S. Apoptosis: A review of programmed cell death. *Toxicol. Pathol.* **2007**, *35*, 495–516. [CrossRef] [PubMed]
19. Gao, X.; Liu, Y.; Deeb, D.; Arbab, A.S.; Gautam, S.C. Anticancer activity of pristimerin in ovarian carcinoma cells is mediated through the inhibition of prosurvival Akt/NF-kappaB/mTOR signaling. *J. Exp. Ther. Oncol.* **2014**, *10*, 275–283.
20. Deeb, D.; Gao, X.; Liu, Y.B.; Pindolia, K.; Gautam, S.C. Pristimerin, a quinonemethide triterpenoid, induces apoptosis in pancreatic cancer cells through the inhibition of pro-survival Akt/NF-kappaB/mTOR signaling proteins and anti-apoptotic Bcl-2. *Int. J. Oncol.* **2014**, *44*, 1707–1715. [CrossRef]
21. Yan, Y.Y.; Bai, J.P.; Xie, Y.; Yu, J.Z.; Ma, C.G. The triterpenoid pristimerin induces U87 glioma cell apoptosis through reactive oxygen species-mediated mitochondrial dysfunction. *Oncol. Lett.* **2013**, *5*, 242–248. [CrossRef] [PubMed]
22. Downard, J.S.; Kim, S.H.; Kil, K.S. Localization of the cis-acting regulatory DNA sequences of the Myxococcus xanthus tps and ops genes. *J. Bacteriol.* **1988**, *170*, 4931–4938. [CrossRef] [PubMed]
23. Yousef, B.A.; Hassan, H.M.; Guerram, M.; Hamdi, A.M.; Wang, B.; Zhang, L.Y.; Jiang, Z.Z. Pristimerin inhibits proliferation, migration and invasion, and induces apoptosis in HCT-116 colorectal cancer cells. *Biomed. Pharmacother.* **2016**, *79*, 112–119. [CrossRef] [PubMed]
24. Liu, Y.B.; Gao, X.; Deeb, D.; Arbab, A.S.; Gautam, S.C. Pristimerin Induces Apoptosis in Prostate Cancer Cells by Down-regulating Bcl-2 through ROS-dependent Ubiquitin-proteasomal Degradation Pathway. *J. Carcinog. Mutagen.* **2013**, (Suppl. 6), 005. [CrossRef] [PubMed]
25. Byun, J.Y.; Kim, M.J.; Eum, D.Y.; Yoon, C.H.; Seo, W.D.; Park, K.H.; Hyun, J.W.; Lee, Y.S.; Lee, J.S.; Yoon, M.Y.; et al. Reactive oxygen species-dependent activation of Bax and poly(ADP-ribose) polymerase-1 is required for mitochondrial cell death induced by triterpenoid pristimerin in human cervical cancer cells. *Mol. Pharmacol.* **2009**, *76*, 734–744. [CrossRef] [PubMed]
26. Costa, P.M.; Ferreira, P.M.; Bolzani, V.d.S.; Furlan, M.; de Freitas Formenton Macedo Dos Santos, V.A.; Corsino, J.; de Moraes, M.O.; Costa-Lotufo, L.V.; Montenegro, R.C.; Pessoa, C. Antiproliferative activity of pristimerin isolated from Maytenus ilicifolia (Celastraceae) in human HL-60 cells. *Toxicol. In Vitro* **2008**, *22*, 854–863. [CrossRef] [PubMed]
27. Wu, C.C.; Chan, M.L.; Chen, W.Y.; Tsai, C.Y.; Chang, F.R.; Wu, Y.C. Pristimerin induces caspase-dependent apoptosis in MDA-MB-231 cells via direct effects on mitochondria. *Mol. Cancer Ther.* **2005**, *4*, 1277–1285. [CrossRef] [PubMed]
28. Zhao, Q.; Liu, Y.; Zhong, J.; Bi, Y.; Liu, Y.; Ren, Z.; Li, X.; Jia, J.; Yu, M.; Yu, X. Pristimerin induces apoptosis and autophagy via activation of ROS/ASK1/JNK pathway in human breast cancer in vitro and in vivo. *Cell Death Discov.* **2019**, *5*, 125. [CrossRef] [PubMed]
29. Cheng, S.; Zhang, Z.; Hu, C.; Xing, N.; Xia, Y.; Pang, B. Pristimerin Suppressed Breast Cancer Progression via miR-542-5p/DUB3 Axis. *Onco Targets Ther.* **2020**, *13*, 6651–6660. [CrossRef]
30. Lee, J.S.; Yoon, I.S.; Lee, M.S.; Cha, E.Y.; Thuong, P.T.; Diep, T.T.; Kim, J.R. Anticancer activity of pristimerin in epidermal growth factor receptor 2-positive SKBR3 human breast cancer cells. *Biol. Pharm. Bull.* **2013**, *36*, 316–325. [CrossRef]
31. Zhao, Q.; Bi, Y.; Zhong, J.; Ren, Z.; Liu, Y.; Jia, J.; Yu, M.; Tan, Y.; Zhang, Q.; Yu, X. Pristimerin suppresses colorectal cancer through inhibiting inflammatory responses and Wnt/beta-catenin signaling. *Toxicol. Appl. Pharmacol.* **2020**, *386*, 114813. [CrossRef] [PubMed]
32. Park, J.H.; Kim, J.K. Pristimerin, a naturally occurring triterpenoid, attenuates tumorigenesis in experimental colitis-associated colon cancer. *Phytomedicine* **2018**, *42*, 164–171. [CrossRef] [PubMed]
33. Liu, Y.; Ren, Z.; Li, X.; Zhong, J.; Bi, Y.; Li, R.; Zhao, Q.; Yu, X. Pristimerin Induces Autophagy-Mediated Cell Death in K562 Cells through the ROS/JNK Signaling Pathway. *Chem. Biodivers.* **2019**, *16*, e1900325. [CrossRef] [PubMed]
34. Lei, X.; Zhong, Y.; Huang, L.; Li, S.; Fu, J.; Zhang, L.; Zhang, Y.; Deng, Q.; Yu, X. Identification of a novel tumor angiogenesis inhibitor targeting Shh/Gli1 signaling pathway in Non-small cell lung cancer. *Cell Death Dis.* **2020**, *11*, 232. [CrossRef] [PubMed]
35. Wang, Y.; Zhou, Y.; Zhou, H.; Jia, G.; Liu, J.; Han, B.; Cheng, Z.; Jiang, H.; Pan, S.; Sun, B. Pristimerin causes G1 arrest, induces apoptosis, and enhances the chemosensitivity to gemcitabine in pancreatic cancer cells. *PLoS ONE* **2012**, *7*, e43826. [CrossRef] [PubMed]
36. Deeb, D.; Gao, X.; Liu, Y.; Pindolia, K.; Gautam, S.C. Inhibition of hTERT/telomerase contributes to the antitumor activity of pristimerin in pancreatic ductal adenocarcinoma cells. *Oncol. Rep.* **2015**, *34*, 518–524. [CrossRef]
37. Liu, Y.B.; Gao, X.; Deeb, D.; Brigolin, C.; Zhang, Y.; Shaw, J.; Pindolia, K.; Gautam, S.C. Ubiquitin-proteasomal degradation of antiapoptotic survivin facilitates induction of apoptosis in prostate cancer cells by pristimerin. *Int. J. Oncol.* **2014**, *45*, 1735–1741. [CrossRef]

38. Liu, Y.B.; Gao, X.; Deeb, D.; Pindolia, K.; Gautam, S.C. Role of telomerase in anticancer activity of pristimerin in prostate cancer cells. *J. Exp. Ther. Oncol.* **2015**, *11*, 41–49.
39. Yang, H.; Landis-Piwowar, K.R.; Lu, D.; Yuan, P.; Li, L.; Reddy, G.P.; Yuan, X.; Dou, Q.P. Pristimerin induces apoptosis by targeting the proteasome in prostate cancer cells. *J. Cell Biochem.* **2008**, *103*, 234–244. [CrossRef]
40. Wu, H.; Li, L.; Ai, Z.; Yin, J.; Chen, L. Pristimerin induces apoptosis of oral squamous cell carcinoma cells via G(1) phase arrest and MAPK/Erk1/2 and Akt signaling inhibition. *Oncol. Lett.* **2019**, *17*, 3017–3025. [CrossRef]
41. Mu, X.M.; Shi, W.; Sun, L.X.; Li, H.; Wang, Y.R.; Jiang, Z.Z.; Zhang, L.Y. Pristimerin inhibits breast cancer cell migration by up-regulating regulator of G protein signaling 4 expression. *Asian Pac. J. Cancer Prev.* **2012**, *13*, 1097–1104. [CrossRef] [PubMed]
42. Deng, Q.; Bai, S.; Gao, W.; Tong, L. Pristimerin inhibits angiogenesis in adjuvant-induced arthritic rats by suppressing VEGFR2 signaling pathways. *Int. Immunopharmacol.* **2015**, *29*, 302–313. [CrossRef] [PubMed]
43. Eum, D.Y.; Byun, J.Y.; Yoon, C.H.; Seo, W.D.; Park, K.H.; Lee, J.H.; Chung, H.Y.; An, S.; Suh, Y.; Kim, M.J.; et al. Triterpenoid pristimerin synergizes with taxol to induce cervical cancer cell death through reactive oxygen species-mediated mitochondrial dysfunction. *Anticancer Drugs* **2011**, *22*, 763–773. [CrossRef]
44. Yousef, B.A.; Hassan, H.M.; Zhang, L.Y.; Jiang, Z.Z. Pristimerin exhibits in vitro and in vivo anticancer activities through inhibition of nuclear factor-small ka, CyrillicB signaling pathway in colorectal cancer cells. *Phytomedicine* **2018**, *40*, 140–147. [CrossRef] [PubMed]
45. Zhao, Q.; Bi, Y.; Guo, J.; Liu, Y.; Zhong, J.; Liu, Y.; Pan, L.; Guo, Y.; Tan, Y.; Yu, X. Effect of pristimerin on apoptosis through activation of ROS/endoplasmic reticulum (ER) stress-mediated noxa in colorectal cancer. *Phytomedicine* **2021**, *80*, 153399. [CrossRef] [PubMed]
46. Lu, Z.; Jin, Y.; Chen, C.; Li, J.; Cao, Q.; Pan, J. Pristimerin induces apoptosis in imatinib-resistant chronic myelogenous leukemia cells harboring T315I mutation by blocking NF-kappaB signaling and depleting Bcr-Abl. *Mol. Cancer* **2010**, *9*, 112, Erratum in *Mol. Cancer* **2021**, *20*, 172. [CrossRef]
47. Zhang, Y.; Wang, J.; Hui, B.; Sun, W.; Li, B.; Shi, F.; Che, S.; Chai, L.; Song, L. Pristimerin enhances the effect of cisplatin by inhibiting the miR-23a/Akt/GSK3beta signaling pathway and suppressing autophagy in lung cancer cells. *Int. J. Mol. Med.* **2019**, *43*, 1382–1394. [CrossRef] [PubMed]
48. Tang, Y.; Lei, Y.; Huang, S.; Li, Z.; Chen, X.; Luo, H.; Cheng, C.; Chen, J.; Zou, X.; Chen, X. Pristimerin Exacerbates Cellular Injury in Conditionally Reprogrammed Patient-Derived Lung Adenocarcinoma Cells by Aggravating Mitochondrial Impairment and Endoplasmic Reticulum Stress through EphB4/CDC42/N-WASP Signaling. *Oxid. Med. Cell. Longev.* **2020**, *2020*, 7409853. [CrossRef] [PubMed]
49. Huang, S.; He, P.; Peng, X.; Li, J.; Xu, D.; Tang, Y. Pristimerin Inhibits Prostate Cancer Bone Metastasis by Targeting PC-3 Stem Cell Characteristics and VEGF-Induced Vasculogenesis of BM-EPCs. *Cell. Physiol. Biochem.* **2015**, *37*, 253–268. [CrossRef]
50. Yun, C.W.; Lee, S.H. The Roles of Autophagy in Cancer. *Int. J. Mol. Sci.* **2018**, *19*, 3466. [CrossRef]
51. Mizushima, N.; Yoshimori, T.; Ohsumi, Y. The role of Atg proteins in autophagosome formation. *Annu. Rev. Cell Dev. Biol.* **2011**, *27*, 107–132. [CrossRef] [PubMed]
52. Levy, J.M.M.; Towers, C.G.; Thorburn, A. Targeting autophagy in cancer. *Nat. Rev. Cancer* **2017**, *17*, 528–542. [CrossRef] [PubMed]
53. Huang, P.; Sun, L.Y.; Zhang, Y.Q. A Hopeful Natural Product, Pristimerin, Induces Apoptosis, Cell Cycle Arrest, and Autophagy in Esophageal Cancer Cells. *Anal. Cell. Pathol.* **2019**, *2019*, 6127169. [CrossRef] [PubMed]
54. Cevatemre, B.; Erkisa, M.; Aztopal, N.; Karakas, D.; Alper, P.; Tsimplouli, C.; Sereti, E.; Dimas, K.; Armutak, E.I.I.; Gurevin, E.G.; et al. A promising natural product, pristimerin, results in cytotoxicity against breast cancer stem cells in vitro and xenografts in vivo through apoptosis and an incomplete autopaghy in breast cancer. *Pharmacol. Res.* **2018**, *129*, 500–514. [CrossRef] [PubMed]
55. Valastyan, S.; Weinberg, R.A. Tumor metastasis: Molecular insights and evolving paradigms. *Cell* **2011**, *147*, 275–292. [CrossRef] [PubMed]
56. Bakir, B.; Chiarella, A.M.; Pitarresi, J.R.; Rustgi, A.K. EMT, MET, Plasticity, and Tumor Metastasis. *Trends Cell Biol.* **2020**, *30*, 764–776. [CrossRef] [PubMed]
57. Mittal, V. Epithelial Mesenchymal Transition in Tumor Metastasis. *Annu. Rev. Pathol.* **2018**, *13*, 395–412. [CrossRef] [PubMed]
58. Li, J.; Guo, Q.; Lei, X.; Zhang, L.; Su, C.; Liu, Y.; Zhou, W.; Chen, H.; Wang, H.; Wang, F.; et al. Pristimerin induces apoptosis and inhibits proliferation, migration in H1299 Lung Cancer Cells. *J. Cancer* **2020**, *11*, 6348–6355. [CrossRef] [PubMed]
59. Zuo, J.; Guo, Y.; Peng, X.; Tang, Y.; Zhang, X.; He, P.; Li, S.; Wa, Q.; Li, J.; Huang, S.; et al. Inhibitory action of pristimerin on hypoxia-mediated metastasis involves stem cell characteristics and EMT in PC-3 prostate cancer cells. *Oncol. Rep.* **2015**, *33*, 1388–1394. [CrossRef]
60. Shu, C.; Yu, X.; Cheng, S.; Jing, J.; Hu, C.; Pang, B. Pristimerin Suppresses Trophoblast Cell Epithelial-Mesenchymal Transition via miR-542-5p/EGFR Axis. *Drug Des. Dev. Ther.* **2020**, *14*, 4659–4670. [CrossRef]
61. Liu, S.; Dong, Y.; Wang, Y.; Hu, P.; Wang, J.; Wang, R.Y. Pristimerin exerts antitumor activity against MDA-MB-231 triple-negative breast cancer cells by reversing of epithelial-mesenchymal transition via downregulation of integrin beta3. *Biomed. J.* **2021**, *44* (Suppl. 1), S84–S92. [CrossRef] [PubMed]
62. Kessenbrock, K.; Plaks, V.; Werb, Z. Matrix metalloproteinases: Regulators of the tumor microenvironment. *Cell* **2010**, *141*, 52–67. [CrossRef] [PubMed]

63. Tu, Y.; Tan, F.; Zhou, J.; Pan, J. Pristimerin targeting NF-kappaB pathway inhibits proliferation, migration, and invasion in esophageal squamous cell carcinoma cells. *Cell Biochem. Funct.* **2018**, *36*, 228–240. [CrossRef] [PubMed]
64. Chae, Y.C.; Kim, J.H. Cancer stem cell metabolism: Target for cancer therapy. *BMB Rep.* **2018**, *51*, 319–326. [CrossRef]
65. Singh, P.; Augustine, D.; Rao, R.S.; Patil, S.; Awan, K.H.; Sowmya, S.V.; Haragannavar, V.C.; Prasad, K. Role of cancer stem cells in head-and-neck squamous cell carcinoma—A systematic review. *J. Carcinog.* **2021**, *20*, 12. [CrossRef] [PubMed]
66. Nishida, N.; Yano, H.; Nishida, T.; Kamura, T.; Kojiro, M. Angiogenesis in cancer. *Vasc. Health Risk Manag.* **2006**, *2*, 213–219. [CrossRef] [PubMed]
67. Mu, X.; Shi, W.; Sun, L.; Li, H.; Jiang, Z.; Zhang, L. Pristimerin, a triterpenoid, inhibits tumor angiogenesis by targeting VEGFR2 activation. *Molecules* **2012**, *17*, 6854–6868. [CrossRef]
68. Lee, S.O.; Kim, J.S.; Lee, M.S.; Lee, H.J. Anti-cancer effect of pristimerin by inhibition of HIF-1alpha involves the SPHK-1 pathway in hypoxic prostate cancer cells. *BMC Cancer* **2016**, *16*, 701. [CrossRef] [PubMed]
69. Zhang, B.; Zhang, J.; Pan, J. Pristimerin effectively inhibits the malignant phenotypes of uveal melanoma cells by targeting NF-kappaB pathway. *Int. J. Oncol.* **2017**, *51*, 887–898. [CrossRef]
70. Mabuchi, S.; Kuroda, H.; Takahashi, R.; Sasano, T. The PI3K/AKT/mTOR pathway as a therapeutic target in ovarian cancer. *Gynecol. Oncol.* **2015**, *137*, 173–179. [CrossRef]
71. Yan, F.; Liao, R.; Silva, M.; Li, S.; Jiang, Y.; Peng, T.; Lazarovici, P.; Zheng, W. Pristimerin-induced uveal melanoma cell death via inhibiting PI3K/Akt/FoxO3a signalling pathway. *J. Cell. Mol. Med.* **2020**, *24*, 6208–6219. [CrossRef]
72. Rezatabar, S.; Karimian, A.; Rameshknia, V.; Parsian, H.; Majidinia, M.; Kopi, T.A.; Bishayee, A.; Sadeghinia, A.; Yousefi, M.; Monirialamdari, M.; et al. RAS/MAPK signaling functions in oxidative stress, DNA damage response and cancer progression. *J. Cell. Physiol.* **2019**, *234*, 14951–14965. [CrossRef]
73. Huang, H.D.; Yao, B.G. Analysis of 1,698 cases of elderly gastric disease diagnosed by gastroscope. *Chin. Med. J.* **1987**, *100*, 685–687. [PubMed]
74. Guo, Y.; Zhang, W.; Yan, Y.Y.; Ma, C.G.; Wang, X.; Wang, C.; Zhao, J.L. Triterpenoid pristimerin induced HepG2 cells apoptosis through ROS-mediated mitochondrial dysfunction. *J. BUON* **2013**, *18*, 477–485. [PubMed]
75. Hayashi, D.; Shirai, T.; Terauchi, R.; Tsuchida, S.; Mizoshiri, N.; Mori, Y.; Arai, Y.; Mazda, O.; Kubo, T. Pristimerin inhibits the proliferation of HT1080 fibrosarcoma cells by inducing apoptosis. *Oncol. Lett.* **2020**, *19*, 2963–2970. [CrossRef] [PubMed]
76. Zhao, H.; Wang, C.; Lu, B.; Zhou, Z.; Jin, Y.; Wang, Z.; Zheng, L.; Liu, K.; Luo, T.; Zhu, D.; et al. Pristimerin triggers AIF-dependent programmed necrosis in glioma cells via activation of JNK. *Cancer Lett.* **2016**, *374*, 136–148. [CrossRef] [PubMed]
77. Oeckinghaus, A.; Hayden, M.S.; Ghosh, S. Crosstalk in NF-kappaB signaling pathways. *Nat. Immunol.* **2011**, *12*, 695–708. [CrossRef] [PubMed]
78. Yadav, V.R.; Prasad, S.; Sung, B.; Kannappan, R.; Aggarwal, B.B. Targeting inflammatory pathways by triterpenoids for prevention and treatment of cancer. *Toxins* **2010**, *2*, 2428–2466. [CrossRef] [PubMed]
79. Rosa, A.; Ballarino, M.; Sorrentino, A.; Sthandier, O.; De Angelis, F.G.; Marchioni, M.; Masella, B.; Guarini, A.; Fatica, A.; Peschle, C.; et al. The interplay between the master transcription factor PU.1 and miR-424 regulates human monocyte/macrophage differentiation. *Proc. Natl. Acad. Sci. USA* **2007**, *104*, 19849–19854. [CrossRef]
80. Mori, Y.; Shirai, T.; Terauchi, R.; Tsuchida, S.; Mizoshiri, N.; Hayashi, D.; Arai, Y.; Kishida, T.; Mazda, O.; Kubo, T. Antitumor effects of pristimerin on human osteosarcoma cells in vitro and in vivo. *Onco Targets Ther.* **2017**, *10*, 5703–5710. [CrossRef]
81. Rankin, E.B.; Giaccia, A.J. Hypoxic control of metastasis. *Science* **2016**, *352*, 175–180. [CrossRef] [PubMed]
82. Vaupel, P. The role of hypoxia-induced factors in tumor progression. *Oncologist* **2004**, *9* (Suppl. 5), 10–17. [CrossRef] [PubMed]
83. Wei, W.; Wu, S.; Wang, X.; Sun, C.K.; Yang, X.; Yan, X.; Chua, M.S.; So, S. Novel celastrol derivatives inhibit the growth of hepatocellular carcinoma patient-derived xenografts. *Oncotarget* **2014**, *5*, 5819–5831. [CrossRef] [PubMed]
84. Mofers, A.; Pellegrini, P.; Linder, S.; D'Arcy, P. Proteasome-associated deubiquitinases and cancer. *Cancer Metastasis Rev.* **2017**, *36*, 635–653. [CrossRef] [PubMed]
85. Tiedemann, R.E.; Schmidt, J.; Keats, J.J.; Shi, C.X.; Zhu, Y.X.; Palmer, S.E.; Mao, X.; Schimmer, A.D.; Stewart, A.K. Identification of a potent natural triterpenoid inhibitor of proteosome chymotrypsin-like activity and NF-kappaB with antimyeloma activity in vitro and in vivo. *Blood* **2009**, *113*, 4027–4037. [CrossRef] [PubMed]
86. Tao, L.; Xia, X.; Kong, S.; Wang, T.; Fan, F.; Wang, W. Natural pentacyclic triterpenoid from Pristimerin sensitizes p53-deficient tumor to PARP inhibitor by ubiquitination of Chk1. *Pharmacol. Res.* **2024**, *201*, 107091. [CrossRef] [PubMed]
87. Iijima, T.; Taira, N. Modification by manganese ions and verapamil of the responses of the atrioventricular node to norepinephrine. *Eur. J. Pharmacol.* **1976**, *37*, 55–62. [CrossRef] [PubMed]
88. Jafri, M.A.; Ansari, S.A.; Alqahtani, M.H.; Shay, J.W. Roles of telomeres and telomerase in cancer, and advances in telomerase-targeted therapies. *Genome Med.* **2016**, *8*, 69. [CrossRef] [PubMed]
89. Wu, Q.; Yang, Z.; Nie, Y.; Shi, Y.; Fan, D. Multi-drug resistance in cancer chemotherapeutics: Mechanisms and lab approaches. *Cancer Lett.* **2014**, *347*, 159–166. [CrossRef]
90. Dewanjee, S.; Dua, T.K.; Bhattacharjee, N.; Das, A.; Gangopadhyay, M.; Khanra, R.; Joardar, S.; Riaz, M.; Feo, V.; Zia-Ul-Haq, M. Natural Products as Alternative Choices for P-Glycoprotein (P-gp) Inhibition. *Molecules* **2017**, *22*, 871. [CrossRef]

91. Choi, Y.H.; Yu, A.M. ABC transporters in multidrug resistance and pharmacokinetics, and strategies for drug development. *Curr. Pharm. Des.* **2014**, *20*, 793–807. [CrossRef] [PubMed]
92. Yan, Y.Y.; Wang, F.; Zhao, X.Q.; Wang, X.K.; Chen, Y.F.; Liu, H.; Xie, Y.; Fu, L.W. Degradation of P-glycoprotein by pristimerin contributes to overcoming ABCB1-mediated chemotherapeutic drug resistance in vitro. *Oncol. Rep.* **2017**, *37*, 31–40. [CrossRef] [PubMed]

pharmaceuticals

MDPI

Review

Vatairea Genus as a Potential Therapeutic Agent—A Comprehensive Review of Ethnobotanical, Phytochemical, and Pharmacological Properties

Sarah Andrade Toledo, Laryssa Danielle da Silva Reis, Brenda Costa da Conceição, Lucas Villar Pedrosa da Silva Pantoja, Fábio José Coelho de Souza-Junior, Flávia Cristina Santos Garcez, Cristiane Socorro Ferraz Maia and Eneas Andrade Fontes-Junior *

Laboratory of Pharmacology of Inflammation and Behavior, Institute of Health Sciences, Federal University of Pará, Belém 66075110, Brazil
* Correspondence: efontes@ufpa.br

Abstract: The *Vatairea* genus (Fabaceae family) is widespread in the Amazon rainforest. Some species of this genus are known for their ethnobotanical significance and biological potential. The present study explores the pharmacological and promising therapeutic activities, ethnobotanical profile, and phytochemical prospection of *Vatairea* sp., a monophyletic group of flowering plants, which includes economically and culturally important genera due to their diverse uses, including medicinal applications. *V. lundellii*, *V. guianensis*, *V. erythrocarpa*, *V. fusca*, *V. heteroptera*, *V. paraensis*, *V. sericea*, and *V. macrocarpa* are included in the *Vatairea* sp., also recognized for its high wood quality and potential medicinal properties. Studies show significant antibacterial activity in *V. guianensis* extracts against Gram-positive and Gram-negative bacteria, whereas *V. macrocarpa* lectin exhibits broad-spectrum antibacterial effects, including modulation of antibiotic resistance. Additionally, *V. macrocarpa* and *V. guianensis* have demonstrated antifungal properties, with compounds like Vatacarpan exhibiting potent activity against *Candida* sp. In vivo studies highlight the neurotoxic effects of *V. macrocarpa* lectin, suggesting a dual role in the central nervous system. Despite these findings, research on Vatairea's toxicological aspects is limited, with only a few studies on *V. macrocarpa* and *V. guianensis* extracts indicating a need for further exploration of this genus' pharmacological and therapeutic potential.

Keywords: *Vatairea* sp.; folk medicine; phytochemical; pharmacology; ethnobotany

1. Introduction

Traditional medicine has supplied a foundation for pharmacology for decades, contributing to drug discovery and development. The Amazon rainforest, rich in biodiversity and folk medicine, is a crucial resource for discovering bioactive compounds [1].

In Amazon plants, the *Vatairea* genus has received significant prominence. The genus is a non-endemic common plant in Brazil, composed of eight species and classified in the family Leguminosae (Fabaceae). *Vatairea* sp. is also present in other Amazon countries, such as Peru, Venezuela, and Colombia. Plants of *Vatairea* sp. are popularly known as amargoso (bitter), angelim-amargoso (bitter angelim), angelim-do-igapó, guáboa, angelim [2]. In traditional communities, these botanical species' heartwood and bark are prepared by maceration and utilized for gastrointestinal diseases, insulin control, and other functions; however, solely two of the eight species have been studied for pharmacological activities

 https://doi.org/10.3390/ph18030422

(i.e., V. *guianensis* and *V. macrocarpa*). Their ethnopharmacological therapeutic uses in Brazil involve treating digestive and circulatory systems diseases [3,4].

This comprehensive review aims to systematize the existing knowledge and provide an in-depth and critical analysis of the genus *Vatairea*, highlighting its pharmacological and therapeutic potential, ethnobotanical significance, and phytochemical properties. Our pioneering approach also highlights existing gaps, providing insights into future research. For this purpose, studies on PubMed, Scopus, and Web of Science platforms were selected without language restrictions. The scientific names of the *Vatairea* species and their scientific synonyms (World Flora Online database) were used as search keys. Articles related to the plant's therapeutic, pharmacological, ethnobiological, and phytochemical aspects were selected.

2. Ethnobotanical Features

2.1. Taxonomy and Botanical Aspects

Recognized as the most diversified family in terms of Brazilian flora and one of the largest angiosperm families, the Fabaceae family comprises 19,325 species divided into 727 genera worldwide, with 2807 species across 222 genera found in Brazil [5]. The Fabaceae family is also a monophyletic group of flowering plants, popularly known as leguminous, ranging from trees to shrubs. It plays a pivotal role in nitrogen fixation through its relationship with the soil. The family is divided into three subfamilies: Caesalpinioideae, Mimosoideae, and Faboideae [6]. Some genera within the Fabaceae family stand out for economic and cultural reasons due to their high diversity and versatile uses, ranging from food and construction to medicinal purposes [7].

Vatairea is one of the primary genera in the family, known for its neotropical origin and excellent wood quality, comprising eight species: *Vatairea lundellii*, *V. erythrocarpa*, *V. fusca*, *V. guianensis*, *V. heteroptera*, *V. macrocarpa*, *V. paraensis*, and *V. sericea* [8] (Figure 1). These species share some similarities, such as spirally grouped leaves at the top of their branches and petals ranging from shades of blue to purple, with their primary life form being trees [9]. The genus has garnered scientific interest due to its diverse applications, including its potential medicinal uses, reflecting the significant subject for this comprehensive review.

V. heteroptera is endemic to Brazil and unique in distribution in the Atlantic Forest. It is also a predominantly large tree, averaging 20–30 m in height, and heartwood tends towards brown, with a trunk that has barely perceptible sapwood at the beginning. *V. erythrocarpa* grows more towards the central side of the Amazon. It presents a red epithet commonly over 20–30 m tall, with a more yellowish-brown interior [8].

V. fusca also varies between 20 and 30 m in height, with its brown heartwood, seed, and embryo difficult to identify. Such species are abundant in the lower Amazon region and southern Pará state. *V. lundellii* is over 20 m tall, with yellowish-brown heartwood, and blooms relatively during drier periods, such as January to March, with its fruit growing soon afterward. Its geographical occupation is also characteristic of southern Mexico, predominantly in rainforests [8].

V. guianensis is recurrent throughout the Amazon River region, accompanied by floodplain forests; it is of medium size, 8–25 m; has easy recognition through the size of its flowers, which reach up to 3.5 cm; and huge sapopemas at the beginning of the trunk, being considered the most geographically distributed. *V. macrocarpa* is 5–12 m high, geographically native with greater predominance in the Brazilian Cerrado region. This plant presents a slightly thinner bark, associated with a brown heartwood, and enormous phenotypic plasticity, with specific variations related to the soil [8].

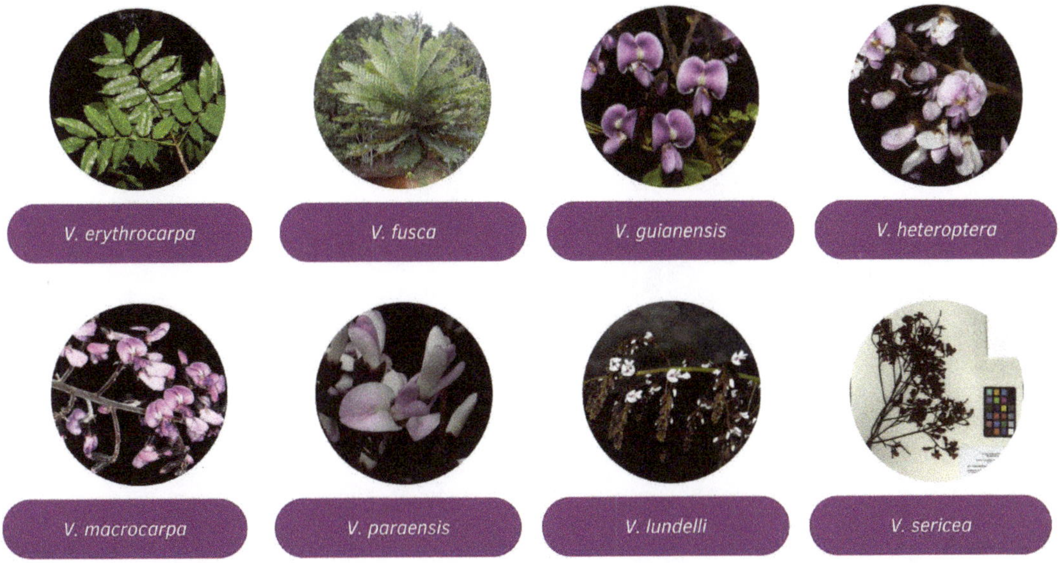

Figure 1. Photographs of the *Vatairea* species. The images of *V. erythrocarpa*, *V. fusca*, *V. guianensis*, *V. heteroptera*, and *V. macrocarpa* were provided by Domingos Cardoso and are sourced from the Reflora website [2]. The photograph of *V. paraensis* is credited to L. O. A. Teixeira, also from the *Reflora* website [2]. Images of *V. lundelli* and *V. sericea* were obtained from the *Trópicos* website, with photos by Aguilar Fernandez [10] and MBG [11].

V. paraensis, the largest tree (30–40 m in height) in the *Vatairea* genus, presents huge sapopemas on the trunk base and rougher bark, resembling *V. fusca*. Other trees differ from this, however, due to its more turbocharged hypanthus [8]. Finally, predominantly located in the rainforest, *V. sericea* is also a large tree (20–40 m), with uncommonly sharper leaflets, small sapopemas on the trunk, a rougher surface, and more yellowish heartwood [8].

2.2. Distribution and Traditional Uses

Vatairea sp. are native to Brazil and endemic in Guyana and the Atlantic coast of Central America and Mexico [8]. In Brazil, the species are found in the Amazon (*V. erythroderma*, *V. fusca*, *V. guianensis*, *V. macrocarpa*, *V. paraensis*, and *V. sericea*), Cerrado, Caatinga (*V. macrocarpa*), and in the Atlantic Forest (*V. heteroptera* and *V. lundellii*) [8,12].

Plants of the genus are commonly known in Brazil as 'faveira', 'fava', 'fava-amarela', 'sucupira', 'sucupira-amarela', 'sucupira-preta', 'sucupira-amargosa', 'bittersa', 'andiroba-amargos', 'angelim-de-igapó', 'angelim', 'angelim-amargoso', 'angelim-do-cerrado', 'pau-roxo' (Figure 2) [2,13].

According to ethnopharmacological information, plants of the *Vatairea* genus are universally used for dermatological treatments. *V. guianensis* is used in the form of juice, tincture, or maceration of the fruit, bark, stem, or root, to treat superficial mycoses and skin diseases [13–16]. It also corresponds to the most cited species in the reviewed literature, accompanied by the species *V. macrocarpa* and *V. lundellii*, which also have antimicrobial potential [16–22].

Anti-inflammatory and antiproliferative activities have also been associated with the *V. guianensis* and *V. macrocarpa* species [22–25]. *V. macrocarpa* also helps to control diabetes and treat stomach problems [23,26–28].

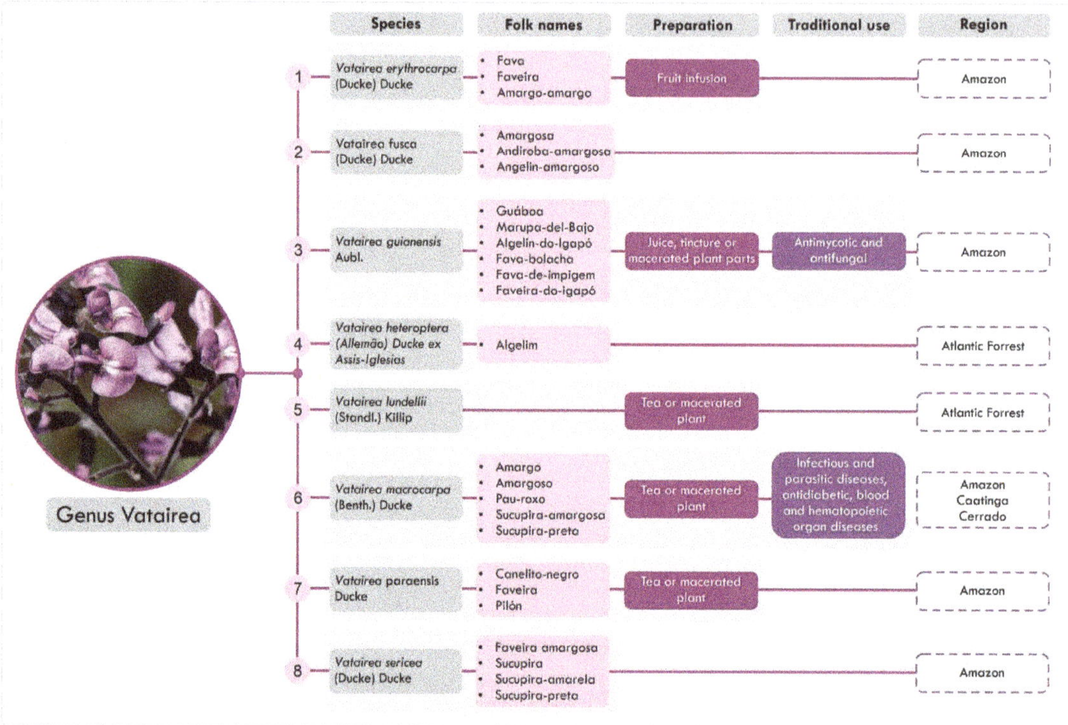

Figure 2. Popular names, preparation, traditional uses, and geographical distribution of *Vatairea* sp.

Thus, the eight species of *Vatairea*, native to Brazil, often have similar popular names and applications in traditional medicine, related to treating infections and inflammatory processes, but also applied to treating endocrine diseases. The preparation forms observed are also diverse, including juices, tinctures, teas, and macerations, which may indicate different solubility patterns to the diverse medicinal properties reported by traditional people [2,4,13,22–24].

3. Phytochemical Aspects

Only three of eight *Vatairea* species were subjected to phytochemical studies, namely *V. guianensis*, *V. macrocarpa*, and *V. heteroptera*, whose findings are summarized in Table 1 and are discussed below.

Table 1. Phytochemical aspects of *Vatairea* genus.

Species	Collection Sites	Plant Parts	Type of Extraction	Phytoconstituents Identified	Reference
V. guianensis	Unspecified	Heartwood	Hot extraction Solvent: benzene	Chrysophanic acid-9-anthrone, physcion-9-anthrone and physcion-10-anthrone	[29]
	Ilha do Marapatá, Manaus—Brazil	Stem bark	Soxhlet extraction. Solvent: ethanol	Chrysophanol, physcion, emodin, and triterpenes	[14]
	Parque Ecológico de Porto Velho, Rondônia—Brazil	Fruits	Essential oil hydrodistillation with ethanol	Aldehydes (hexanal, (2Z)-heptenal, (2E,4E)-decadienal, undecenal, dodecanal) and carboxylic acids (docosahexaenoic acid, hexadecanoic acid, and stearic acid)	[18]
	Belém, Pará—Brazil	Leaves	Maceration extraction; Solvent: ethanol	Chrysophanol and physcion	[19]
			Maceration extraction; Solvent: ethanol	5,3′-dihydroxy-4′-methoxy-2″, 2″-dimethylpyrano-(5″,6″:8,7)-isoflavone; 5,7-dihydroxy-3′, 4′-methylenedioxy-8-prenyl-isoflavone; 5,3′-dihydroxy-4′-methoxy-7-O-β-glucopyranoside-8-prenyl-isoflavone; and derrone	
	Belém, Pará—Brazil	Sapwood	Maceration extraction; Solvent: ethanol	Crysophanol, physcion, formononetin, bolusantol D, betulinic acid, sitosterol, and stigmasterol	[30]
	Belém, Pará—Brazil	Leaves	Maceration extraction; Solvent: ethanol	5,7,3′-trihydroxy-4′-methoxy-8-prenyl-isoflavone; upiwighteone; and 5,7,4′-trihydroxy-3′-methoxy-8-prenyl isoflavone	[22]
V. heteroptera	Linhares Forest Reserve, Rio Doce, Espírito Santo—Brazil	Trunk wood	Maceration extraction; Solvent: benzene	Chrysophanol, sitosterol, stigmasterol, emodin, (2S)-7-hydroxiflavone, and formononetin	[31]
V. macrocarpa	Campo Grande, Mato Grosso—Brazil	Leaves	Maceration extraction; Solvent: ethanol	Catechin, epicatechin, kaempferol-3-O-α-l-rhamnopyranoside, tannins	[24]

3.1. *Vatairea guianensis*

Simatupang et al. [29] conducted an illuminating phytochemical investigation of *V. guianensis* to identify potential chemical compounds related to the skin-irritating effects of the wood derived from this species. It is worth highlighting that species of the genus *Vatairea* have significant economic value due to the commercialization of trunk wood, which was extensively exported to Europe in past decades. Simatupang and colleagues [29] identified three anthrone compounds in the benzene extract of the heartwood of *V. guianensis* for the first time, namely chrysophanic acid-9-anthrone, physcion-9-anthrone, and physcion-10-anthrone (Table 1). Some anthrone derivatives have been shown to cause skin irritation [32].

Following Simatupang et al. [29]'s study, Piedade and Wolter Filho [14] identified a new anthraquinone from *V. guianensis*, called physcion. The authors employed a different phytochemical approach, using a hot extraction with a Soxhlet apparatus to obtain an ethanolic extract, fractionated with organic solvents (e.g., hexane, benzene, and methanol). The benzene fraction allowed the isolation of physcion, chrysophanol, emodin, and dihydromacarfinic acid (a triterpene compound). This successful phytochemical approach led to the isolation of significant quantities of these compounds (Table 1).

The first phytochemical study with the species *V. guianensis* was published only in 2011, based on the essential oil of its fruits. Chemical analysis identified the prevalence of aldehydes and carboxylic acids, including docosahexaenoic acid (DHA), an omega-3 fatty acid known for its role in neurodevelopment [18,33]. On the other hand, analysis of the ethanolic extract demonstrated the presence of anthraquinone compounds, chrysophanol, and physcion, confirming the previously identified species [18].

In addition, four new isoflavonoid compounds from *V. guianensis* leaves were identified: 5,3′-dihydroxy-4′-methoxy-2″,2″-dimethylpyrano-(5″,6″:8,7)-isoflavone,5,7-dihydroxy-3′,4′-methylenedioxy-8-prenyl-isoflavone, 5,3′-dihydroxy-4′-methoxy-7-O-β-glucopyranoside-8-prenyl-isoflavone, and derrone [19]. The authors suggested that this phytochemical profile was closely related to the significant antioxidant properties exhibited by this plant. In this context, Souza and coworkers [30] also assessed the chemical profile of the ethanolic extract of *V. guianensis*, investigating the sapwood part. Fractionation of the ethanolic extract with hexane yielded the isolation of chrysophanol, physcion, formononetin, bolusantol D, betulinic acid, sitosterol, and stigmasterol. It is important to highlight that formononetin and bolusantol D had been previously reported for species of the Fabaceae family, but this was the first report of their occurrence in the *Vatairea* genus.

The most recent scientific report on the phytochemical profile of *V. guianensis* was also conducted by Souza and colleagues [22]. In a scenario focused on flavonoid identification, they revealed a novel isoflavonoid obtained from the ethanolic extract of *V. guianensis* leaves, which was fractionated with ethyl acetate. The identified isoflavonoid compounds were 5,7,3′-trihydroxy-4′-methoxy-8-prenyl-isoflavone (a new compound identified in the species), lupiwighteone, and 5,7,4′-trihydroxy-3′-methoxy-8-prenylisoflavone.

Albeit lectins are not part of the secondary metabolism in plants, their pivotal role in biological systems has increased scientific interest, particularly in species of the genus *Vatairea*. Remarkably, these proteins can recognize and bind to specific carbohydrates, mediating essential immunological processes such as pathogen defense and cell signaling. Lectins are present in plants and animals and can have various applications in medical research, such as in diagnosis, antiviral, antitumor drugs, and drug delivery systems [34–37]. Thus, new lectins with benefits in these areas have been extensively investigated. Lectins from the *Vatairea* genus, specifically *V. guianensis*, have been successfully isolated and studied, revealing key structural and functional properties. The *V. guianensis* lectin exhibits high thermal stability and remains stable across all-around acidic and basic pH levels. Its glycoprotein structure resembles known lectins, including *V. macrocarpa* [38,39].

3.2. *Vatairea macrocarpa*

The limited phytochemical investigations of *V. macrocarpa* reveal a predominant presence of phenolic compounds, particularly catechin, epicatechin, kaempferol-3-O-α-l-rhamnopyranoside, tannins, and other phenolic substances [23]. Santana et al. [19] conducted a comprehensive phytochemical analysis, preparing eight extracts from various parts of the plant using hexane, ethyl acetate, and ethanol as solvents. The extracts were obtained from root wood (hexane and ethyl acetate), root bark (ethyl acetate), stem wood (hexane, ethyl acetate, and ethanol), stem bark (ethyl acetate), and leaves (ethyl acetate). From the ethyl acetate extract of the root bark, several compounds were isolated following fractionation with hexane, ethyl acetate, and methanol. Notably, a new pterocarpan was identified and named Vatacarpan by the authors, along with musizin, a naphthoquinone previously reported in the literature.

The lectin from *V. macrocarpa* has also been a focus of the investigation. This lectin was identified with a 22 kDa N-terminal sequence, a structural feature comparable to other endogenous protein fragments, suggesting potential shared functional roles [38,39].

3.3. *Vatairea heteroptera*

Formiga et al. [30] investigated the phytochemical composition of *V. heteroptera*, focusing on the trunk wood, which was extracted using benzene. The study identified several key compounds: chrysophanol, sitosterol, stigmasterol, emodin, (2S)-7-hydroxyflavone, and formononetin. This report is notable for being the first to document phytochemicals with potential medicinal value in the genus *Vatairea*. Specifically, the study identified anthraquinones (chrysophanol and emodin), flavonoids ((2S)-7-hydroxyflavone and formononetin), and triterpenoids (sitosterol and stigmasterol) in the genus.

Thus, there is a marked lack of information on the phytochemical composition of *Vatairea* sp. In the few studies carried out, aldehydes and carboxylic acids (essential oil) were identified: lectins (seeds) [18,40–42], which will be discussed in more detail later, given the interest in the literature on these substances; anthraquinones, flavonoids, triterpenes, and tannins (extracts from various parts of plants), related to the antioxidant potential of some of these species [14,19,22,24,30]. These elements need to be further investigated, and new studies need to be conducted to increase knowledge of these species' potential and the safety of their use.

4. Pharmacological Properties

There are limited studies on the safety of using *Vatairea* species for therapeutic purposes. Despite this, its effects on microorganisms and diseases related to the central nervous, endocrine, immune, cardiovascular, and renal systems have already been explored. The investigation, however, is still in its initial stages. Studies related to the biological properties of *Vatairea* species are summarized in Table 2 and will be discussed below.

Table 2. Pharmacological properties of Vatairea genus.

Experimental Model	Specie	Extract (Part)	Dose/Concentration (via)	Key Outcomes	Ref.
Toxicity Studies					
In vitro toxicity					
Leukocyte viability (mice)	*V. macrocarpa*	Ethanolic (leaves)	3–90 μg/mL	No cytotoxicity (MTT).	[24]
Lymphocyte culture (human)	*V. macrocarpa*	Lectin (seed)	0.5–45 μM	Trypan blue assay—concentration-dependent cytotoxicity (≥1 μM)	[43]
			0.5–8 μM	Comet assay: 8 μM—increases DNA damage 0.5–2 μM—decreases doxorubicin-induced DNA damage	
In vivo toxicity					
Acute (male mice)	*V. guianensis*	Hydroethanolic (seed)	2000 and 5000 mg/kg (oral)	No signals of toxicity, or death. LD_{50} > 5000 mg/kg	[16]
	V. macrocarpa	Methanolic (heartwood)	100–5000 mg/kg (oral)	No behavioral changes, or death. LD_{50} > 5000 mg/kg	[44]
		Ethanolic (stembark)	250–5000 mg/kg (oral)	No signals of toxicity, or death. LD_{50} > 5000 mg/kg	[26]
Subchronic 30 days (male rats)	*V. macrocarpa*	Methanolic (heartwood)	20–500 mg/kg (oral)	No behavioral, anatomical, or histological changes, either death ↑ Segmented neutrophils (500 mg/kg). ↑ Alkaline phosphatase ↑ Plasma protein ↓ γ-glutamyl transferase (100 mg/kg). ↓ Triacylglyceride	[44]
Communicable diseases					
In vitro antibacterial test					
Enterococcus faecalis	*V. guianensis*	Hydroalcoholic (seed) Hexane (seed) Chloroform (seed) Methanolic (seed)	0.4–100 μg/mL	MIC 12.5 μg/mL; MBC 25 μg/mL MIC 12.5 μg/mL; MBC 25 μg/mL MIC 3.12 μg/mL; MBC 12.5 μg/mL MIC 12.5 μg/mL; MBC 50 μg/mL	[45]
Escherichia coli	*V. macrocarpa*	Lectin (seed)	1.0–1024 μg/mL	No antibiotic activity (MIC ≥ 1024 μg/mL) Decrease norfloxacin antibiotic activity	[42]
Klebsiella oxytoca	*V. macrocarpa*	Lectin (seed)	31.25–250 μg/mL	No antibiotic activity (MIC > 250 μg/mL)	[40]
Pseudomonas aeruginosa	*V. macrocarpa*	Lectin (seed)	31.25–250 μg/mL	Weakly inhibition of planktonic growth (250 μg/mL).	[40]
	V. guianensis	Hydroalcoholic (seed) Hexane (seed) Chloroform (seed) Methanolic (seed)	0.4–100 μg/mL	MIC 25 μg/mL; MBC 100 μg/mL MIC 25 μg/mL; MBC 100 μg/mL MIC 25 μg/mL; MBC 100 μg/mL MIC 25 μg/mL; MBC 50 μg/mL	[45]
Salmonella sp.	*V. guianensis*	Hydroalcoholic (seed) Hexane (seed) Chloroform (seed) Methanolic (seed)	0.4–100 μg/mL	No activity No activity MIC 50 μg/mL; MBC 100 μg/mL MIC 50 μg/mL; MBC 100 μg/mL	[45]

Table 2. *Cont.*

Experimental Model	Specie	Extract (Part)	Dose/Concentration (via)	Key Outcomes	Ref.
Staphylococcus aureus	*V. guianensis*	Aqueous (leaves)	2.275 mg/mL (30 µL/hole)	Antibacterial activity at 44.4% of ciprofloxacin (agar diffusion test).	[17]
		Hydroalcoholic (seed)	0.4–100 µg/mL	MIC 3.12 µg/mL; MBC 6.25 µg/mL	[45]
		Hexane (seed)		MIC 6.25 µg/mL; MBC 12.5 µg/mL	
		Chloroform (seed)		MIC 3.12 µg/mL; MBC 12.5 µg/mL	
		Methanolic (seed)		MIC 6.25 µg/mL; MBC 12.5 µg/mL	
	V. macrocarpa	Lectin (seed)	1.0–1024 µg/mL	No antibiotic activity (MIC ≥ 1024 µg/mL) Increase in norfloxacin, penicillin, and gentamicin antibiotic activity	[42]
	V. macrocarpa	Lectin (seed)	31.25–250 µg/mL	Complete inhibition of planktonic growth (250 µg/mL) Inhibition of biomass formation in biofilms Decrease in the number of viable cells in the biofilm	[40]
S. epidermidis	*V. macrocarpa*	Lectin (seed)	31.25–250 µg/mL	Complete inhibition of planktonic growth (250 µg/mL) Influence in biofilm formation Decrease in the number of viable cells in the biofilm	[40]
Streptococcus sanguis	*V. macrocarpa*	Lectin (seed)	100 µg/mL	Inhibition of bacterial adhesion to the acquired pellicle on tooth enamel	[41]
In vivo antibacterial test					
Mycobacterium bovis	*V. macrocarpa*	Ethanolic (leaves)	30–300 mg/kg	Antimycobacterial activity	[24]
In vitro antifungal test					
Candida albicans	*V. macrocarpa*	Ethyl acetate (root bark)	-	MIC 0.98 µg/mL	[20]
		Vatacarpan (root bark)		MIC 0.98 µg/mL	
		Lectin (seed)	31.25–250 µg/mL	Weakly inhibition of planktonic growth (250 µg/mL)	[40]
	V. guianensis	Ethanolic extract (leaves)	0.125–1024 µg/mL	MIC 128 µg/mL; MFC 512 µg/mL	[22]
		Hexanic fraction		No activity	
		Ethyl acetate fraction		MIC 16 µg/mL; MFC 32 µg/mL.	
		Methanol/H_2O fraction		No activity	
		5,7,3′-trihydroxy-4′-methoxy-8-prenylisoflavone	0.125–256 µg/mL	No activity	
C. dubliniensis	*V. guianensis*	Ethanolic extract (leaves)	0.125–1024 µg/mL	MIC 32 µg/mL	[22]
		Hexanic fraction		MIC 64 µg/mL	
		Ethyl acetate fraction		MIC 8 µg/mL; MFC 16 µg/mL	
		Methanol/H_2O fraction		No activity	
		5,7,3′-trihydroxy-4′-methoxy-8-prenylisoflavone	0.125–256 µg/mL	MIC 8 µg/mL	

Table 2. *Cont.*

Experimental Model	Specie	Extract (Part)	Dose/Concentration (via)	Key Outcomes	Ref.
C. krusei	*V. guianensis*	Ethanolic extract (leaves) Hexanic fraction Ethyl acetate fraction Methanol/H_2O fraction	0.125–1024 μg/mL	MIC 128 μg/mL MIC 512 μg/mL; MFC 512 μg/mL MIC 8 μg/mL; MFC 32 μg/mL No activity	[22]
		5,7,3′-trihydroxy-4′-methoxy-8-prenylisoflavone	0.125–256 μg/mL	No activity	
C. parapsilosis	*V. macrocarpa*	Ethyl acetate	-	MIC 0.98 μg/mL	[20]
	V. guianensis	Ethanolic extract (leaves) Hexanic fraction Ethyl acetate fraction Methanol/H_2O fraction		No activity MIC 64 μg/mL MIC 8 μg/mL; MFC 32 μg/mL No activity	[22]
		5,7,3′-trihydroxy-4′-methoxy-8-prenylisoflavone	0.125–256 μg/mL	MIC 32 μg/mL	
In vitro antiprotozoal test					
Leishmania amazonensis	*V. macrocarpa*	Ethyl acetate (root bark)	-	Antileishmanial activity (IC_{50} 71.47 μg/mL)	[20]
Non-communicable diseases					
Endocrine system					
Type 2 diabetes (streptozotocin; male rats)	*V. macrocarpa*	Ethanolic (stembark)	250 and 500 mg/kg (oral, 22 days)	Reductions observed include postprandial glycemia, food and fluid intake, urinary volume, and the excretion of glucose and urea in urine Improvement in weight gain Reduction in HOMA-R index	[26]
			500 mg/kg (oral, 21 days)	Increase insulin receptor and AKT phosphorylation in the liver, extensor digitorum longus muscles, and retroperitoneal white adipose tissue	[27]
Cardiovascular and renal systems					
Ex vivo aortic contraction (rat)	*V. guianensis*	Lectin (seed)	1–100 μg/mL	Concentration-dependent relaxation of phenylephrine-induced aortic contraction This effect appears to involve the release of nitric oxide (NO) by the vascular endothelium Galactose abolishes the lectin's vasorelaxant effect	[38]
In situ kidney perfusion (rat)	*V. macrocarpa*	Lectin (seed)	10 μg/mL	Increase perfusion pressure, renal vascular resistance, urinary flow, and glomerular filtration rate Galactose abolishes the lectin's kidney effect Moderate protein buildup in tubules and urinary spaces Renal tubules with eosinophilic casts	[46]

Table 2. *Cont.*

Experimental Model	Specie	Extract (Part)	Dose/Concentration (via)	Key Outcomes	Ref.
Angiogenic activity Embryo chorioallantoic membrane (chicken)	*V. macrocarpa*	Lectin (seed)	0.5–8 μM	↑ Vascularization and number of blood vessels (angiogenesis) ↑ Length, size, number of complexes, and blood vessel junctions ↑ Inflammatory cells and fibroblasts ↑ Thickening of CAM ↑ VEGF and TNF-α expression Lactose reduced the lectin's effects	[43]
Immune system					
In vitro inflammation					
Neutrophil phagocytic activity	*V. macrocarpa*	Ethanolic (leaves)	3–30 μg/mL	Reduction in neutrophil phagocytic activity	[24]
In vivo inflammation					
Carrageenan-induced pleurisy, BCG-induced pleurisy, CFA-induced paw edema	*V. macrocarpa*	Ethanolic (leaves)	10–300 mg/kg (oral)	Dose-dependent reduction in leukocyte migration and protein concentration in pleural exudate CFA-induced paw edema: no effect in hyperalgesia, reduction in paw edema, and cold sensitivity	[24]
Neutrophil migration (female rat)	*V. macrocarpa*	Lectin (seed)	9.6×10^{-7}, 1.9×10^{-6}, or 3.8×10^{-6} M (1 mL, intraperitoneal)	Neutrophil and mononuclear cell migration to the peritoneal cavity is induced in a dose-dependent manner through macrophage-mediated mechanisms (cytokine release) Galactose abolishes the lectin's proinflammatory effect, suggesting it acts via its carbohydrate-binding site.	[47]
	V. macrocarpa	Lectin (seed)	4.8×10^{-7}, 9.6×10^{-7}, or 1.9×10^{-6} mol	Lectin induces cultured macrophages to release a neutrophil chemotactic mediator	[48]
Paw edema (rat)	*V. guianensis*	Lectin (seed)	0.01, 0.1, and 1 mg/kg	Time- and dose-dependent paw edema, with polymorphonuclear infiltrate Indomethacin (COX blocker) partially inhibits this effect, but L-NAME (NOS inhibitor) does not	[49]
Central nervous system					
Neuroinflammation (male mice)	*V. macrocarpa*	Lectin (seed)	0.3–3 μg/site (intracerebroventricular)	Depressive-like effect (forced swimming test) Proinflammatory effect in the hippocampus: (↑ COX-2, GFAP, and S100B)	[50]
Nociception					
Orofacial nociception (zebrafish)	*V. macrocarpa*	Lectin (seed)	0.025, 0.05 or 0.1 mg/mL (20 μL; intraperitoneal)	No pain relief effect	[51]
Wound-healing					
Dorsal wound (rat)	*V. guianensis*	Hydroethanolic (seed)	100–500 mg/kg (topical)	Improve wound contraction from the third day of treatment (100 mg/kg) Inflammatory response reduction Stimulation of collagen synthesis	[16]

4.1. Toxicity Studies

As mentioned above, only two species (*V. macrocarpa* and *V. guianensis*) have been evaluated for their toxicity. *V. macrocarpa* leaves' ethanolic extract did not show cytotoxicity in neutrophils culture [24]. No adverse effects in rodents, such as relevant behavioral changes or deaths, were observed at subchronic doses [44]. On the other hand, the lectin from *V. macrocarpa* showed in vitro cytotoxicity in human lymphocytes at concentrations above 0.5 μM and demonstrated genotoxicity at concentrations above 8.0 μM [43].

For *V. guianensis*, the hydroethanolic extract obtained by maceration showed no acute oral toxicity at doses below 2000 mg/kg [16]. Thus, the studies indicate that extracts of *V. macrocarpa* and *V. guianensis* are relatively safe, noting that they only cover in vitro tests and murine models. It is also important to highlight the cytotoxic and genotoxic effects of the *V. macrocarpa* lectin. Therefore, there is a need for more in-depth investigations to validate the safety of its use, since they are widely used in traditional medicine. It is also important to highlight the need to investigate the toxicity of the other six species of the genus, for which no studies were identified.

4.2. Pharmacological Studies

Although the *Vatairea* genus comprises diverse species, most studies investigating pharmacological activity primarily focused on *V. macrocarpa* and *V. guianensis*. Numerous models have been used to investigate their pharmacological activities and therapeutic potential. In vitro studies gathered findings that underscore the importance of studying medicinal plants, such as, in this case, species of the *Vatairea* genus.

It is noted that predominantly in vivo studies have demonstrated the pharmacological activities derived from various species of the genus *Vatairea*. Molecules such as lectins, found in several species including *V. macrocarpa* and *V. guianensis*, present numerous opportunities for modulating biological systems [52].

4.2.1. Antibacterial Activity

Antibacterial activity of several *V. guianensis* extracts (e.g., hydroalcoholic, hexane, chloroform, and methanolic) against Gram-positive (*Staphylococcus aureus* and *Enterococcus faecalis*) and Gram-negative (*Pseudomonas aeruginosa* and *Salmonella* sp.) bacteria have been reported [45]. All extracts demonstrated such activity, with minimum inhibitory concentration (MIC) ranging from 3.12 to 50 μg/mL and minimum bactericidal concentration (MBC) ranging from 6.25 to 100 μg/mL. Additionally, Oliveira et al. [17] confirmed the effectiveness of *V. guianensis* against *S. aureus*, further supporting its antibacterial properties.

Anthraquinones are well-documented for their significant antimicrobial potential [53]. Within the *Vatairea* genus, particularly in *V. guianensis*, notable anthraquinone compounds such as chrysophanol, physcion, and their derivatives have been identified, likely contributing to the antimicrobial activity reported [22,30,31]. Physcion, a natural anthraquinone derivative, exhibits remarkable antibacterial activity against *S. aureus*, *S. epidermidis*, and *P. aeruginosa*. At the same time, chrysophanol has also been consistently highlighted for its potent antimicrobial properties against various bacterial and fungal strains [54–56]. These findings revealed how phytochemical investigations are essential for advancing pharmacological research on natural products, as they enable the identification of bioactive compounds and provide critical insights into their therapeutic potential, paving the way for the discovery of novel antimicrobial agents.

Unlike *V. guianensis*, for which research focuses on antibacterial activity in extracts, *V. macrocarpa* has been extensively studied for its lectin, a protein extracted from the seed. Vasconcelos et al. [40] demonstrate the broad-spectrum antibacterial activity of *V. macrocarpa* lectin against several pathogens, including S. *epidermidis*, *S. aureus*, *Klebsiella oxytoca*, and

P. aeruginosa. Similarly, Teixeira [41] found that lectins from different plant species, including *V. macrocarpa*, reduced the adhesion of *Streptococcus* sp. to the salivary components of dental plaque. These findings suggest that the *V. macrocarpa* lectin, like the lectins from other species, can disrupt bacterial adhesion, potentially preventing biofilm formation. This potential antibacterial activity of *V. macrocarpa* seed lectins was tested against multi-drug-resistant bacteria strains of *S. aureus* and *E. coli* [42]. The *V. macrocarpa* lectin demonstrated the ability to modulate antibiotic activity [57]. When combined with antibiotics, such as gentamicin, norfloxacin, and penicillin, the lectin increased the effectiveness against *S. aureus*, but not against *E. coli* [42]. In silico predictions suggest that this interaction between the lectin and gentamicin involves residues within the lectin's carbohydrate-binding site [58]. This finding reinforces the potential of *V. macrocarpa* lectins as a promising strategy for combating multi-resistant bacteria.

4.2.2. Antifungal Activity

In addition to antibacterial properties, *V. guianensis* and *V. macrocarpa* have also been explored for their antifungal potential. Santana et al. [20] investigated in vitro the antifungal activity of several Fabaceae species, including *V. macrocarpa*. In this study, the authors explore the ethyl acetate extract of *V. macrocarpa* and evaluate fractions and isolated compounds. Notably, the isolated compound vatacarpan demonstrated significant in vitro activity against *Candida albicans* (MIC = 0.98 μg/mL), a remarkably low concentration compared to established antifungal drugs, such as fluconazole and amphotericin B. This finding highlights the potential of *V. macrocarpa* as a source for developing new antifungal agents. Recently, in a study on antifungal activity focusing on *V. guianensis*, Souza et al. [22] isolated a new compound, 5,7,3′-trihydroxy-4′-methoxy-8-prenylisoflavone, from leaves, and evaluated its antifungal properties. The authors employed the ethanolic extract of *V. guianensis* leaves against several *Candida* species, including *C. dubliniensis*, *C. albicans*, *C. parapsilosis*, and *C. krusei*. The results demonstrated the antifungal activity of the extract against *C. dubliniensis*, *C. albicans*, and *C. krusei*. Remarkably, the extract fraction exhibited significant activity against all fungi investigated, while the isolated compound showed more potent activity against *C. parapsilosis* and *C. dubliniensis*.

The evidence gathered demonstrates the potential of *V. macrocarpa* and *V. guianensis* for treating infectious conditions, presenting a broad spectrum of action, combating bacteria and fungi, and enhancing the activity of conventional antibiotics. These findings are interestingly aligned with the traditional use of these plants to treat skin diseases, conditions that can be explored in in vitro and murine models, to expand the pharmacological characterization of the species and elucidate its potential benefits [52]. No studies were identified regarding the possible antibiotic properties of the other *Vatairea* species, highlighting yet another gap that must be filled.

4.2.3. Endocrine System

Among the species of the *Vatairea* genus, *V. macrocarpa* stands out for its endocrine-modulating effects. In streptozotocin-challenged rats, ethanolic extracts of *V. macrocarpa* demonstrated significant anti-diabetic activity by improving insulin resistance, with authors suggesting a possible modulation of pancreatic beta-cell function [26]. A recent study employing refined pharmacological techniques found that *V. macrocarpa* stem bark ethanolic extract attenuated diabetes-like parameters by reducing glycemia, urinary glucose, and urea levels. The extract improved insulin signaling by enhancing GLUT4 receptor translocation to the cell membrane and decreasing phosphoenolpyruvate carboxykinase (PEPCK) activity, thereby reducing gluconeogenesis [27]. These findings, combined with the phenolic-rich composition of *V. macrocarpa*, highlight its potential as a source of endocrine-active compounds.

4.2.4. Cardiovascular and Renal Systems

V. macrocarpa galactose-binding lectin from seeds significantly increases perfusion pressure, renal vascular resistance, urinary flow, and glomerular filtration rate, not altering the tubular transport of sodium, potassium, or chloride in isolated Wistar rats' kidneys [46]. Pretreatment with a lectin–galactose complex blocked these renal parameters' increase, suggesting that the lectin specifically interacts with carbohydrate-binding sites in the renal system. Additionally, kidneys treated with the lectin showed moderate deposits of proteinaceous material in the tubules and urinary space, while those pretreated with the lectin–galactose complex showed only small amounts of this material, with no abnormalities in the renal tubules. These results indicate that *V. macrocarpa* lectin significantly affects renal function, modulated by its interaction with carbohydrates [46].

V. guianensis lectin exhibits vasorelaxant ex vivo activity in contracted rat aortas. This effect is strictly endothelium-dependent and involves nitric oxide production and the lectin domain [38]. Interestingly, despite the structural similarity, *V. macrocarpa* and *V. guianensis* lectins demonstrated divergent effects on the vascular bed. *V. macrocarpa* lectin demonstrated vasoconstrictive properties on the renal artery, whereas *V. guianensis* lectin exhibited a vasorelaxant effect on the aorta. This peculiarity should be further explored to elucidate the structure–activity relationship and the mechanisms that trigger such effects [38,46].

4.2.5. Immune System

Anti-inflammatory properties of the ethanolic leaf extract of *V. macrocarpa* in experimental in vitro models were also described. The extract exhibits phenolic compounds and flavonoids, such as catechin, epicatechin, and kaempferol-3-O-a-l-rhamnopyranoside. The in vivo model was effective in reducing leukocyte migration and protein exudation in carrageenan-induced pleurisy, as well as inhibiting inflammatory parameters in models of persistent paw inflammation and bacillus Calmette–Guérin (BCG)-induced pleurisy. These findings suggest that *V. macrocarpa* extract has potential as a natural agent for treating inflammatory diseases [24].

Interestingly, Alencar et al. [47] showed that *V. macrocarpa* seed lectins can induce an inflammatory response. The lectin was injected into the peritoneum of rats to investigate how it triggers this effect, resulting in increased neutrophil migration into the peritoneal cavity. However, adding α-D-galactose to the lectin solution partially inhibited this effect. Neutrophil migration was also reduced when the peritoneal cavity was depleted from resident cells previously, suggesting an indirect mechanism of neutrophil migration, possibly mediated by resident macrophages. The authors propose that galactose-binding lectins' effects are not linked to inflammatory mediators like lipoxygenase, cyclooxygenase, or platelet-activating factor (PAF). On the other hand, they observed that dexamethasone and thalidomide reduce lectin-induced neutrophil migration, indicating the possible involvement of cytokines in their proinflammatory effects [47].

Furthermore, aiming to confirm their hypothesis of the involvement of macrophage signaling in the proinflammatory effect of lecithin, Alencar et al. [48] injected *V. macrocarpa* seed lectin into a primary culture of rat macrophages. The culture supernatant was collected and injected into rats' peritoneal cavities, increasing neutrophil migration proportionally to the lectin concentration. They therefore concluded that *V. macrocarpa* seed lectin can induce cultured macrophages to release a neutrophil chemotactic mediator. These findings highlight the *V. macrocarpa* seed lectin as an important tool for studying pathological conditions associated with excess leukocytes at inflammatory sites causing tissue damage [48]. This also demonstrates an important divergence between the anti-inflammatory effects promoted by the *V. macrocarpa* leaf extract and the proinflammatory effects induced by the seed lectin [24,47,48].

Still investigating the proinflammatory property of lectin, this time obtained from *V. guianensis* seeds, Marques et al. [49] administered it to the rat's paws, observing the formation of edema in a time- and dose-dependent manner. The researchers suggest that *V. guianensis* lectin binds to specific glycans on targets, triggering inflammatory responses. The COX inhibitor indomethacin and interleukin-1β inhibitor thalidomide partially blocked the edematogenic effect, while the NOS inhibitor L-NAME did not. While pointing to the involvement of prostaglandins and interleukins in lectin-induced edema, this finding excludes the nitric oxide pathway, contrasting with its vasorelaxation mechanism previously discussed [38,49].

4.2.6. Central Nervous System

Notably, lectins are the most studied molecules in glycobiology, and plant lectins can serve as important tools for studying the role of carbohydrate–protein interactions in cellular function modulation. In the central nervous system (CNS) context, it was recently demonstrated that the *V. macrocarpa* seed lectin can alter neural function, eliciting depressive effects and activating neuroinflammatory markers [50]. The study highlights that although it has a carbohydrate affinity, like galactose-1 (gal-1), the lectin can exert neurotoxic effects in the hippocampus of mice, in contrast to the neuroprotective action already reported for gal-1. These findings suggest a possible dual role of galactose-binding lectins in the modulation of CNS function [50]. Lectins can be utilized in both basic and applied research, offering new alternatives for understanding neurological diseases, such as mental disorders, neurodegenerative diseases, and neuro-oncological conditions, as well as driving the search for new therapies for the diagnosis and treatment of these conditions [50,52].

4.2.7. Nociception

Leite et al. [51] studied the effects of *V. macrocarpa* lectin on nociception using menthol- or capsaicin-induced orofacial pain models in zebrafish, the only identified study of this activity for the genus. However, *V. macrocarpa* seed lectin pretreatment failed to demonstrate orofacial antinociception [51].

4.2.8. Wound-Healing

Research on the wound-healing properties of *V. guianensis* has demonstrated its potential to modulate the healing process by affecting the inflammatory response's intensity and promoting collagen synthesis pathways. This capability indicates that compounds found in the plant may influence tissue regeneration and decrease inflammation related to the healing process [16]. This effect would not be linked only to the pro/anti-inflammatory effect, but also to the antioxidant and antimicrobial activities of the plants. The correlation between these aspects suggests that the modulation of the inflammatory response by *V. guianensis* during the healing process may be partly mediated by the interaction of lectin with glycans on lesioned tissues. This interaction influences the production of essential inflammatory mediators for the initial response to injury that regulates the synthesis of structural components such as collagen, which is crucial to adequate scar tissue formation [16,49]. These hypotheses should be tested in the future, as they may contribute to developing new therapeutic agents and a better understanding of scar modulation strategies.

5. Final Considerations

This review is the first to highlight the potential of the *Vatairea* genus, which is utilized in traditional Amazonian medicine and systematizing knowledge about its ethnobotany, traditional knowledge, and uses, but also concerning the scientific evidence regarding its phytochemical composition, pharmacological properties, and safety of its use.

Beginning with its traditional applications, which emphasize its role in treating various skin conditions, it can address numerous pathological states, irritations, wound care, or superficial infections. Interestingly, it has been found that some plant components, such as the lectins present in the seeds, can irritate and stimulate inflammatory processes in peripheral contexts and the central nervous system. However, this stimulating activity of the inflammatory response appears to contribute positively to the evolution of the healing process [13,14,16].

The ability to inhibit the growth of various Gram-positive and Gram-negative bacteria and fungi is an interesting property for treating wounds and skin infections. This effect is likely associated with the antioxidant and anti-inflammatory properties of the phenolic compounds present in the extracts, which could contribute synergistically to the treatment's overall benefit. This multi-target pattern of drug action has been frequently explored in the search for more effective and safe therapeutic agents and appears to be the case for the *Vatairea* species studied [16,20,22].

In the context of diabetes, for example, the incidence of wounds and skin diseases is critical, given the difficulty in healing associated with the risk of infections that often lead to amputations, and even death. *V. macrocarpa*, in addition to its antimicrobial and anti-inflammatory effects and antioxidant potential, also showed benefits in diabetes models, reducing insulin resistance and glycemia. These effects can be used in isolation and synergistically [26].

Considering also the low toxicity of the extracts of *V. macrocarpa* and *V. guianensis*, it is important to advance in the pharmacological research of the *Vatairea* species, to elucidate their constitutions and properties in the various associated contexts and favor the development of safe and effective therapeutic agents.

Author Contributions: S.A.T.: conceptualization, formal analysis, investigation, methodology, writing—original draft; L.D.d.S.R.: formal analysis, investigation, writing—original draft; F.J.C.d.S.-J.: formal analysis, investigation, writing—original draft; B.C.d.C.: formal analysis, investigation, writing—original draft; F.C.S.G.: formal analysis, investigation, writing—original draft; L.V.P.d.S.P.: formal analysis, investigation, writing—original draft; C.S.F.M.: writing, data curation—review and editing; E.A.F.-J.: conceptualization, data curation, funding acquisition, methodology, project administration, writing—original draft, writing—review and editing. All authors have read and agreed to the published version of the manuscript.

Funding: Amazon Foundation for Research Support (FAPESPA)—scholarships to B.C.d.C., L.V.P.d.S.P. (grant number 02/2023); Foundation for the Coordination of Improvement of Higher Education Personnel (CAPES)—scholarship to S.A.T.

Institutional Review Board Statement: Not applicable.

Data Availability Statement: No new data were created or analyzed in this study. Data sharing is not applicable to this article.

Conflicts of Interest: The authors declare that this research was conducted in the absence of any commercial or financial relationships that could be construed as a potential conflict of interest.

References

1. Braga, F.C. Brazilian traditional medicine: Historical basis, features and potentialities for pharmaceutical development. *J. Tradit. Chin. Med. Sci.* **2021**, *8*, S44–S50. [CrossRef]
2. REFLORA. Public Search of Virtual Herbarium. Available online: https://reflora.jbrj.gov.br/reflora/herbarioVirtual/ (accessed on 29 June 2024).
3. Miguéis, G.d.S.; da Silva, R.H.; Júnior, G.A.D.; Guarim-Neto, G. Plants used by the rural community of Bananal, Mato Grosso, Brazil: Aspects of popular knowledge. *PLoS ONE* **2019**, *14*, e0210488. [CrossRef] [PubMed]
4. Ribeiro, R.V.; Bieski, I.G.C.; Balogun, S.O.; Martins, D.T.d.O. Ethnobotanical study of medicinal plants used by Ribeirinhos in the North Araguaia microregion, Mato Grosso, Brazil. *J. Ethnopharmacol.* **2017**, *205*, 69–102. [CrossRef]
5. de Amorim, L.D.M.; Sousa, L.d.O.F.d.; Oliveira, F.F.M.; Camacho, R.G.V.; de Melo, J.I.M. Fabaceae na Floresta Nacional (FLONA) de Assú, semiárido potiguar, nordeste do Brasil. *Rodriguésia* **2016**, *67*, 105–124. [CrossRef]
6. Silveira, F.S.; Miotto, S. A família Fabaceae no Morro Santana, Porto Alegre, Rio Grande do Sul, Brasil: Aspectos taxonômicos e ecológicos. *Rev. Bras. Biociências* **2013**, *11*, 93–114.
7. Ferreira, G.C.; Gomes, J.I.; Hopkins, M.J.G. Estudo anatômico das espécies de Leguminosae comercializadas no estado do Pará como "angelim". *Acta Amaz.* **2004**, *34*, 387–398. [CrossRef]
8. Cardoso, D.B.O.S.; Ramos, G.; Lima, H.C. Flora e Funga do Brasil. 2020. Available online: https://floradobrasil.jbrj.gov.br/FB23208 (accessed on 29 June 2024).
9. De Lima, H.C. Revisão Taxonômica Do Gênero Vataireopsis Ducke (LEG. FAB.). *Rodriguésia* **1980**, *32*, 21–40. [CrossRef]
10. Tropicos. Available online: https://tropicos.org/image/101098123 (accessed on 20 December 2024).
11. Tropicos. Available online: https://tropicos.org/image/100495992 (accessed on 20 December 2024).
12. Plants of the World Online. Plants of the World Online | Kew Science. Available online: http://www.plantsoftheworldonline.org/ (accessed on 20 December 2024).
13. Grenand, P.; Moretti, C.; Jacquemin, H.; Prévost, M.-F. Pharmacopées Traditionnelles en Guyane. In *IRD Éditions eBooks*; IRD Éditions; Elsevier: Amsterdam, The Netherlands, 2004; p. 186. [CrossRef]
14. Filho, W. Antraquinonas de *Vatairea guianensis* AUBI. (FABACEAE). Available online: https://repositorio.inpa.gov.br/bitstream/1/13726/1/artigo-inpa.pdf (accessed on 29 June 2024).
15. Araújo, G.d.M.L.d.; de Araújo, N.D.; de Farias, R.P.; Cavalcanti, F.C.N.; Lima, M.D.L.F.; Braz, R.A.F.d.S. Micoses superficiais na Paraíba: Análise comparativa e revisão literária. *An. Bras. Dermatol.* **2010**, *85*, 943–946. [CrossRef]
16. da Silva, C.T.L.; Medeiros, B.J.S.; dos Santos, K.C.; Pereira-Filho, R.; de Albuquerque-Júnior, R.L.C.; Sousa, P.J.d.C.; Carvalho, J.C.T. Topical healing activity of the hydroethanolic extract from the seeds of *Vatairea guianensis* (AUBLET) Research Article. *Int. J. Pharm. Sci. Rev. Res.* **2011**, *8*, 1–8.
17. Oliveira, A.A.; Segovia, J.F.; Sousa, V.Y.; Mata, E.C.; Gonçalves, M.C.; Bezerra, R.M.; Junior, P.O.; Kanzaki, L.I. Antimicrobial activity of amazonian medicinal plants. *SpringerPlus* **2013**, *2*, 371. [CrossRef]
18. Ottobelli, I.; Facundo, V.A.; Zuliani, J.; Luz, C.C.; Brasil, H.O.B.; Militão, J.S.L.T.; Braz-Filho, R. Estudo químico de duas plantas medicinais da amazônia: *Philodendron scabrum* k. Krause (araceae) e *Vatairea guianensis* aubl. (fabaceae). *Acta Amaz.* **2011**, *41*, 393–400. [CrossRef]
19. de Souza, R.F.; Marinho, V.H.S.; da Silva, G.A.; Costa-Júnior, L.M.; da Silva, J.K.R.; Bastos, G.N.T.; Arruda, A.C.; da Silva, M.N.; Arruda, M.S.P. New Isoflavones from the Leaves of *Vatairea guianensis* Aublé. *J. Braz. Chem. Soc.* **2013**, *24*, 1857–1863. [CrossRef]
20. Santana, D.B.; Da Costa, R.C.; Araújo, R.M.; De Paula, J.E.; Silveira, E.R.; Filho, R.B.; Espíndola, L.S. Activity of Fabaceae species extracts against fungi and Leishmania: Vatacarpan as a novel potent anti-Candida agent. *Rev. Bras. Farmacogn.* **2015**, *25*, 401–406. [CrossRef]
21. Mendoza-Cruz, E.; Sánchez-Gutiérrez, F.; Valdez-Hernández, J.I.; Mendoza-Cruz, E.; Sánchez-Gutiérrez, F.; Valdez-Hernández, J.I. Actividad de la guacamaya escarlata *Ara macao cyanoptera* (Psittaciformes: Psittacidae) y características estructurales de su hábitat en Marqués de Comillas, Chiapas. *Acta Zool. Mex.* **2017**, *33*, 169–180. [CrossRef]
22. Souza, R.; da Silva, G.; Arruda, A.; da Silva, M.; Santos, A.; Grisólia, D.; Silva, M.; Salgado, C.; Arruda, M.S. A New Prenylisoflavone from the Antifungal Extract of Leaves of *Vatairea guianensis* Aubl. *J. Braz. Chem. Soc.* **2016**, *28*, 1132–1136. [CrossRef]
23. de Jesus, N.Z.T.; Lima, J.C.d.S.; da Silva, R.M.; Espinosa, M.M.; Martins, D.T.d.O. Levantamento etnobotânico de plantas popularmente utilizadas como antiúlceras e antiinflamatórias pela comunidade de Pirizal, Nossa Senhora do Livramento-MT, Brasil. *Rev. Bras. Farm.* **2009**, *19*, 130–139. [CrossRef]
24. dos Santos, E.; Silva-Filho, S.E.; Radai, J.A.S.; Arena, A.C.; Fraga, T.L.; Cardoso, C.A.L.; Croda, J.; Kassuya, C.A.L. Anti-inflammatory properties of ethanolic extract from *Vatairea macrocarpa* leaves. *J. Ethnopharmacol.* **2021**, *278*, 114308. [CrossRef] [PubMed]

25. Costa, A.R.; Santos, A.M.; Barreto, F.S.; Costa, P.M.; Roma, R.R.; Rocha, B.A.; Oliveira, C.V.; Duarte, A.E.; Pessoa, C.; Teixeira, C.S. In vitro antiproliferative effects of *Vatairea macrocarpa* (Benth.) Ducke lectin on human tumor cell lines and in vivo evaluation of its toxicity in Drosophila melanogaster. *Food Chem. Toxicol.* **2024**, *190*, 114815. [CrossRef]
26. Oliveira, H.C.; dos Santos, M.P.; Grigulo, R.; Lima, L.L.; Martins, D.T.; Lima, J.C.; Stoppiglia, L.F.; Lopes, C.F.; Kawashita, N.H. Antidiabetic activity of *Vatairea macrocarpa* extract in rats. *J. Ethnopharmacol.* **2008**, *115*, 515–519. [CrossRef]
27. Baviloni, P.D.; dos Santos, M.P.; Aiko, G.M.; Reis, S.R.d.L.; Latorraca, M.Q.; da Silva, V.C.; Dall'oglio, E.L.; Júnior, P.T.d.S.; Lopes, C.F.; Baviera, A.M.; et al. Mechanism of anti-hyperglycemic action of *Vatairea macrocarpa* (Leguminosae): Investigation in peripheral tissues. *J. Ethnopharmacol.* **2010**, *131*, 135–139. [CrossRef]
28. Eddouks, M.; Bidi, A.; El Bouhali, B.; Hajji, L.; Zeggwagh, N.A. Antidiabetic plants improving insulin sensitivity. *J. Pharm. Pharmacol.* **2014**, *66*, 1197–1214. [CrossRef]
29. Simatupang, M.H.; Dietrichs, H.H.; Gottwald, H. Über die hautreizenden Stoffe in *Vatairea guianensis* Aubl. *Holzforschung* **1967**, *21*, 89–94. [CrossRef]
30. de Souza, R.F.; da Silva, J.K.R.; da Silva, G.A.; Arruda, A.C.; da Silva, M.N.; Arruda, M.S.P. Chemical Study and Evaluation of the Antioxidant Potential of Sapwood of *Vatairea guianensis* Aubl. *Rev. Virtual Quim.* **2015**, *7*, 1893–1906. [CrossRef]
31. Formiga, M.D.; Gottlieb, O.R.; Mendes, P.H.; Koketsu, M.; de Almieda, M.L.; Pereira, M.O.d.S.; Magalhães, M.T. Constituents of Brazilian leguminosae. *Phytochemistry* **1975**, *14*, 828–829. [CrossRef]
32. Sehgal, V.N.; Verma, P.; Khurana, A. Anthralin/dithranol in dermatology. *Int. J. Dermatol.* **2014**, *53*, e449–e460. [CrossRef] [PubMed]
33. Carvalho, P.O.; Campos, P.R.b.; Noffs, M.A.; Oliveira, J.G.; Shimizu, M.T.; da Silva, D.M. Application of microbial lipases to concentrate polyunsaturated fatty acids. *Química Nova* **2003**, *26*, 75–80. [CrossRef]
34. Vandenborre, G.; Smagghe, G.; Van Damme, E.J. Plant lectins as defense proteins against phytophagous insects. *Phytochemistry* **2011**, *72*, 1538–1550. [CrossRef]
35. Gemeiner, P.; Mislovičová, D.; Tkáč, J.; Švitel, J.; Pätoprstý, V.; Hrabárová, E.; Kogan, G.; Kožár, T. Lectinomics. *Biotechnol. Adv.* **2009**, *27*, 1–15. [CrossRef]
36. Zwierzina, H.; Bergmann, L.; Fiebig, H.; Aamdal, S.; Schöffski, P.; Witthohn, K.; Lentzen, H. The preclinical and clinical activity of aviscumine: A potential anticancer drug. *Eur. J. Cancer* **2011**, *47*, 1450–1457. [CrossRef]
37. Bies, C.; Lehr, C.-M.; Woodley, J.F. Lectin-mediated drug targeting: History and applications. *Adv. Drug Deliv. Rev.* **2003**, *56*, 425–435. [CrossRef]
38. Silva, H.C.; Nagano, C.S.; Souza, L.A.; Nascimento, K.S.; Isídro, R.; Delatorre, P.; Rocha, B.A.M.; Sampaio, A.H.; Assreuy, A.M.S.; Pires, A.F.; et al. Purification and primary structure determination of a galactose-specific lectin from *Vatairea guianensis* Aublet seeds that exhibits vasorelaxant effect. *Process. Biochem.* **2012**, *47*, 2347–2355. [CrossRef]
39. Cavada, B.S.; Osterne, V.J.S.; Pinto-Junior, V.R.; Souza, L.A.G.; Lossio, C.F.; Silva, M.T.L.; Correia-Neto, C.; Oliveira, M.V.; Correia, J.L.A.; Neco, A.H.B.; et al. Molecular dynamics and binding energy analysis of *Vatairea guianensis* lectin: A new tool for cancer studies. *J. Mol. Model.* **2020**, *26*, 22. [CrossRef]
40. Vasconcelos, M.A.; Arruda, F.V.S.; Carneiro, V.A.; Silva, H.C.; Nascimento, K.S.; Sampaio, A.H.; Cavada, B.; Teixeira, E.H.; Henriques, M.; Pereira, M.O. Effect of Algae and Plant Lectins on Planktonic Growth and Biofilm Formation in Clinically Relevant Bacteria and Yeasts. *BioMed Res. Int.* **2014**, *2014*, 365272. [CrossRef]
41. Teixeira, E.; Napimoga, M.; Carneiro, V.; de Oliveira, T.; Cunha, R.; Havt, A.; Martins, J.; Pinto, V.; Goncalves, R.; Cavada, B. In vitro inhibition of Streptococci binding to enamel acquired pellicle by Plant Lectins. *J. Appl. Microbiol.* **2006**, *101*, 111–116. [CrossRef]
42. Santos, V.F.; Costa, M.S.; Campina, F.F.; Rodrigues, R.R.; Santos, A.L.E.; Pereira, F.M.; Batista, K.L.R.; Silva, R.C.; Pereira, R.O.; Rocha, B.A.M.; et al. The Galactose-Binding Lectin Isolated from *Vatairea macrocarpa* Seeds Enhances the Effect of Antibiotics Against *Staphylococcus aureus*–Resistant Strain. *Probiotics Antimicrob. Proteins* **2019**, *12*, 82–90. [CrossRef]
43. Véras, J.H.; Cardoso, C.G.; Puga, S.C.; Bisneto, A.V.d.M.; Roma, R.R.; Silva, R.R.S.; Teixeira, C.S.; Chen-Chen, L. Lactose-binding lectin from *Vatairea macrocarpa* seeds induces in vivo angiogenesis via VEGF and TNF-α expression and modulates in vitro doxorubicin-induced genotoxicity. *Biochimie* **2022**, *194*, 55–66. [CrossRef] [PubMed]
44. Jesus, N.Z.T.; Júnior, I.F.S.; Lima, J.C.S.; Colodel, E.M.; Martins, D.T.O. Hippocratic screening and subchronic oral toxicity assessments of the methanol extract of *Vatairea macrocarpa* heartwood in rodents. *Rev. Bras. Farm.* **2012**, *22*, 1308–1314. [CrossRef]
45. da Silva, C.T.L.; Mendonça, L.C.; Chagas Monteiro, M.; Carvalho, J.C.T. Antimicrobial activity of extracts obtained from the seeds of *Vatairea guianensis* (Aublet). *Bol. Latinoam. Caribe Plantas Med. Aromát.* **2011**, *10*, 456–462.
46. Monteiro, A.M.O.; Havt, A.; Barbosa, P.S.F.; Soares, T.F.; Evangelista, J.S.A.M.; Alencar, N.M.N.; Monteiro, H.S.A.; Martins, A.M.C.; de Menezes, D.B.; Fonteles, M.C.; et al. Renal effects induced by the lectin from *Vatairea macrocarpa* seeds. *J. Pharm. Pharmacol.* **2005**, *57*, 1329–1333. [CrossRef]

47. Alencar, N.M.; Assreuy, A.M.; Alencar, V.B.; Melo, S.C.; Ramos, M.V.; Cavada, B.S.; Cunha, F.Q.; Ribeiro, R.A. The galactose-binding lectin from *Vatairea macrocarpa* seeds induces in vivo neutrophil migration by indirect mechanism. *Int. J. Biochem. Cell Biol.* **2003**, *35*, 1674–1681. [CrossRef]
48. Alencar, N.M.N.; Assreuy, A.M.S.; Havt, A.; Benevides, R.G.; de Moura, T.R.; de Sousa, R.B.; Ribeiro, R.A.; Cunha, F.Q.; Cavada, B.S. *Vatairea macrocarpa* (Leguminosae) lectin activates cultured macrophages to release chemotactic mediators. *Naunyn-Schmiedeberg's Arch. Pharmacol.* **2006**, *374*, 275–282. [CrossRef] [PubMed]
49. Marques, G.F.; Osterne, V.J.; Almeida, L.M.; Oliveira, M.V.; Brizeno, L.A.; Pinto-Junior, V.R.; Santiago, M.Q.; Neco, A.H.; Mota, M.R.; Souza, L.A.; et al. Contribution of the carbohydrate-binding ability of *Vatairea guianensis* lectin to induce edematogenic activity. *Biochimie* **2017**, *140*, 58–65. [CrossRef]
50. Gonçalves, F.M.; Freitas, A.E.; Peres, T.V.; Rieger, D.K.; Ben, J.; Maestri, M.; Costa, A.P.; Tramontina, A.C.; Gonçalves, C.A.; Rodrigues, A.L.S.; et al. *Vatairea macrocarpa* Lectin (VML) Induces Depressive-like Behavior and Expression of Neuroinflammatory Markers in Mice. *Neurochem. Res.* **2013**, *38*, 2375–2384. [CrossRef] [PubMed]
51. Leite, G.d.O.; Santos, S.A.A.R.; Bezerra, F.M.D.H.; de Silva, F.E.S.; Ribeiro, A.D.d.C.; Roma, R.R.; Silva, R.R.S.; Santos, M.H.C.; Santos, A.L.E.; Teixeira, C.S.; et al. Is the orofacial antinociceptive effect of lectins intrinsically related to their specificity to monosaccharides? *Int. J. Biol. Macromol.* **2020**, *161*, 1079–1085. [CrossRef] [PubMed]
52. Araújo, J.R.C.; Coelho, C.B.; Campos, A.R.; Moreira, R.d.A.; Monteiro-Moreira, A.C.d.O. Animal Galectins and Plant Lectins as Tools for Studies in Neurosciences. *Curr. Neuropharmacol.* **2020**, *18*, 202–215. [CrossRef]
53. Fosso, M.Y.; Chan, K.Y.; Gregory, R.; Chang, C.-W.T. Library Synthesis and Antibacterial Investigation of Cationic Anthraquinone Analogs. *ACS Comb. Sci.* **2012**, *14*, 231–235. [CrossRef]
54. Liu, X.; Hu, H.; Liu, J.; Chen, J.; Chu, J.; Cheng, H. Physcion, a novel anthraquinone derivative against *Chlamydia psittaci* infection. *Vet. Microbiol.* **2023**, *279*, 109664. [CrossRef]
55. Comini, L.R.; Vieyra, F.E.M.; Mignone, R.A.; Páez, P.L.; Mugas, M.L.; Konigheim, B.S.; Cabrera, J.L.; Montoya, S.C.N.; Borsarelli, C.D. Parietin: An efficient photo-screening pigment in vivo with good photosensitizing and photodynamic antibacterial effects in vitro. *Photochem. Photobiol. Sci.* **2016**, *16*, 201–210. [CrossRef]
56. García-Sosa, K.; Villareal-Alvarez, N.; Lübben, P.; Peña-Rodríguez, L.M. Chrysophanol, an Antimicrobial Anthraquinone from the Root Extract of *Colubrina greggii*. *J. Mex. Chem. Soc.* **2020**, *50*, 76–78. [CrossRef]
57. Fonseca, S.; dos Santos, N.S.S.; Torres, A.; Siqueira, M.; da Cunha, A.; Manzoni, V.; Provasi, P.F.; Gester, R.; Canuto, S. Role of the Solvent and Intramolecular Hydrogen Bonds in the Antioxidative Mechanism of Prenylisoflavone from Leaves of *Vatairea guianensis*. *J. Phys. Chem. A* **2023**, *127*, 10807–10816. [CrossRef]
58. Santos, J.V.d.O.; Porto, A.L.F.; Cavalcanti, I.M.F. Potential Application of Combined Therapy with Lectins as a Therapeutic Strategy for the Treatment of Bacterial Infections. *Antibiotics* **2021**, *10*, 520. [CrossRef] [PubMed]

pharmaceuticals

Review

Current Utilization and Research Status of Herbal Medicine Sipjeondaebotang for Anemia: A Scoping Review

Gyeongmuk Kim [1,†], Han-Gyul Lee [2,†], Won Jung Ha [1] and Seungwon Kwon [2,*]

[1] Department of Clinical Korean Medicine, Graduate School, Kyung Hee University, Seoul 02447, Republic of Korea; kkm156@naver.com (G.K.); new_mon@naver.com (W.J.H.)

[2] Department of Cardiology and Neurology, Kyung Hee University College of Korean Medicine, Kyung Hee University Medical Center, Seoul 02447, Republic of Korea; gyulee0614@hanmail.net

* Correspondence: kkokkottung@hanmail.net; Tel.: +82-02-958-9127

† These authors contributed equally to this work.

Abstract: Background/Objectives: Anemia is a global health issue affecting diverse populations, particularly older adults, and conventional treatments often show limited efficacy. This study aimed to evaluate the utilization and effectiveness of Sipjeondaebotang (SDT), a prescription drug used in traditional East Asian medicine, in treating various types of anemia. Methods: A scoping review was conducted following Arksey and O'Malley's framework and PRISMA-ScR guidelines. Six electronic databases were searched for clinical studies on SDT, while focusing on human participants and excluding animal and cellular studies. Sixteen studies, including nine randomized controlled trials, two controlled clinical trials, two case series, and three case reports, involving 863 participants, were analyzed. These studies were primarily conducted in China, Korea, and Japan. Results: According to the analysis, SDT improved hemoglobin levels across all types of anemia studied, with all controlled studies showing significant improvements compared with the control groups. Additionally, SDT reduced blood loss, improved recovery times, and decreased transfusion requirements in patients with post-operative anemia, with lower adverse event rates than those in the control groups. These findings suggest that SDT may enhance hematological parameters and improve overall patient outcomes. Conclusions: In conclusion, SDT may be an effective treatment for anemia that improves hemoglobin levels and patient outcomes. However, further high-quality, large-scale studies are necessary to standardize SDT prescriptions, confirm the optimal treatment duration, and validate its efficacy and safety across different anemia types.

Keywords: anemia; Sipjeondaebotang; Shiquan Dabu tang; Juzentaihoto; hemoglobin; hematocrit

1. Introduction

Anemia is a condition characterized by a decrease in the number of red blood cells (RBCs) or hemoglobin levels, leading to an inadequate oxygen supply to body tissues [1,2]. Anemia is a global public health problem that affects people of all ages in both developing and developed countries [3,4]. Especially in individuals aged $\geq$ 65 years, anemia significantly contributes to morbidity and mortality and affects the quality of life. In the context of global aging, anemia is a burden on individuals, society, and healthcare providers [5,6].

Anemia is classified based on its etiology, including types such as iron deficiency anemia, which results from defects in the differentiation and maturation of erythroid cells; vitamin deficiency anemia, caused by deficiencies in vitamin B12 and folic acid; anemia due to bleeding; hemolytic anemia; aplastic anemia; chronic disease-related anemia due to conditions such as renal failure or malignant tumors; and hereditary diseases such as sickle cell anemia [7].

Iron deficiency anemia is treated with oral or intravenous iron supplements such as iron sucrose [8]. Pernicious anemia due to vitamin B12 or folate deficiency is managed with vitamin B12 and folate supplements [9]. Anemia in chronic kidney disease (CKD) patients is treated with iron supplements and erythropoietin receptor activators [10]. These conventional Western treatments improve hemoglobin levels and alleviate symptoms. However, these treatments may not be effective in all cases. In the case of anemia in CKD patients, even when erythropoietin receptor activators are used at appropriate doses, 5–10% of CKD patients show insufficient clinical response [11]. Additionally, for the treatment of iron deficiency anemia, only approximately 10% of orally administered iron supplements are absorbed in the intestine, indicating several clinical limitations [12].

In East Asia, herbal medicine prescriptions from traditional East Asian medicine (TEAM) have been orally administered to manage clinical symptoms associated with anemia, which is recognized as a clinical syndrome known as "blood deficiency" in TEAM theory [13,14]. Herbal prescriptions for the treatment of this condition have been developed over time, and their indications and effects have been documented in medical texts and clinical case studies [15–17].

Among these, Sipjeondaebotang (SDT; Shiqua Dabu Tang in Chinese and Juzentaihoto in Japanese) is a prescription composed of 10 herbal medicines (Table 1). SDT is a herbal prescription that tonifies blood deficiency. In a previous systematic review of anemia [17], it was noted that Astragali Radix (Root of *Astragalus membranaceus* Bunge), Atractylodis Rhizoma Alba (Rhizome of *Atractylodis Rhizoma* Alba), and Angelicae Gigantis Radix (Root of *Angelica gigas* Nakai) were the most commonly used herbal medicines in the analyzed studies. Since SDT contains these herbal medicines, it raises the possibility of improving anemia by tonifying the blood effects of SDT. Recently, clinical reports on the use of SDT for anemia were published. Chen et al. and Ai et al. conducted randomized controlled trials (RCT) on SDT in patients with post-operative anemia and reported that the combination of SDT and conventional therapy was more beneficial than conventional therapy alone in improving anemia [18,19]. However, there is limited comprehensive clinical information on the effects of SDT on anemia.

Table 1. The 10 Herbal medicines that constitute Sipjeondaebotang.

Herbal Medicine	Scientific Name (Family)
Ginseng Radix	*Panax ginseng* C. A. Meyer (Araliaceae)
Astragali Radix	*Astragalus membranaceus* Bunge (Fabaceae)
Hoelen alba	*Poria cocos* Wolf (Polyporaceae)
Atractylodis Rhizoma Alba	*Atractylodes japonica* Koidzumi (Asteraceae)
Glycyrrhizae Radix	*Glycyrrhiza uralensis* Fischer (Fabaceae)
Rehmanniae Radix preparate *	*Rehmannia glutinosa* (Liboschitz ex Steudel) (Plantaginaceae)
Angelicae gigantis Radix	*Angelica gigas* Nakai (Apiaceae)
Cnidii Rhizoma	*Cnidium officinale* Makino (Apiaceae)
Paeoniae Radix alba	*Paeonia lactiflora* Pallas (Paeoniaceae)
Cinnamomi Cortex	*Cinnamomum cassia* Presl (Lauraceae)

* *Rehmanniae Radix preparata* is the steamed and dried root of *Rehmannia glutinosa* (Liboschitz ex Steudel).

To clarify the effects and indications of SDT for anemia, we reviewed all clinical reports and reviews on SDT for anemia. This review aimed to evaluate comprehensively the current evidence supporting the use of SDT in treating anemia, determine its significance in clinical practice and identify knowledge gaps. This review will help establish a clearer understanding of SDT clinical efficacy, guiding future research to enhance its clinical application.

2. Results

2.1. Literature Search and Selection Process

Seventy documents published up to 30 June 2024 were identified. Finally, 16 studies [18–33] were selected using a literature selection process (Figure 1). A total of 22 duplicate studies were excluded from the analysis. In addition, 31 studies were excluded based on their titles and abstracts because they were not directly related to SDT or anemia, were not conducted in human patients, or were not related to herbal medicines. Following a professional review, one study was excluded because the original text could not be located.

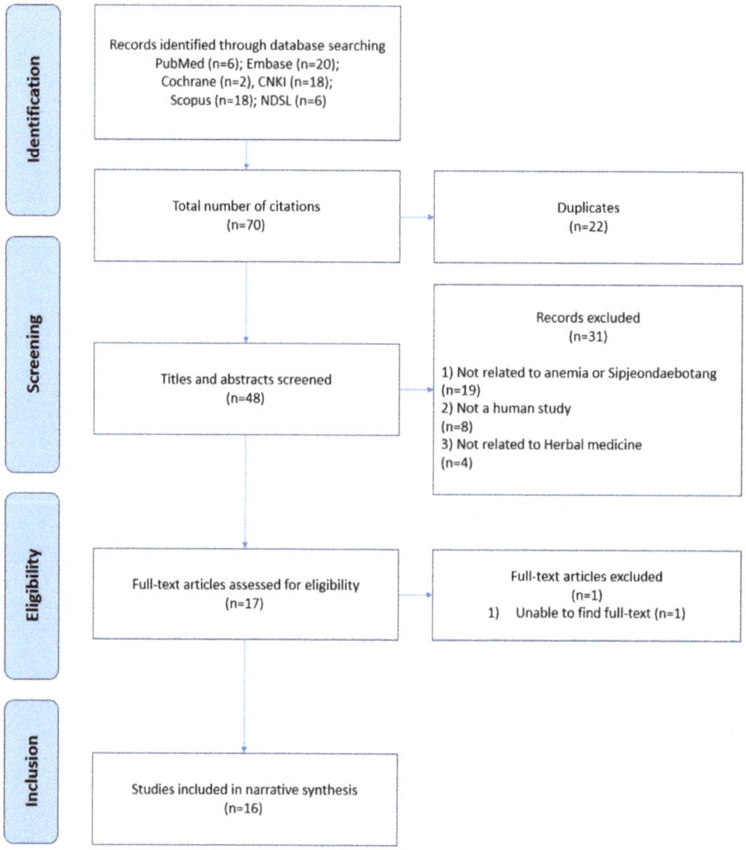

Figure 1. Study flow chart.

2.2. General Characteristics of the Identified Literature

The relevant literature was published over the past 26 years (1999–2024). Except for one Chinese paper published in 1999 [20], all publications date from 2000 onward (Table 2).

Table 2. General characteristics of the included studies (n = 16).

Variables	Categories	N (%)
Publication year	1990–1999	1 (6.25%)
	2000–2009	3 (18.75%)
	2010–2024	12 (75%)
Research Methodology	Case series	2 (12.5%)
	Case report	3 (18.75%)
	Randomized controlled trial	9 (56.25)
	Non-randomized controlled trial	2 (12.5%)
Location	China	10 (62.5%)
	South Korea	2 (12.5%)
	Japan	4 (25%)

2.3. Study Designs

Of the 16 studies reviewed, five were observational studies (31.25%) [20,21,24,30,31] and 11 were interventional studies (68.75%) [18,19,22,23,25–29,32,33]. Among the observational studies, three were case reports [24,30,31] and two were case series [20,21]. The interventional studies included nine RCTs [18,19,25–29,32,33] and two controlled clinical trials [22,23].

Of the nine RCTs, six focused on interventions for anemia resulting from post-operative bleeding, all of which were related to orthopedic surgeries [18,19,27,29,32,33]. Two studies addressed patients receiving erythropoietin for CKD anemia [25,26], while one study investigated anemia due to gastrointestinal bleeding [28].

One of the two case series examined hemolytic anemia after interferon/ribavirin therapy in patients with hepatitis C [21]. The three case reports addressed treatments for CKD anemia [30], anemia due to gastrointestinal hemorrhage [31], and myelodysplastic syndrome, respectively [24].

2.4. Research Regions

The studies were conducted across three countries, with the majority of studies conducted in China (n = 10/16, 62.5%) [18–20,25–29,32,33]. Two case studies were conducted in Korea (n = 2/16, 12.5%) [30,31], and two controlled clinical trials, one case study, and one case series were conducted in Japan (n = 4/16, 25%) [21–24].

2.5. Demographic Characteristics of Study Participants

2.5.1. Participant Number, Sex, and Age

After excluding literature reviews, 863 participants were involved in the included studies (Table 2). Among these, 112 patients were included in case reports and case series, while 751 patients participated in RCTs or controlled clinical trials. Yao et al. (2012) did not report the sex of the participants. Of the remaining 809 participants in the other studies, 425 (52.53%) were male and 384 (47.47%) were female. Patient ages ranged from 18 to 67 years, with one study not mentioning the age [25]. Interventional studies expressed age as a mean value.

2.5.2. Types of Anemia

Classified by the type of anemia, there were seven studies on post-operative anemia [18,19,23,27,29,32,33], four studies on CKD anemia [22,25,26,30], two studies on gastrointestinal bleeding anemia [28,31], one study on hemolytic anemia [21], one study on myelodysplastic syndrome [24], and one study on an unspecified type of anemia [20]. Among the nine RCTs, six addressed post-operative anemia [18,19,27,29,32,33], two focused on CKD anemia [25,26], and one investigated gastrointestinal bleeding anemia [28]. There was one case report each for CKD anemia [30], gastrointestinal bleeding anemia [30], and myelodysplastic syndrome [24]. In controlled clinical trials, there was one case each of post-operative anemia [23] and CKD anemia [22]. The case series included one of hemolytic anemia [21] and one of unknown anemia [20] (Figure 2, Table 3).

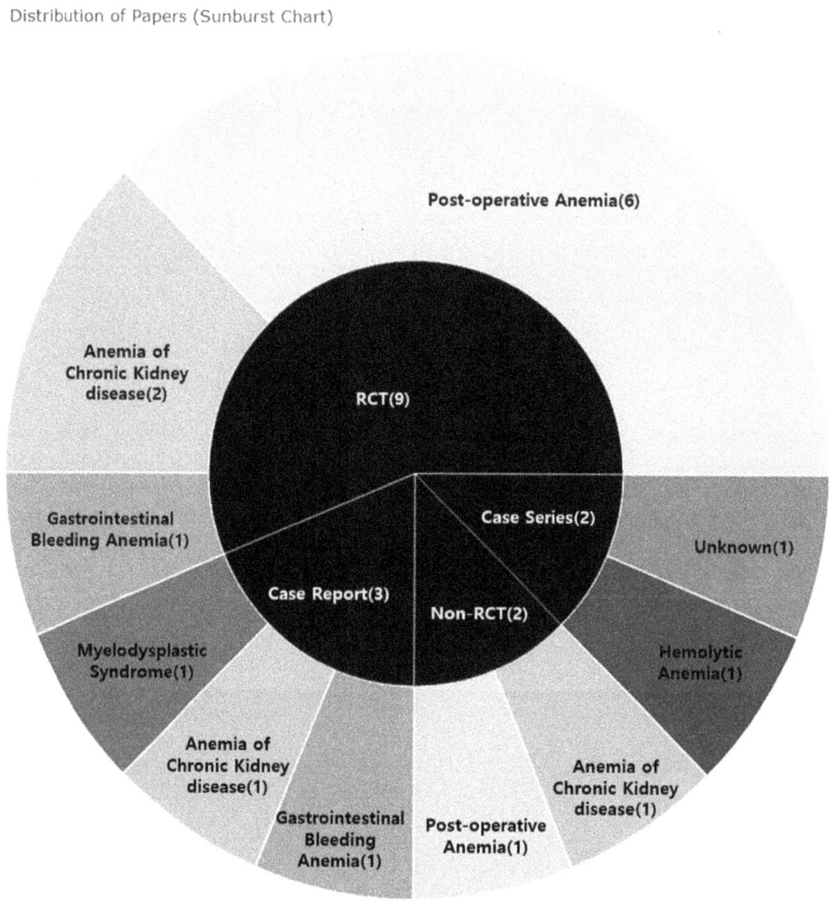

Figure 2. Distribution of studies by type of research. RCT—randomized controlled trial.

Table 3. Demographic and clinical characteristics of patients.

Location/ Design	Sample Size (Male/Female)	Age (Treatment/Control)	Types of Anemia	Author (Year)
South Korea/ Case report	1(0/1)	76	Gastrointestinal bleeding anemia	Kim (2020) [31]
South Korea/ Case report	1(1/0)	47	CKD anemia	Kim (2019) [30]
China/RCT	54	Not mentioned	CKD anemia	Yao (2012) [25]
China/RCT	120(70/50)	40.3 ± 2.8	CKD anemia	Yao (2016) [26]
China/RCT	60(31/29)	(64.21 ± 2.29 /66.21 ± 1.86)	Post-operative anemia (knee joint replacement)	Fang (2018) [29]
China/RCT	120(73/47)	71.47 ± 4.66	Post-operative anemia (proximal femur nail antirotation)	Li (2020) [32]

Table 3. *Cont.*

Location/ Design	Sample Size (Male/Female)	Age (Treatment/Control)	Types of Anemia	Author (Year)
China/RCT	100(57/43)	(48.46 ± 3.66 /48.14 ± 3.27)	Gastrointestinal bleeding anemia	Li (2018) [28]
China/ Case series	42(23/19)	18~67	Unknown (no mention)	Wang (1999) [20]
China/RCT	45(22/23)	(66.32 ± 8.09 /63.57 ± 6.32)	Post-operative anemia (total hip arthroplasty)	Tian (2020) [33]
China/RCT	40(13/27)	65~82 (68.7 ± 5.33 /70.7 ± 4.68)	Post-operative anemia (total hip arthroplasty)	Sheng (2017) [27]
China/RCT	80(34/46)	75~95(83.6 ± 7.2) /76~93(82.4 ± 5.8)	Post-operative anemia (proximal femur nail antirotation)	Ai (2022) [19]
Japan/ Case report	1(0/1)	76	Myelodysplastic syndrome	Beinu (2011) [24]
China/RCT	72(26/46)	(67.36 ± 6.38 /67.89 ± 7.47)	Post-operative anemia (total knee arthroplasty)	Chen (2024) [18]
Japan/ Controlled clinical trial	18(0/18)	(49.4 ± 9.4 /52.1 ± 3.1)	Post-operative anemia (total hip arthroplasty or rotational acetabular osteotomy)	Kishida (2009) [23]
Japan/ Controlled clinical trial	42(33/9)	(67 ± 12/62 ± 12)	CKD anemia	Nakamoto (2008) [22]
Japan/ Case series	67(42/25)	(54.8 ± 9.0/54.6 ± 7.8)	Hemolytic anemia	Sho (2004) [21]

2.5.3. Types of Treatment and Medication

Research on post-operative anemia focused on orthopedic surgeries, with five studies related to hip surgery [19,23,27,32,33] and two studies related to knee surgery [18,29]. Blood transfusions were administered in the research on myelodysplastic syndrome [24]. In four studies on CKD anemia, erythropoietin was used in all cases [25,26,28,30]. Iron supplements [18,20,25,26,31], folic acid [18,20,25,26,28], and vitamin B12 [20,25,26,28] were concurrently administered. In two case reports, acupuncture was performed alongside the administration of SDT [30,31] (Table 4).

2.6. Details in Intervention

2.6.1. Dosage, Frequency, and Treatment Period of Herbal Medicine

In this context, "dosage" refers to the total combined quantity of the listed herbal medicines administered in a unit. For example, administering one dosage twice daily indicates that the specified amount is divided into two separate administrations within a 24 h period. Regarding the dosage (Table 5), when the composition was considered as one dosage unit, two case reports indicated two doses per day [30,31]. In nine RCTs conducted in China, as well as in two controlled clinical trials and a case series from Japan, the prescribed dosage was one dose per day [18,19,21–23,25–29,32,33]. One case report from Japan did not specify the dosage [24].

Table 4. Summary of the included studies.

Intervention	Other Treatment	Other Medications	Outcomes	Significant Findings	Adverse Events	References
SDT variants 1	Acupuncture	Beta-blocker Vasodilator Analgesics Antiemetic Iron supplements Statin Proton pump inhibitor	Hb RBC WBC Hct Intensity of dizziness (VAS)	The major blood parameters returned to normal ranges Hb 8.8 g/dL $\rightarrow$ 11.8 g/dL RBC 2.68 $\times$ 10^6/µL $\rightarrow$ 3.86 $\times$ 10^6/µL WBC 2.21 $\times$ 10^3/µL $\rightarrow$ 3.16 $\times$ 10^3/µL Hct 26% $\rightarrow$ 35.9% The patient's subjective symptom of dizziness VAS 5 $\rightarrow$ 1	Not mentioned	Kim (2020) [31]
SDT	Acupuncture	Antacid Amino acid rHuEPO	Hb Fatigue severity scale(FSS)	The patient's hemoglobin levels improved after taking the medicine Hb 9.6 g/dL $\rightarrow$ 12.7 g/dL The patient's fatigue severity scale (FSS) was improved 35 $\rightarrow$ 15	Not mentioned	Kim (2019) [30]
SDT variants 2	(-)	rHuEPO Iron Folic acid Vitamin B12	Hb Hct	The patient's hemoglobin and hematocrit level of the treatment group were significantly increased Treatment group: Hb 64.68 $\pm$ 9.11 $\rightarrow$ 105.82 $\pm$ 13.66 Hct 20.87 $\pm$ 2.18 $\rightarrow$ 32.51 $\pm$ 3.11 Control group: Hb 64.42 $\pm$ 7.50 $\rightarrow$ 95.23 $\pm$ 12.50 Hct 20.47 $\pm$ 2.23 $\rightarrow$ 28.57 $\pm$ 2.68	Not mentioned	Yao (2012) [25]
SDT variants 3	(-)	rHuEPO Iron Folic acid Vitamin B12	Treatment effective rate Hb Hct	Total effective rate of treatment group was significantly higher and the patient's hemoglobin and hematocrit level of the treatment group were significantly increased Treatment group: Total effective rate Hb 62.46 $\pm$ 12.64 $\rightarrow$ 106.21 $\pm$ 11.61 Hct 21.52 $\pm$ 3.20 $\rightarrow$ 31.51 $\pm$ 4.21 Control group Total effective rate 81.67 Hb 63.13 $\pm$ 14.01 $\rightarrow$ 87.07 $\pm$ 12.21 Hct 20.17 $\pm$ 3.27 $\rightarrow$ 25.81 $\pm$ 4.67	Not mentioned	Yao (2016) [26]

Table 4. *Cont.*

Intervention	Other Treatment	Other Medications	Outcomes	Significant Findings	Adverse Events	References
SDT	Knee joint replacement	Tranexamic Acid Sodium Chloride Morphine Epinephrine Ropivacaine	Amount of bleeding and drainage Hb Knee resting pain score(VAS)	The Hb in the treatment group was significantly improved compared to the control group The knee resting pain score (VAS) of treatment group was significantly lower than that of control group Treatment group: The patient satisfaction of treatment group was significantly higher than that of control group Treatment group: Hb $104.36 \pm 8.83 \rightarrow 117.72 \pm 6.07$ VAS 6.31 ± 0.52 Satisfaction 96.0 Control group: Hb $107.83 \pm 9.08 \rightarrow 109.62 \pm 5.38$ VAS 8.02 ± 0.81 Satisfaction 82.0	Not mentioned	Fang (2018) [29]
SDT variants 4	Proximal femur nail antirotation	Not mentioned	Hb Hct Hidden blood loss Fasting blood glucose level Hospitalization and fracture healing times Hip joint function recovery rates	The Hb, Hct was significantly improved and hidden blood loss was reduced, and hospitalization and fracture healing time were shorter than control group. Treatment group Hb $122.85 \pm 15.24 \rightarrow 100.85 \pm 13.28$ Hct $33.65 \pm 5.41 \rightarrow 27.96 \pm 3.25$ Hidden blood loss $245.74 \pm 88.26 \rightarrow 188.26 \pm 70.12$ Hospitalization time 8.72 ± 2.37 Fracture healing time 12.65 ± 1.34 Control group Hb $120.96 \pm 16.31 \rightarrow 90.41 \pm 11.27$ Hct $32.98 \pm 6.13 \rightarrow 25.47 \pm 4.52$ Hidden blood loss $288.67 \pm 90.94 \rightarrow 245.94 \pm 75.36$ Hospitalization time 15.12 ± 3.41 Fracture healing time 15.27 ± 5.78	Not mentioned	Li (2020) [32]
SDT	No treatment	Erythropoietin Vitamin B12 Folic acid Somatostatin Pantoprazole sodium	Hb Reticulocytes Platelets White blood cells	The Hb was significantly improved and reticulocytes, platelets, white blood cell counts were significantly increased. Treatment group Hb $42.86 \pm 5.41 \rightarrow 95.47 \pm 6.98$ Reticulocytes $0.95 \pm 0.25 \rightarrow 2.48 \pm 1.63$ Platelets: $28.95 \pm 5.42 \rightarrow 59.74 \pm 9.85$ White blood cells: $2.44 \pm 0.52 \rightarrow 4.85 \pm 1.6$	Total adverse event rate Treatment group: 4.00% Control group: 34.00%	Li (2018) [28]

Table 4. *Cont.*

Intervention	Other Treatment	Other Medications	Outcomes	Significant Findings	Adverse Events	References
SDT	No treatment	Iron Folic acid Vitamin B12	Hb	The total effect rates were 95.2%	Not mentioned	Wang (1999) [20]
SDT	Total hip arthroplasty	Tranexamic acid	RBC Hb Hct D-dimer Total blood loss Patient blood volume Dominant blood loss Hidden blood loss Transfusion rate and average transfusion volume Harris hip score Traditional Chinese medicine (TCM) Syndrome score and efficacy	The treatment group's RBC, Hb, Hct were significantly improved and D-dimer, total blood loss, hidden blood loss were significantly lower than control group. The Harris hip score and TCM syndrome efficacy were significantly higher in treatment group.	Total adverse event rate Treatment group: 13.64% Control group: 30.43%	Tian (2020) [33]
SDT variants 5	Total hip arthroplasty	Not mentioned	Hb Hct Total blood loss Intra-operative blood loss Post-operative drainage Hidden blood loss Transfusion rate	The treatment group's Hb and Hct were significantly improved and total, post-operative drainage, hidden blood loss were significantly reduced. Transfusion rate was also lower in treatment group. Treatment group Hb $131.5 \pm 15.1 \rightarrow 93.5 \pm 17.9$ Hct $0.42 \pm 0.05 \rightarrow 0.29 \pm 0.05$ Post-operative drainage 456.2 ± 147.3 Hidden blood loss 796.7 ± 354.6 Transfusion rate 15% Control group Hb $130.5 \pm 13.9 \rightarrow 83.5 \pm 9.6$ Hct $0.41 \pm 0.06 \rightarrow 0.24 \pm 0.04$ Post-operative drainage 612.4 ± 161.5 Hidden blood loss 1064.6 ± 335.7 Transfusion rate 35%	No adverse effect	Sheng (2017) [27]

Table 4. *Cont.*

Intervention	Other Treatment	Other Medications	Outcomes	Significant Findings	Adverse Events	References
SDT	Proximal femur nail antirotation	Antibiotics Ribaroxaban Albumin	Hb Serum albumin Transfusion rate Transfusion volume Serum albumin infusion rate Serum albumin infusion volume	The treatment group's Hb level was significant increased and transfusion rates and volume were significantly lower than control group. Treatment group Hb 115.24± 6.13 → 80.45 ± 9.48 Transfusion rate 20.0% Transfusion volume 1.94 ± 0.44 Control group Hb 116.43 ± 3.64 → 71.81 ± 12.43 Transfusion rate 40.0% Transfusion volume 3.86 ± 2.62	Total adverse event rate Treatment group: 30% Control group: 47.5%	Ai (2022) [19]
① SDT ② SDT variants 6 ③ SDT variants 7	Transfusion	Vitamin K2 Hwangigunjung-tang Samul-tang	WBC RBC Hb Platelet	After adding malt sugar to Sipjeondaebotang, hemoglobin and platelet levels significantly increased. Bone marrow findings showed a reduction in erythroblasts.	No adverse effect	Beinu (2011) [24]
SDT	Total knee arthroplasty	Iron sucrose injection	Hb RBC Hct Platelet Interleukin-6 Tumor necrosis factor-alpha C-reactive protein Hospital for special surgery knee score(HSS) Visual analogue scale (VAS) Perioperative blood loss and transfusion rate Post-operative complication rate	The effective rate of the treatment group and the HSS score were significantly higher than that of the control group, and the levels of Hb, RBC, Hct were significantly increased. The levels of protein and CRP and the VAS score, and the perioperative blood transfusion rate were significantly lower than that in the control group. Treatment group Effective rate 91.7% Hb 130.44 ± 7.13 → 121.39 ± 6.05 RBC 4.30 ± 0.25 → 3.96 ± 0.19 Hct 39.88 ± 3.30 IL-6 97.52 ± 5.89 → 31.80 ± 2.58 TNF-a 17.51 ± 2.18 → 7.16 ± 1.11 CRP 26.87 ± 3.38 → 11.70 ± 1.87 HSS score 61.92 ± 2.87 → 85.86 ± 2.65 VAS score 6.87 ± 1.10 → 1.17 ± 0.43 Perioperative transfusion rate 8.33% Control group Hb 130.44 ± 7.13 → 121.39 ± 6.05 RBC 4.30 ± 0.25 → 3.96 ± 0.19 Hct 39.88 ± 3.30 IL-6 98.22 ± 6.08 → 34.52 ± 2.79 TNF-a 17.32 ± 2.39 → 8.31 ± 1.30 CRP 26.34 ± 5.53 → 13.37 ± 2.11 Perioperative transfusion rate 27.78% HSS score 61.53 ± 3.08 → 84.67 ± 2.08 VAS score 6.81 ± 1.12 → 1.93 ± 0.47	Total adverse event rate Treatment group: 5.56% Control group: 27.78%	Chen (2024) [18]

Table 4. *Cont.*

Intervention	Other Treatment	Other Medications	Outcomes	Significant Findings	Adverse Events	References
SDT	Total hip arthroplasty or rotational acetabular osteotomy Autologous donation	Not mentioned	Hb blood loss post-operative recovery rate laboratory tests (serum creatinine, AST, ALT, Na, K)	The Hb levels were significantly improved during the preoperative period. At the last autologous donation, the levels of Hb were higher in treatment group than control group. Treatment group Reduction of Hb at last autologous donation 0.7 g/dL Control group Reduction of Hb at last autologous donation 1.5 g/dL	No adverse effect	Kishida (2009) [23]
SDT	Not mentioned	Erythropoietin	Hb CRP	The Hb levels of treatment group were significantly increased, and the CRP levels were significantly decreased compared to the control group. Treatment group Hb $8.4 \pm 1.10 \rightarrow 9.5 \pm 1.3$ CRP $1.4 \pm 1.7 \rightarrow 0.6 \pm 0.8$ Control group Hb $8.3 \pm 0.7 \rightarrow 8.5 \pm 0.5$ CRP did not significantly change	No adverse effect in treatment group	Nakamoto (2008) [22]
SDT	Not mentioned	Interferon plus ribavirin(IFN/Rib)	Hb ALT	The Hb levels of treatment group showed significant reduction in HB decrease, and requirement for ribavirin dose reduction or withdrawal were significantly lower than that of the control group. Treatment group Requirement for ribavirin dose reduction/withdrawal 13% (4/32) Control group Requirement for ribavirin dose reduction/withdrawal 13% (4/32)	Not mentioned	Sho (2004) [21]

SDT, Sipjeondaebotang. Hb, Hemoglobin, RBC, Red blood cell. WBC, White blood cell. Hct, Hematocrit. rHuEPO, Recombinant human erythropoietin. AST, aspartate transaminase. ALT, Alanine aminotransferase. CRP, C-reactive protein.

Table 5. Summary of the ingredients, dosage, frequency, and treatment duration of the included studies. The family name of the plant of origin of the herbal medicine is in parentheses.

Intervention	Composition	Dosage	Frequency	Treatment Duration	References
SDT variants 1	*Panax ginseng* C. A. Meyer (Araliaceae) 6 g, *Astragalus membranaceus* Bunge (Fabaceae) 3 g, *Wolfiporia extensa* (Peck) Ginns (as *Poria cocos* Wolf) (Polyporaceae) 6 g, *Atractylodes japonica* Koidzumi (Asteraceae) 6 g, *Glycyrrhiza uralensis* Fischer (Fabaceae) 6 g, *Rehmannia glutinosa* (Liboschitz ex Steudel) (Plantaginaceae) 3 g, *Angelica gigas* Nakai (Apiaceae) 3 g, *Cnidium officinale* Makino (Apiaceae) 3 g, *Paeonia lactiflora* Pallas (Paeoniaceae) 3 g, *Cinnamomum cassia* Presl (Lauraceae) 3 g, *Zingiber officinale* Roscoe (Zingiberaceae) 6 g, *Ziziphus jujuba* Mill. (Rhamnaceae) 4 g, *Pinellia ternata* (Thunb.) Makino ex Breitenbach (Araceae) 4 g, *Citrus reticulata* Blanco (Rutaceae) 4 g.	2 doses per day	Three times per day p.o	41 days	Kim (2020) [31]
SDT	*P. ginseng* 6 g, *A. membranaceus* 6 g, *W. extensa* 5 g, *A. japonica* 5 g, *G. uralensis* 5 g, *R. glutinosa* 5 g, *A. gigas* 5 g, *C. officinale* 5 g, *P. lactiflora* 5 g, *C. cassia* 6 g, *Z. jujuba* 6 g, *Z. officinale* 6 g	2 doses per day	Three times per day p.o	16 days	Kim (2019) [30]
SDT variants 2	*P. ginseng* 9 g, *A. membranaceus* 30 g, *W. extensa* 12 g, *A. japonica* 10 g, *G. uralensis* 6 g, *R. glutinosa* 20 g, *A. gigas* 15 g, *C. officinale* 9 g, *P. lactiflora* 10 g, *C. cassia* 5 g, *Rheum palmatum* L. (Polygonaceae) 9 g.	1 dose per day	Two times per day p.o	3 months	Yao (2012) [25]
SDT variants 3	*A. membranaceus* 30 g, *W. extensa* 12 g, *A. japonica* 10 g, *G. uralensis* 6 g, *R. glutinosa* 20 g, *A. gigas* 15 g, *C. officinale* 9 g, *P. lactiflora* 10 g, *C. cassia* 5 g, *R. palmatum* 9 g.	1 dose per day	Two times per day p.o	3 months	Yao (2016) [26]
SDT	*A. membranaceus* 50 g, *W. extensa* 10 g, *A. japonica* 13 g, *G. uralensis* 6 g, *A. gigas* 10 g, *C. officinale* 8 g, *P. lactiflora* 13 g, *Equus asinus* L. (Equidae) (*as Asini Corri* Colla) 10 g.	1 dose per day	Two times per day p.o	1 day	Fang (2018) [29]
SDT variants 4	*A. membranaceus* 15 g, *A. japonica* 15 g, *C. officinale* 10 g, *R. glutinosa* 10 g, *A. gigas* 10 g, *W. extensa* 10 g, *P. lactiflora* 10 g, *C. cassia* 3 g, *G. uralensis* 3 g, *Codonopsis pilosula* (Franch.) Nannf. (Campanulaceae) 15 g.	1 dose per day	Two times per day p.o	3 days	Li (2020) [32]
SDT	*P. ginseng* 6 g, *A. membranaceus* 12 g, *W. extensa* 9 g, *A. japonica* 9 g, *G. uralensis* 3 g, *R. glutinosa* 12 g, *A. gigas* 9 g, *C. officinale* 6 g, *P. lactiflora* 9 g, *C. cassia* 3 g.	1 dose per day	Two times per day p.o	10 days	Li (2018) [28]
SDT	*P. ginseng* 6 g, *A. membranaceus* 20 g, *W. extensa* 15 g, *A. japonica* 20 g, *G. uralensis* 6 g, *R. glutinosa* 20 g, *A. gigas* 20 g, *C. officinale* 12 g, *P. lactiflora* 20 g, *C. cassia* 5 g, *R. glutinosa* 20 g, *Leonurus japonicus* (Lamiaceae) 15 g, *Crataegus pinnatifida* (Rosaceae) 10 g, *Triticum aestivum* L. 10 g, *Hordeum vulgare* (Poaceae) 10 g.	1 dose per day	Not mentioned	3 months~4 years (mean 18 months)	Wang (1999) [20]
SDT	*A. membranaceus* 12 g, *W. extensa* 9 g, *A. japonica* 9 g, *G. uralensis* 3 g, *R. glutinosa* 12 g, *A. gigas* 9 g, *C. officinale* 6 g, *P. lactiflora* 9 g, *C. cassia* 3 g, *C. pilosula* 9 g.	1 dose per day	Two times per day p.o	7 days	Tian (2020) [33]

Table 5. *Cont.*

Intervention	Composition	Dosage	Frequency	Treatment Duration	References
SDT variants 5	*A. membranaceus* 15 g, *W. extensa* 10 g, *A. japonica* 15 g, *G. uralensis* 3 g, *R. glutinosa* 15 g, *A. gigas* 10 g, *C. officinale* 10 g, *P. lactiflora* 10 g, *C. cassia* 3 g, *C. pilosula* 15 g, *Selaginella doederleinii* (Selaginellaceae) 15 g, *Coix lacryma-jobi* (Poaceae) 30 g, *Salvia miltiorrhiza* (Lamiaceae) 20 g, *Polygonatum odoratum* (Asparagaceae) 15 g, *Polygonum multiflorum* (Polygonaceae) 15 g, *Ligustrum lucidum* (Oleaceae) 10 g, *Eucommia ulmoides* (Eucommiaceae) 15 g.	1 dose per day	Two times per day p.o	14 days	Sheng (2017) [27]
SDT	*A. membranaceus* 20 g, *W. extensa* 15 g, *A. japonica* 20 g, *G. uralensis* 3 g, *R. glutinosa* 15 g, *A. gigas* 15 g, *C. officinale* 15 g, *P. lactiflora* 15 g, *C. cassia* 3 g, *C. pilosula* 20 g.	1 dose per day	Two times per day p.o	14 days	Ai (2022) [19]
① SDT ② SDT variants 6 ③ SDT variants 7	①: *P. ginseng* 3 g, *A. membranaceus* 3 g, *W. extensa* 3 g, *A. japonica* 3 g, *G. uralensis* 1.5 g, *R. glutinosa* 3 g, *A. gigas* 5 g, *C. officinale* 3 g, *P. lactiflora* 3 g, *C. cassia* 3 g ②: in ①, *R. glutinosa, C. officinale, P. lactiflora, A. gigas* were changed to 6 g. ③: in ②, add *Oryza sativa* L. (Poaceae) 10 g	Not mentioned	Not mentioned	31 months	Beinu (2011) [24]
SDT	*P. ginseng* 6 g, *A. membranaceus* 20 g, *W. extensa* 15 g, *A. japonica* 15 g, *G. uralensis* 6 g, *R. glutinosa* 15 g, *A. gigas* 15 g, *C. officinale* 6 g, *P. lactiflora* 6 g, *C. cassia* 6 g, *Drynaria fortunei* J.Smith (Polypodiaceae) 10 g, *Pyritum* 10 g	1 dose per day	Two times per day p.o	14 days	Chen (2024) [18]
SDT	*P. ginseng* 3 g, *A. membranaceus* 3 g, *W. extensa* 3 g, *A. japonica* 3 g, *G. uralensis* 1.5 g, *R. glutinosa* 3 g, *A. gigas* 5 g, *C. officinale* 3 g, *P. lactiflora* 3 g, *C. cassia* 3 g	7.5 g per day	Not mentioned	21 days	Kishida (2009) [23]
SDT	*P. ginseng* 3 g, *A. membranaceus* 3 g, *W. extensa* 3 g, *A. japonica* 3 g, *G. uralensis* 1.5 g, *R. glutinosa* 3 g, *A. gigas* 5 g, *C. officinale* 3 g, *P. lactiflora* 3 g, *C. cassia* 3 g	7.5 g per day	Not mentioned	12 weeks	Nakamoto (2008) [22]
SDT	*P. ginseng* 3 g, *A. membranaceus* 3 g, *W. extensa* 3 g, *A. japonica* 3 g, *G. uralensis* 1.5 g, *R. glutinosa* 3 g, *A. gigas* 5 g, *C. officinale* 3 g, *P. lactiflora* 3 g, *C. cassia* 3 g	7.5 g per day	Not mentioned	2 weeks	Sho (2004) [21]

Regarding the frequency of SDT administration investigated in studies, it was not described in two case series [20,21], one case report [24], and two controlled clinical trials [22,23]. It was described as twice per day in nine RCTs [18,19,25–29,32,33] and three times per day in two case reports [30,31].

The treatment duration across the studies varied from 1 day to 4 years. When considering only interventional studies, the treatment duration varied from 1 day to 3 months [18, 19,22,23,25–29,32,33]. The most common treatment duration was 14 days [18,19,21,27], and six of the 16 studies had a treatment duration of 14–21 days [18,19,21,23,27,30].

2.6.2. Composition of SDT and Herbal Medicines Included in Its Variants

In ten studies [18–23,28–30,33], the original SDT was employed, whereas six studies [24–27,31,32] applied variants of SDT. The herbal medicines added to the original SDT in these variants included Zingiberis Rhizoma Crudus, Jujubae Fructus, Pinelliae Rhizoma, Citri Pericarpium, Rhei Radix et Rhizoma, Codonopsis Pilosulae Radix, Selaginellae herba, Coicis Semen, Salviae Radix, Polygonati Rhizoma, Reynoutriae Multiflorae Radix, Ligustri Fructus, Eucommia ulmoides Oliver, and Oryzae Gluten. Among these, Rhei Radix et Rhizoma [28,29] and Codonopsis Pilosulae Radix [30,34] were the most frequently used, each appearing in two studies, whereas the other herbs were used only once. Additionally, Codonopsis Pilosulae Radix was used in two studies that reported the use of the original SDT formula [19,33]. The dosage of each herb varied widely, ranging from 1.5 g to 50 g.

Among the three studies addressing CKD anemia, two RCTs [25,26] included the addition of Rhei Radix et Rhizoma. For post-operative anemia, Codonopsis Pilosulae Radix was added in three [19,27,32] out of six RCTs, making it the most frequently added herbal medicine. Other herbal additives were added or removed according to the patient's specific condition.

2.7. Evaluation Methods

Evaluation Tools

The evaluation tools are listed in order of frequency of use as follows: Hemoglobin levels were analyzed in all 16 studies. This was followed by hematocrit (Hct) in seven studies [18,25–27,31–33], RBC count in four studies [18,24,31,33], platelet count in three studies [18,24,28], and white blood cell (WBC) count in two studies [24,31]. In addition to Hb and Hct levels and RBC, platelet, and WBC counts, other blood tests included fasting blood glucose [32], reticulocyte [28], D-dimer [33], interleukin-6, tumor necrosis factor-alpha, C-reactive protein [18], serum creatinine, AST, ALT, sodium, and potassium levels [23]. In cases of post-operative anemia, blood loss [23,27,32,33] and transfusion volume were assessed [18,27,33].

2.8. Treatment Outcomes

In nine RCTs [18,19,25–29,32,33], hemoglobin levels were significantly improved in the patients compared with those in the control groups. Two controlled clinical trials [22,23] also demonstrated significant improvements in hemoglobin levels of patients compared with those of the controls. In three case reports [24,30,31], hemoglobin levels were restored to normal ranges in patients. Additionally, one case series [21] reported a significant reduction in hemoglobin levels in the treatment group.

Among the seven studies that measured Hct levels [18,25–27,31–33], six with control groups [18,25–27,32,33] showed significant improvements in Hct levels, and one case report [31] indicated a return to the normal range.

All studies focusing on post-operative anemia [18,19,23,27,29,32,33] reported significant improvements in hemoglobin levels. Additional significant improvements were observed in visual analog scale VAS scores, patient satisfaction, total blood loss, hidden blood loss, length of hospital stay, fracture healing time, post-operative drainage volume, transfusion rate, and transfusion volume.

Among the studies targeting CKD anemia, in three controlled studies [22,25,26], both hemoglobin and Hct levels showed significant increase, accompanied by a reduction in C-reactive protein levels and an improved total effective rate. A case report noted improvements in fatigue severity [30].

In a single case report of anemia following gastrointestinal bleeding, hemoglobin, Hct, RBC, and WBC levels were restored and VAS scores decreased. In one RCT [28], significant increases were observed in hemoglobin levels and reticulocyte, platelet, and WBC counts.

For myelodysplastic syndrome, a single case report [24] documented significant increases in hemoglobin and platelet levels.

Finally, in a case series focusing on hemolytic anemia [21], the reduction in hemoglobin levels was significantly less pronounced, and the requirement for dose reduction or discontinuation of ribavirin, an anemia-inducing treatment drug, was lower.

2.9. Safety

Adverse events were reported in four studies [18,19,28,33]. The total incidence of adverse events was lower in the treatment groups than in the control groups in each study, with rates of 4%/34%, 13.64%/30.43%, 30%/47.5%, and 5.56%/27.78%, respectively.

3. Discussion

This study aimed to investigate the status of studies applying SDT to various types of anemia. The analysis was conducted based on four detailed questions: (1) what type of studies have been conducted? (2) what types of anemia has SDT been used for? (3) what improvements did SDT make when applied to patients? and (4) what is the level of evidence supporting the efficacy of herbal medicines?

3.1. Research Status

All the 16 studies included in the analysis were conducted in East Asian countries, specifically South Korea, China, and Japan. Although a worldwide database was selected for the search, the papers selected for analysis were limited to East Asia, likely because research utilizing SDT was predominantly published in this region. Among the 16 studies that applied SDT to anemia, nine were RCTs, constituting the highest proportion (56.25%), and all RCTs were conducted in China. Anemia can be easily diagnosed through blood tests that measure hemoglobin and Hct levels. Therefore, it is plausible that conducting RCTs for anemia is easier than for other diseases. All RCTs compared a control group undergoing conventional Western medical treatment for anemia with an experimental group receiving the same conventional treatment combined with SDT, regardless of the etiology of anemia.

Post-operative anemia accounted for the highest proportion of the analyzed studies, with six RCTs and one controlled clinical trial representing a significant number of high evidence level studies. In contrast, CKD anemia had two RCTs and one case report, gastrointestinal bleeding anemia had one RCT and one case report, hemolytic anemia had one case series, and myelodysplastic syndrome had one case report, indicating relatively fewer studies.

3.2. Types of Anemia

The most common type of anemia treated with SDT was post-operative anemia (43.75%). Studies on post-operative anemia showed significant improvements in hemoglobin and RBC levels and reductions in intra-operative transfusion requirements and hidden blood loss post-surgery with SDT administration. Intra-operative transfusions can be used to correct anemia or anticoagulant imbalances during and after surgery; surgery itself can increase the risk of venous thromboembolism (VTE), which can be dose-dependent on the amount of transfused blood [35]. Therefore, reducing the amount of transfusion through SDT administration may help lower the risk of VTE. The second most frequently studied type was CKD anemia, and recombinant human erythropoietin was chosen as the basic treatment in all the included studies.

3.3. Significance of SDT Treatment

All studies included in the analysis examined changes in hemoglobin levels. All 11 interventional studies (nine RCTs and two controlled clinical trials) showed significant increases in hemoglobin levels in the treatment group compared with the control group. Additionally, three case reports and one case series demonstrated a return to normal hemoglobin levels, indicating that SDT administration increased hemoglobin levels in different types of anemia, such as post-operative anemia, CKD anemia, myelodysplastic syndrome, gastrointestinal bleeding anemia, and hemolytic anemia. Studies on post-operative anemia reported significant increases in hemoglobin levels and overall patient condition improvements, including VAS pain scores, patient satisfaction, total blood loss, hidden blood loss, length of hospital stay, fracture healing time, post-operative drainage volume, transfusion rate, and transfusion volume, suggesting that SDT is effective in improving anemia during the post-operative recovery process. In studies on CKD anemia, significant increases in Hb and Hct levels were observed, indicating that SDT may contribute to the improvement of anemia caused by reduced kidney function. Furthermore, studies on anemia following gastrointestinal bleeding showed recovery in Hb, Hct, RBC, and WBC levels and a decrease in VAS scores, whereas studies on myelodysplastic syndrome and hemolytic anemia reported significant therapeutic effects. This suggests that SDT may be useful for treating anemia under various pathological conditions.

3.4. Proposed Treatment Mechanisms for SDT in Anemia

The studies included in the analysis examined the effects of various herbal medicines of SDT on the hematopoietic system, bone marrow, and erythrocytes. Experimental research showed that Rehmanniae Radix preparata, a component of SDT, stimulates the hematopoietic system and increases the secretion of various hematopoietic factors [34]. Additionally, SDT was shown to be effective in restoring hematopoietic function in damaged bone marrow [36]. Another study highlighted that SDT contains substances that promote the growth of hematopoietic stem cells and play a crucial role in bone marrow stimulation, including essential fatty acids [37]. Research on Palmultang (Ba Bao Tang in Chinese and Hachimotsuto in Japanese), which includes components of SDT, demonstrated that it stimulates the transcription of erythropoietin mRNA in the liver and kidneys and enhances serum erythropoietin expression [38]. Moreover, extracts of Paeoniae Radix alba and Astragali Radix, which are constituents of SDT, were reported to increase hemoglobin levels and RBC volume [39].

Based on these findings, the multi-compound formulation of SDT appears to influence the hematopoietic system by enhancing serum erythropoietin expression and stimulating the bone marrow, which could benefit patients with anemia. However, to elucidate these effects more clearly, additional well-designed clinical and experimental studies are required.

3.5. Limitations of This Study and Suggestions for Further Studies

Based on the analysis of the reviewed studies, applying SDT for anemia generally improved hemoglobin and Hct levels in anemia patients. However, the amount of the included herbs varied across studies, and the dosages also differed, with some studies using one dose and others using two doses. Additionally, in terms of herbal composition, some studies addressing CKD anemia included the addition of Rhei Radix et Rhizoma, whereas studies on post-operative anemia often added Codonopsis Pilosulae Radix to the SDT. This suggests the need to standardize SDT prescription and format based on the type of anemia.

The analysis showed that hemoglobin and Hct levels significantly improved in controlled studies and returned to normal ranges in case reports, indicating their reliability as measures. Therefore, it is essential to include blood tests for assessing hemoglobin and Hct levels in study designs, and efforts should be made to standardize these measures. The treatment duration in the included studies varied from 1 day to 4 years, but the most commonly used treatment period was 14 days, with 6 out of 16 studies having a duration of 14 to 21 days. Therefore, a 2 to 3 weeks administration period seems to be the most appropriate; however, additional studies are required to confirm the treatment period.

Finally, although all studies demonstrated improvements in hemoglobin levels and significant enhancements in outcome measures, there were limitations due to small sample sizes, varied follow-up periods, the risk of publication bias, and heterogeneous study designs. Therefore, once well-controlled RCTs and other clinical studies are conducted, systematic reviews and meta-analyses with higher levels of evidence will be necessary to validate the effects of SDT on each type of anemia.

4. Materials and Methods

In this study, a scoping review design was adopted to investigate the status of studies that used SDT for anemia. A scoping review is a research approach that methodically searches for, collects, and synthesizes available knowledge to outline essential concepts, evidence types, and gaps in relevant research areas [40]. This method is useful for obtaining a broad understanding of the current state of research on a particular topic by examining the scope and characteristics of available studies [40,41].

This study adhered to the methodology outlined by Arksey and O'Malley [40] and the Expanded Reporting Items for Systematic Reviews and Meta-Analyses (PRISMA-ScR) for scoping reviews. The research was executed across the following five stages: (1) establishment of research questions; (2) identification of relevant studies; (3) selection of studies; (4) organization of data; and (5) collection, summary, and reporting of results.

4.1. Identifying the Research Questions

Before starting the research, we posed the question: "What studies have applied SDT to anemia?" Therefore, the primary objective of this review was to analyze the existing literature on the clinical outcomes of SDT for anemia. To clarify the objectives of this review, we present the following research questions. (1) What types of studies have been conducted? (2) What types of anemia have SDT been used for? (3) What improvements did SDT make when applied to patients? (4) What is the level of evidence supporting the efficacy of herbal medicines?

4.2. Literature Search

The PICO framework guided the formulation of the search query, which focused on the use of SDT to treat anemia. The search specifically included clinical studies involving human participants. Studies conducted at the cellular level or utilizing animal models were excluded. The scope of the intervention was confined exclusively to the herbal formula, SDT, as it pertains to TEAM. The etiology of anemia treatment included all types. SDT variants (Gamisipjeondaebotang in Korean, Jiawei Shiquan Dabu Tang in Chinese, and Kamijuzentaihoto in Japanese), which adjust some of the ten ingredients based on the patient's condition or symptoms, were also included in the study. Formulations, such as decoctions, pills, powders, and capsules, were included without restrictions. Studies that used non-oral administration methods, including acupoints or intravenous injections, were excluded. No specific constraints were imposed on the types of controls or outcomes considered. Eligible studies were focused exclusively on clinical research and encompassed a variety of research designs, including case reports, case series, prospective and retrospective observational studies, before-and-after studies, RCTs, integrative literature reviews, and systematic reviews. The selection was limited to studies fully published in academic journals, and unpublished manuscripts while conference abstracts were not considered.

Six electronic databases were used for the literature review: MEDLINE (PubMed), Embase, Cochrane Library, National Digital Science Library, China National Knowledge Infrastructure, and SCOPUS. In addition to the databases, relevant studies, previously identified but not captured through the search strategy, were also included in the analysis. A comprehensive search of all titles, abstracts, subject headings, and studies published up to 30 June 2024, was conducted on 11 July 2024, using the specified term combinations detailed in Appendix A.

4.3. Literature Selection

All literature search results were organized using EndNote version 21. Two reviewers (GK and HL) independently reviewed the titles, abstracts, and full texts of the studies, and selected the appropriate literature based on their understanding of the process and purpose of this study. The second reviewer (HL) re-evaluated the literature through a primary review. Disagreements during the literature selection process were resolved through discussion between the two reviewers. If a consensus could not be reached, the final decision was made by a third reviewer (SK).

After eliminating duplicates, studies were selected based on their titles and abstracts, while adhering to the inclusion and exclusion criteria. The introductory sections of the selected studies were then reviewed to finalize the selection for inclusion.

4.4. Data Extraction and Schematization

The studies ultimately included were analyzed and discussed in relation to the primary research questions. To establish the basic characteristics of these studies, we compiled information on the authors, publication year, study field, and design. Each study was catalogued in a structured format that encompassed essential details about the participants, classification of diseases, treatment specifics, methods of assessment, and primary outcomes, facilitating an understanding of the participant demographics and interventions, as well as the impact of the treatments.

The data gathered primarily pertained to observational and interventional studies, with the necessary details documented in systematic reviews. In general, all information was transcribed exactly as it appeared in the source material. Authorship was noted using the surname of the first author, publication year was noted as the year of entry into the bibliographic database, and field of study was defined as the discipline of the first author's affiliated institution. The study designs were categorized according to the methodologies outlined in the Public Health Guidance (2012) issued by the National Institute for Health and Care Excellence [42]. Documents were categorized based on established criteria; if the methodology was not explicitly defined, the most suitable classification was determined based on the document's content. The research designs were broadly segmented into observational, interventional, and literature studies.

For publication year, research design, and research area, a table was compiled, listing the number of documents and their proportion relative to the total document count. Excel 2019 was used to create a chart to examine the distribution of study designs over time. Using Python 3.10.6, a sunburst chart was generated, the inner circle of which categorizes the studies, whereas the outer circle details the specific diseases addressed by these studies.

Furthermore, basic details about the study participants were outlined, including total participant count, sex distribution, age range, duration of treatment, and specific type of anemia. If only the sex ratio was available, approximate numbers were deduced by applying the sex ratio to the total number of participants. Treatment duration was expressed in days or months. In cases where a control group was present, details for both the treatment and control groups were provided separately. Data not specified were labeled as "Not mentioned", and the diagnostic criteria for anemia were explicitly described as per the documents.

For treatment details, the records included both herbal medicine treatments and supplementary therapies used in conjunction with herbal medicine. The specific name of the herbal prescription, its composition, administration methods (frequency and dosage per day), and total duration of treatment were documented. If frequency or dosage was not mentioned, it was labeled as "Not mentioned." If the treatment duration was absent, it was estimated in days from the visit to the treatment end date. In cases where the prescription composition was not detailed, it was recorded according to the original source, with reference to the Korea Pharmaceutical Information Center (www.health.kr). Concurrent treatments, including conventional therapies and other TEAM therapies, such as acupuncture, cupping, and moxibustion, were also summarized.

The evaluation methods employed in each study were analyzed based on the descriptions in the text. Observational studies concentrated on documenting clinical progression. Interventional studies rigorously examined the evaluation methods specified in the research design.

The main findings were derived from the treatment outcomes emphasized in the Discussion and Conclusion Sections of the studies. Improvements were also noted if pretreatment results for the evaluation tools were available. In cases of multiple assessments, both the initial and final results were documented.

Author Contributions: Conceptualization, S.K.; methodology, S.K. and H.-G.L.; validation, S.K., H.-G.L. and W.J.H.; formal analysis, G.K. and H.-G.L.; Investigation, G.K. and H.-G.L.; resources, G.K. and H.-G.L.; funding acquisition, S.K.; data curation, G.K. and H.-G.L.; writing—original draft preparation, G.K. and H.-G.L.; writing—review and editing, S.K. and W.J.H.; visualization, G.K.; supervision, S.K.; project administration, S.K. All authors have read and agreed to the published version of the manuscript.

Funding: This research was supported by a grant from the Korea Health Technology R&D Project through the Korea Health Industry Development Institute, funded by the Ministry of Health and Welfare, Republic of Korea (grant number RS-2023-KH142002).

Institutional Review Board Statement: Not applicable.

Informed Consent Statement: Not applicable.

Data Availability Statement: The original contributions presented in the study are included in the article, further inquiries can be directed to the corresponding author.

Conflicts of Interest: The authors declare no conflicts of interest.

Appendix A. Key Words Used in Searches

[Pubmed]

1. (Anemia[MeSH Terms])
2. (((((((((Sipjeondaebo-tang[Title/Abstract]) OR (sipjeondaebotang[Title/Abstract])) OR (sibjeondaebo-tang[Title/Abstract])) OR (sibjeondaebo-tang[Title/Abstract])) OR (Juzentaiho-to[Title/Abstract])) OR (Juzen-taiho-to[Title/Abstract])) OR (Juzentaihoto[Title/Abstract])) OR (shiquandabutang[Title/Abstract])) OR (shi-quan-da-bu-tang[Title/Abstract])) OR (shiquandabu-tang[Title/Abstract])4 OR 5
3. #1 AND #2

[Embase]

1. 'anemia'/exp OR anemia
2. 'sipjeondaebo tang':ab,ti OR 'sipjeondaebotang:ab,ti OR 'sibjeondaebo tang':ab,ti OR 'juzentaiho to':ab,ti OR 'juzen taiho to':ab,ti OR juzentaihoto:ab,ti OR shiquandabu-tang:ab,ti OR 'Shi quan da bu tang':ab,ti
3. #1 AND #2

[Cochrane]

1. MeSH descriptor: [Anemia] explode all trees
2. Sipjeondaebo-tang OR Sipjeondaebotang OR sibjeondaebo-tang OR Juzentaiho-to OR Juzen-taiho-to OR Juzentaihoto OR Shiquandabutang OR Shi-quan-da-bu-tang
3. #1 AND #2

[CNKI]

1. TKA = Anemia OR TKA = 貧血

2. TI = 'Juzentaiho-to' OR TI = 'Juzen-taiho-to' OR TI = 'Juzentaihoto' OR TI = Shiquandabutang OR TI = 'Shi-quan-da-bu-tang' OR TI = '十全大補湯' OR TI = '十全大补汤'
3. #1 AND #2

[SCOPUS]

1. TITLE-ABS-KEY ("anemia")
2. INDEXTERMS ("anemia")
3. #1 OR #2
4. INDEXTERMS ("Sipjeondaebo-tang" OR "sipjeondaebotang" OR "sibjeondaebo-tang" OR "sibjeondaebo-tang" OR "Juzentaiho-to" OR "Juzen-taiho-to" OR "Juzentaihoto" OR "shiquandabutang" OR "shi-quan-da-bu-tang")
5. TITLE-ABS-KEY ("Sipjeondaebo-tang" OR "sipjeondaebotang" OR "sibjeondaebo-tang" OR "sibjeondaebo-tang" OR "Juzentaiho-to" OR "Juzen-taiho-to" OR "Juzentaihoto" OR "shiquandabutang" OR "shi-quan-da-bu-tang")
6. #4 OR #5
7. #3 AND #6

[NDSL]
"전체 = (빈혈 | "anemia") AND 전체 = (십전대보탕 | 十全大補湯)"

References

1. Shander, A.; Goodnough, L.T.; Javidroozi, M.; Auerbach, M.; Carson, J.; Ershler, W.B.; Ghiglione, M.; Glaspy, J.; Lew, I. Iron Deficiency Anemia-Bridging the Knowledge and Practice Gap. *Transfus. Med. Rev.* **2014**, *28*, 156–166. [CrossRef] [PubMed]
2. Leung, K.C.A.; Lam, M.J.; Wong, H.C.A.; Hon Kam, L.; Li, X. Iron Deficiency Anemia: An Updated Review. *Curr. Pediatr. Rev.* **2024**, *20*, 339–356. [CrossRef] [PubMed]
3. Cappellini, M.D.; Motta, I. Anemia in Clinical Practice—Definition and Classification: Does Hemoglobin Change with Aging? *Semin. Hematol.* **2015**, *52*, 261–269. [CrossRef] [PubMed]
4. Pasaribu, R.D.; Aritonang, E.; Sudaryati, E.; Zuska, F. Anemia in Pregnancy: Study Phenomenology. *Port. J. Public Health* **2023**, *42*, 6–14. [CrossRef]
5. Stauder, R.; Thein, S.L. Anemia in the elderly: Clinical implications and new therapeutic concepts. *Haematologica* **2014**, *99*, 1127–1130. [CrossRef]
6. Savarese, G.; von Haehling, S.; Butler, J.; Cleland, J.G.F.; Ponikowski, P.; Anker, S.D. Iron deficiency and cardiovascular disease. *Eur. Heart J.* **2023**, *44*, 14–27. [CrossRef]
7. Chamoli, S.C. Clinical Evaluation of Different Types of Anemia. *World J. Anemia* **2018**, *2*, 26–30. [CrossRef]
8. Koh, J.S.; Song, I.-C. Pharmacotherapeutics for iron deficiency anemia in adults. *J. Korean Med. Assoc.* **2024**, *67*, 48–53. [CrossRef]
9. Jo, D.Y. Current Clinical Practice: Treatment of pernicious anemia. *Korean J. Med.* **2006**, *71*, 237.
10. Oak, C.Y.; Kim, N.H. Anemia and nutrition in end stage renal disease patient. *J. Korean Med. Assoc.* **2013**, *56*, 592–599. [CrossRef]
11. Fujimoto, D.; Adachi, M.; Miyasato, Y.; Hata, Y.; Inoue, H.; Oda, A.; Kakizoe, Y.; Nakagawa, T.; Shimasaki, A.; Nakamura, K.; et al. Efficacy of continuous erythropoietin receptor activator for end-stage renal disease patients with renal anemia before and after peritoneal dialysis initiation. *Clin. Exp. Nephrol.* **2021**, *25*, 191–199. [CrossRef] [PubMed]
12. Li, A.; Wang, H.; Li, Q.; Dong, W.; Wang, S.; Wang, A.; Wang, X.; Gu, Y. Shengxuebao Mixture for Iron Deficiency Anemia: A Meta-Analysis and Systematic Review. *Complement. Med. Res.* **2022**, *29*, 249–256. [CrossRef]
13. Ding, L.; Xu, L.; Jin, Y.; Wei, Y.; Pan, Y.; Sattar, S.; Tan, Y.; Yang, T.; Zhou, F. Efficacy of SXN in the Treatment of Iron Deficiency Anemia: A Phase IV Clinical Trial. *Evid.-Based Complement. Altern. Med.* **2019**, *2019*, 8796234. [CrossRef] [PubMed]
14. Dang, Z.; Liu, X.; Wang, X.; Li, M.; Jiang, Y.; Wang, X.; Yang, Z. Comparative effectiveness and safety of traditional Chinese medicine supporting Qi and enriching blood for cancer related anemia in patients not receiving chemoradiotherapy: A meta-analysis and systematic review. *Drug Des. Dev. Ther.* **2019**, *13*, 221–230. [CrossRef]
15. Kim, M.; Han, C.-H. Effects of Bojungikgi-tang and its modifications for Anemia: A Systematic Review and Meta-Analysis of Randomized Controlled Trials. *J. Korean Med.* **2023**, *44*, 181–200. [CrossRef]
16. Chiu, M.L.; Hsu, Y.L.; Chen, C.J.; Li, T.M.; Chiou, J.S.; Tsai, F.J.; Lin, T.H.; Liao, C.C.; Huang, S.M.; Chou, C.H.; et al. Chinese Herbal Medicine Therapy Reduces the Risks of Overall and Anemia-Related Mortalities in Patients with Aplastic Anemia: A Nationwide Retrospective Study in Taiwan. *Front. Pharmacol.* **2021**, *12*, 730776. [CrossRef]
17. Jeong, Y.K.; Kim, J.H.; Lee, S.H.; Bang, M.; Chang, G.T. Safety and efficacy of East Asian herbal medicine for iron deficiency anemia in children and adolescents: A systematic review and meta-analysis. *Front. Pharmacol.* **2024**, *15*, 1339486. [CrossRef]
18. Chen, Y.; Ai, J.; Yang, J.; Qi, X.; Zhang, Z. Shiquan Dabu Decoction Combined with Iron Sucrose in Treatment of Perioperative Anemia in Total Knee Arthroplasty. *Acta Chin. Med.* **2024**, *39*, 1098–1103.
19. Ai, J.; Han, Y.; Yao, P.; Zhang, Z.; Zhang, D.; Cao, Y.; Wang, S.; Liu, R. The Effects of Shiquandabu-tang on Postoperative Anemia in Elderly Patients with Intertrochanteric Femur Fractures. *Tradit. Chin. Med. Res.* **2022**, *35*, 54–58.

20. Wang, C.; Yuan, A.; Liu, S. Forty-two cases of moderate-to-severe anemia treated with Shiquandabu-tang. *J. Med. Theory Pract.* **1999**, 286–287.
21. Sho, Y.; Fujisaki, K.; Sakashita, H.; Yamaguchi, K.; Tahara, K.; Kubozono, O.; Ido, A.; Tsubouchi, H. Orally administered Kampo medicine, Juzen-taiho-to, ameliorates anemia during interferon plus ribavirin therapy in patients with chronic hepatitis C. *J. Gastroenterol.* **2004**, *39*, 1202–1204. [CrossRef] [PubMed]
22. Nakamoto, H.; Mimura, T.; Honda, N. Orally administrated Juzen-taiho-to/TJ-48 ameliorates erythropoietin (rHuEPO)-resistant anemia in patients on hemodialysis. *Hemodial. Int.* **2008**, *12*, S9–S14. [CrossRef] [PubMed]
23. Kishida, Y.; Nishii, T.; Inoue, T.; Nishida, S.; Arimitsu, J.; Yoshikawa, H.; Sugano, N. Juzentaihoto (TJ-48), a traditional Japanese herbal medicine, influences hemoglobin recovery during preoperative autologous blood donation and after hip surgery. *Int. J. Clin. Pharmacol. Ther.* **2009**, *47*, 716–721. [CrossRef] [PubMed]
24. Kainuma, M.; Mukae, H.; Furusyo, N.; Unno, M.; Hayashi, J. A Case of Anemia and Thrombocytopenia with Myelodysplastic Syndrome Successfully Treated with Juzentaihoto and Malt Sugar. *Jpn. J. Orient. Med.* **2011**, *62*, 363–368.
25. Yao, S.; Wang, Z.; Ji, H. Clinical observation on treating renal anemia with the Shiquan Dabu decoction plus erythropoietin. *Clin. J. Chin. Med.* **2012**, *4*, 2.
26. Yao, Z. The Effect of Jiawei Shiquandabu Decoction Combined with Erythropoietin in the Treatment of Renal Anemia. *Mod. Diagn. Treat.* **2016**, *27*, 1202–1204.
27. Sheng, L.; Zhou, H.; Fang, Y.; Peng, L.; Dong, G. Effect of Prescription Named "Jiawei Shiquan Dabu Tang" on Hidden Blood Loss After Total Hip Arthroplasty Surgery. *Chin. J. Mod. Appl. Pharm.* **2017**, *34*, 420–422.
28. Li, X. Shiquan Dabu Decoction combined with Western Medicine in the Treatment of Anemia in Late stage of Acute Upper Gastrointestinal Bleeding(Qixue Liangxu) Randomized Parallel Control Study. *J. Pract. Tradit. Chin. Intern. Med.* **2018**, *32*, 46–49.
29. Fang, Y.; Zhou, H. Analysis of Shiquan Dabu decoction in treating recessive blood loss after joint replacement. *China Mod. Dr.* **2018**, *56*, 131–134.
30. Kim, S.-H.; Kim, J.-H.; Lee, H.-K.; Cho, K.-H.; Mun, S.-K.; Jung, W.-S.; Kwon, S.-W. Case of Anemia with Chronic Kidney Disease Using Shipjeondaebo-tang. *J. Intern. Korean Med.* **2019**, *40*, 173–180. [CrossRef]
31. Kyong-lim, K.; Seung-eun, L.; Kyoung-min, K. A Case Report of Elderly Patients with Anemia that Improved with Shipjeondaebo-tang-gami. *J. Intern. Korean Med.* **2020**, *41*, 508–514.
32. Ling, J.; Li, J.; Li, C.; Huang, G. Effects of Jiawei Shiquan Dabu decoction on recessive blood loss and blood glucose levels after operation in the elderly patients with femoral intertrochanteric fracture. *Shaanxi J. Tradit. Chin. Med.* **2020**, *41*, 1254–1257.
33. Tian, H. Clinical Study of Shiquandabu Decoction Combined with Tranexamic Acid on Reducing Perioperative Blood Loss (Syndrome of Qi-Blood Deficiency) in Total Hip Arthroplasty. Master's Thesis, Henan University of Chinese Medicine, Zhengzhou, China, 2020.
34. Wei, D. New Advances in Hidden Blood Loss After Hip Replacement Surgery. *Shenzhen J. Integr. Tradit. Chin. West. Med.* **2017**, *27*, 193–194.
35. Lo, B.D.; Qayum, O.; Penberthy, K.K.; Gyi, R.; Lester, L.C.; Hensley, N.B.; Sciubba, D.M.; Frank, S.M.; Cho, B.C. Dose-dependent effects of red blood cell transfusion and case mix index on venous thromboembolic events in spine surgery. *Vox Sang.* **2023**, *118*, 76–83. [CrossRef]
36. Shi, Y.-P.; Zhu, B.-D.; Huang, Q.; Zheng, T.-F.; Zhao, J.-H. Effect of Shi-Quan-Da-Bu-Granule on routine blood and erythropoietin on myelosuppressed mice. *Lab. Med. Clin.* **2009**, *6*, 1221–1223.
37. Hisha, H.; Yamada, H.; Sakurai, M.H.; Kiyohara, H.; Li, Y.; Yu, C.; Takemoto, N.; Kawamura, H.; Yamaura, K.; Shinohara, S.; et al. Isolation and identification of hematopoietic stem cell-stimulating substances from Kampo (Japanese herbal) medicine, Juzen-taiho-to. *Blood* **1997**, *90*, 1022–1030. [CrossRef]
38. Tian, Y.; Xiang, Y.; Wan, G.; Wan, D.; Zhu, H.; Wang, T.; Yang, X. Effects and mechanisms of Bazhen decoction, Siwu decoction, and Sijunzi decoction on 5-fluorouracil-induced anemia in mice. *J. Tradit. Chin. Med.* **2016**, *36*, 486–495. [CrossRef]
39. Lee, H.W.; Kim, H.; Ryuk, J.A.; Kil, K.J.; Ko, B.S. Hemopoietic effect of extracts from constituent herbal medicines of Samul-tang on phenylhydrazine-induced hemolytic anemia in rats. *Int. J. Clin. Exp. Pathol.* **2014**, *7*, 6179–6185. [PubMed]
40. Arksey, H.; O'Malley, L. Scoping studies: Towards a methodological framework. *Int. J. Soc. Res. Methodol.* **2005**, *8*, 19–32. [CrossRef]
41. Levac, D.; Colquhoun, H.; O'Brien, K.K. Scoping studies: Advancing the methodology. *Implement. Sci.* **2010**, *5*, 69. [CrossRef]
42. National Institute for Health and Care Excellence (NICE). NICE Process and Methods Guides. In Methods for the Development of NICE Public Health Guidance. Available online: https://www.nice.org.uk/process/pmg4/ (accessed on 8 September 2024).

pharmaceuticals

MDPI

Review

Potential of Bitter Medicinal Plants: A Review of Flavor Physiology

Germán Zuluaga [1,2]

[1] Grupo de Estudios en Sistemas Tradicionales de Salud, Escuela de Medicina y Ciencias de la Salud, Universidad del Rosario, Bogotá 111711, Colombia; gzuluaga@cemi.org.co; Tel.: +57-311-2179102
[2] Centro de Estudios Médicos Interculturales, Cota 250010, Colombia

Abstract: The function of the sense of taste is usually confined to the ability to perceive the flavor of food to assess and use the nutrients necessary for healthy survival and to discard those that may be harmful, toxic, or unpleasant. It is almost unanimously agreed that the perception of bitter taste prevents the consumption of toxins from plants, decaying foods, and drugs. Forty years ago, while practicing medicine in a rural area of the Colombian Amazon, I had an unexpected encounter with the Inga Indians. I faced the challenge of accepting that their traditional medicine was effective and that the medicinal plants they used had a real therapeutic effect. Wanting to follow a process of learning about medicinal plants on their terms, I found that, for them, the taste of plants is a primary and fundamental key to understanding their functioning. One of the most exciting results was discovering the therapeutic value of bitter plants. The present review aims to understand whether there is any scientific support for this hypothesis from the traditional world. Can the taste of plants explain their possible therapeutic benefit? In the last 20 years, we have made novel advances in the knowledge of the physiology of taste. Our purpose will be to explore these scientific advances to determine if the bitter taste of medicinal plants benefits human health.

Keywords: physiology of flavor; medicinal bitterness; traditional medicine; medicinal plants

1. Introduction

The function of the sense of taste is usually confined exclusively to the ability to perceive the flavor of food to assess and use the nutrients necessary for healthy survival and to discard those that may be harmful, toxic, or unpleasant.

For many years, four primordial or primary tastes were identified: sweet, salty, sour, and bitter, the combination of which gives rise to the immense mosaic of secondary tastes that we can perceive. Since 1909, Japanese professor Ikeda indicated the existence of another taste modality he called umami, which translates to "tasty", "delicious", or "exquisite" [1]. Currently, most research considers five taste modalities, including umami [2].

There is some unanimity about the biological role of each of the flavors, as summarized by Chandrashekar et al.:

> "Sweet taste enables the identification of energy-rich nutrients, umami enables the recognition of amino acids, salty taste ensures the proper balance of dietary electrolytes, and sour and bitter tastes warn about the ingestion of potentially harmful and/or poisonous chemicals. In humans, taste has the additional value of contributing to the overall pleasure and enjoyment of a meal. Surprisingly, although we can taste a wide range of chemical entities, it is now generally accepted that, qualitatively, they evoke few distinct taste sensations: sweet, bitter, sour, salty and umami. Although this repertoire may seem modest, it has satisfied the evolutionary need for an effective and reliable platform to help recognize and distinguish major dietary components." [3] (p. 288)

In other words, these flavors act synergistically to mediate appetite-protective responses, such as energy regulation, and the intake of salt and protein. They also warn against the consumption of toxic substances and in some cases determine our food preferences [2].

In particular, it is almost unanimously agreed that the perception of bitter taste has the function of preventing the consumption of toxins from plants, decaying foods, and drugs, consistently producing rejection or aversion responses [4]. Similarly, most authors agree that the function of sour taste is to prevent the ingestion of potentially harmful, poisonous, or simply unpleasant chemicals. Indeed, the ability to sense sourness provides an important sensory signal to avoid ingestion of unripe, spoiled, or fermented foods. Taste receptors in the oral cavity trigger aversive behaviors in response to acidic stimuli [5]. Most people respond to the consumption of lemon juice with a violent contortion of the face that clearly indicates a rejection of the sour taste [6].

It does not seem to be disputed that the function of bitter and acidic substances is exclusively to prevent the ingestion of toxic, poisonous, or unpleasant substances. Such a perspective has given rise to the widespread notion that bitter and acidic substances should be avoided. This current scientific knowledge promotes a rejection of anything bitter or acidic, which coincides with a trend that has become widespread in the eating habits of the modern world: acidophobia and bitterphobia, understandable because of the usual initial rejection or aversive behavior that both tastes tend to produce. We can cite a few examples: hardly anyone wants to consume stimulating beverages or foods such as coffee, tea, and chocolate without adding sugar; citrus fruits, which are usually acidic in their natural form, are replaced by genetic varieties that intentionally seek to reduce their acidity and increase their sweetness, as is the case with the new grafted varieties of oranges and lemons; refreshing and thirst quenching drinks offered by the beverage industry are usually nuanced with sugar, sweeteners, flavorings, and fizzy substances. Moreover, most people are abandoning the consumption of medicinal plants, leaving aside mainly bitter plants, and only keeping those that are considered sweet or aromatic. Undoubtedly, the diet of the modern world favors foods and beverages with sweet and salty flavors, abandoning more and more the consumption of substances with bitter and sour flavors. Does this phenomenon of change in the diet have any consequences for human health?

Forty years ago, while I was practicing medicine in a rural area of the Colombian Amazon, I had an unexpected encounter with the Inga Indians. I was faced with the challenge of accepting that their traditional medicine was effective and that the medicinal plants they used had a real therapeutic effect. Obviously, I wanted to approach the study of medicinal plants under the terms and categories of Western medicine, looking for plants with anti-inflammatory, antihypertensive, and hypoglycemic effects and plants for arthritis, collagen diseases, or cancer, among others. And, of course, based on the criteria of phytochemistry and classical pharmacological research, I wanted to find the active principles that would explain the possible therapeutic effect of medicinal plants.

Although this scientific path for the study of medicinal plants continues to be the standard, both in botany and ethnobotany, as well as in phytochemistry and phytopharmacology, our experience has shown us that traditional systems of knowledge respond to other epistemological paths, other methods, other ways of knowing and using plants. To begin with, we were forced to try to understand and interpret the language used by indigenous healers. None of the terms used by our medicine and our western science correspond to the terms used by them. While, for example, I asked for plants for systemic lupus erythematosus or diabetes, they answered with hot or cold plants, purgative or depurative plants, plants for bad air, or for fear and fright. There is, thus, a hermeneutic challenge here that requires us to be willing to engage in an authentic dialogue of sciences.

Accepting this new disposition and wanting to follow a process of learning about medicinal plants, in their own terms, in addition to the predominant category of hot and cold plants (a concept that has been scorned even by anthropologists, ethnobotanists, and pharmacologists), we found that, for them, the taste of plants is a primary and fundamental key to understanding their functioning. Thus, a new ethno-classification of medicinal plants was opened: sweet or aromatic, fresh, acid, and bitter. According to them, flavor is the key to their function and efficacy. During the following years, our studies have tried to follow this new epistemological track. One of the most interesting results was the discovery of the therapeutic value of bitter plants. Indeed, bitter became a key to understand the universe of indigenous and traditional therapeutics [7]. As a result of this experience, we have even come, as physicians, to recommend the consumption of bitter plants for preventive and therapeutic purposes [8]. Although clinical experience has shown its benefits, we are still far from being able to confirm it with experimental epidemiological studies.

As Trius and Moreno state: "Although numerous bitter medicinal plants have been used in folk and traditional medicine and cuisine and inherited by generations, the scientific integration of modern medicine and traditional (ancient) wisdom remain limited." [9]. Indeed, recent ethnobotanical studies report the bitter properties of some medicinal plants. However, they do not usually give the traditional explanation of their efficacy or are associated with benefits related to events such as fever, inflammation, liver, chest diseases, edema, diarrhea, digestion, malaria, and intestinal parasitosis, among others. In Table 1, I cite some bitter medicinal plants reported to be used in cosmopolitan or local communities. Although phytochemical and pharmacological studies have been conducted on most of them, it is rarely reported whether the active ingredients with a physiological or therapeutic effect have a bitter taste themselves.

Table 1. Bitter medicinal plants reported from cosmopolitan or local communities.

Scientific Name	Common Name	Bitter Compounds	Distribution	Ref.
Artemisia absinthium	Ajenjo (span.), Wormwood (eng.)	Thujone, sesquiterpene lactones: absinthin, anabsinthin, anabsin, and artabsin	Cosmopolitan	[10]
Artemisia vulgaris	Altamisa (span.), Mugwort (eng.)	Terpenoids and sesquiterpene lactones	Cosmopolitan	[11]
Azadirachta indica	Nim (span.), Neem (eng.)	Azadirachtin, meliacin, gedunin, nimbidin, nimbolides, salanin, nimbin, valassin, meliacin, limonoid	Indian	[12]
Banisteriopsis caapi	Ayahuasca, yage, capi (span. and indigenous languages)	β-carboline alkaloids	Amazon region	[7]
Coptidis rhizoma	Huang Lian (Chinese)	Alkaloids, lignans, phenylpropanoids, flavonoids, phenolic compounds, and steroids	Traditional Chinese medicine, Japanese traditional herbal medicine (Kampo)	[13]
Garcinia kola	Cola amarga (span.), Orogbo (Yoriba)	Biflavonoids, benzophenones, benzofurans, benzopyran, xanthones, and phytosterols	Traditional African medicine	[14]
Gentiana purpurea	Genciana (span.), Purple Gentian (eng.)	Secoiridoids, amarogentin	Ancient European tradition	[15]
Momordica charantia	Melón amargo (span.), Bitter melon (eng.)	Phenolic components, Kuguaglycoside G, Momordicine	Traditional Chinese medicine	[16]
Phellodendron amurense bark	Amur cork tree (eng.), Huáng bò (Chinese)	Phellodendrine, Berberine	Traditional Chinese medicine	[17]
Verbena officinalis	Verbena (span.), Vervain (eng.)	Iridoids, flavonoids and phenolic acid derivatives	Cosmopolitan	[18]
Vernonia amygdalina	Hoja amarga (span.), Ewuro (Yoruba)	Sesquiterpene lactones: vernodalin, vernolide, hydroxyvernolide	Tongwe (Tanzania)	[19]

The objective of the present review is to understand whether there is any scientific support for this hypothesis from the traditional world. Can the taste of plants really explain their possible therapeutic benefit? Is bitter taste, so little appreciated in our modern world, just an expression of the toxic effect of substances, plants, and foods, or does it have any importance for human health?

In the last 20 years, we have found novel advances in the knowledge of the physiology of taste, for example in the discovery of cell membrane receptors that explain in a fascinating way the way in which these substances activate and generate the chemical and electrical activities involved in the physiology of taste, and in the functional complexity of taste cells, buds and papillae, ions and organic molecules, neurotransmitters and routes or connections of nerve bundles with the different structures of the brain that allow their emission and final interpretation in the cerebral cortex.

Our purpose will be to explore these new scientific advances to determine if the bitter taste of medicinal plants has benefits for human health.

2. The Sense of Taste and Flavor

Taste is recognized as one of the fundamental senses possessed by living beings, thanks to which they can perceive and interact with the outside world. Its importance is recognized even in unicellular and prokaryotic organisms, since it allows them to assess the hydroelectrolytic conditions of the environment and thus obtain nutritive substances or repel those that may be harmful.

The structure and physiology of taste has evolved in the animal kingdom, reaching increasingly complex and well-developed mechanisms in vertebrate animals, mammals, and humans. Whereas in invertebrate organisms the cells responsible for taste sensing are primitive neurons with ciliated dendrites, as identified in the nematode *Caenorhabditis elegans* and the fruit fly *Drosophila melanogaster*, vertebrate taste receptor cells are not neurons but originate in the epithelial covering of the body [20].

In mammals, the taste system is located mainly in the tongue and oral mucosa, from where it is transmitted to the brain via cranial nerves, following a complex route until taste perception is recognized by the cerebral cortex. In simple terms, food chemicals dissolve in saliva and come into contact with taste cells through the taste pore. There, they interact with taste receptors, triggering electrical changes in taste cells, which stimulate the emission of chemical signals, an activity that is translated into impulses sent to the brain [21].

But the sense of taste is much more complex than just receptors for basic flavors and the chemical interactions they generate in taste cells. Despite the tendency to identify taste information in terms of five modalities, the taste system also interprets other attributes derived from chemical stimuli. An intense taste can be pleasant, unpleasant, or neutral. Neurons in the taste pathway register these attributes simultaneously, like the visual system represents shape, brightness, color, and motion. Very often, taste receptors also respond to tactile and thermal stimuli [21].

For this reason, it is important to distinguish between taste and flavor. Taste refers to the capacity of living organisms, from invertebrates to mammals and humans, to perceive an intrinsic biological property of many substances of mineral, vegetable, and animal origin. On the other hand, the final perception of flavor is the result of the activation of several sensory systems: taste, smell, tactile, and thermal sensitivity, among others [22]. Flavor is, therefore, a complex amalgam of sensory information provided by taste, smell, and the tactile sensation of food when it is chewed, a characteristic that scholars usually refer to as mouthfeel. Thus, the word taste is applied, strictly speaking, only to sensations coming from the specialized cells of the mouth, although taste and flavor are commonly used interchangeably [21]. This distinction is also evident in the Spanish language: "Taste (*gusto*) is commonly confused with flavor (*sabor*), the combined sensory experience of olfaction and gustation." [23].

3. The Taste System

Although the physiology of taste has been known with some precision since the beginning of the 20th century, in recent decades, thanks to scientific advances in genetics and immunology, new and more detailed knowledge has been obtained that allows for greater understanding, although many concerns remain to be resolved.

From the phylogenetic point of view, the basic unit of the sense of taste is based on ciliary structures that, from unicellular organisms onwards, develop in certain cells [24], which consequently acquire their specialized character and for this reason are known as taste cells or taste receptor cells (TRCs). In vertebrates, they are small bipolar cells with ciliary properties [2], which have two functionally important connections: microvilli in contact with the oral cavity and synapses with sensory nerve fibers [20].

Taste cells may be alone or in groups of 50 to 100 cells, thus forming the functional units known as taste buds [2]. In each taste bud, there are four morphologically distinguishable cell types. On the one hand, there are the Type IV basal cells confined to the basal surface, which are not involved in taste physiology, serve as support, and are considered progenitors, since they are in charge of cell turnover. On the other hand, there are the three cell groups involved in taste physiology: Type I, Type II, and Type III cells [25] (see Figure 1).

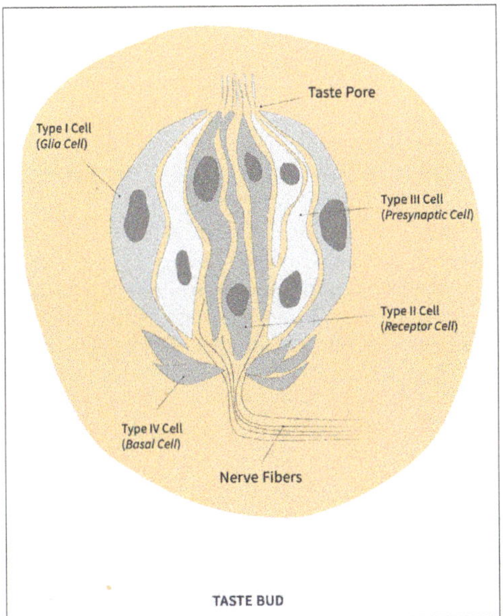

Figure 1. Structure of the taste button.

Taste buds are in turn grouped into larger structures, known as taste papillae, distributed in different geographical areas of the tongue and in some points of the oral mucosa. Four types are distinguished: filiform, fungiform, caliciform, and foliated [26].

Finally, taste papillae are innervated, in a differentiated and apparently specific way for each group of papillae, by nerve bundles and fibers of the cranial nerves, especially the trigeminal (V), facial (VII), glossopharyngeal (IX), and pneumogastric (X) [26], through which gustative sensitivity of the tongue is conveyed to the central nervous system, entering the brain stem, following the hypothalamus, to reach the frontal lobe of the cerebral cortex [27].

4. The Physiology of Taste

The physiological basis of all senses, such as taste, smell, hearing, balance, touch, and vision, has a common biochemical conceptual framework, based on the depolarization of the cell membrane, leading to an ionic exchange that in turn generates electrical and chemical changes inside the cell. However, the initial trigger is different from case to case. This is how the three known mechanisms are described: (a) mechanotransduction, in which the trigger is a pressure change, as occurs in the cochlear and vestibular receptors of the organ of hearing, (b) phototransduction, in which the trigger is light, as occurs in the retinal receptors of the organ of the eye, and (c) chemotransduction, in which the trigger is a chemical substance or molecule, as occurs in the gustatory receptors of the organ of taste [24]. Some authors add a fourth mechanism, thermoreception, in which temperature is the trigger, perhaps also present in the sense of taste [28]. The physiology of taste is mainly chemosensory.

Like neurons, taste cells present at rest a net negative charge inside and a net positive charge outside. The chemicals in the food modify this situation through various mechanisms that increase the concentration of positive ions inside. The result is the suppression of the charge difference between the outside and the inside of these cells. This depolarization causes the taste cells to release neurotransmitters to the exterior—molecules that trigger the transmission of electrical messages in the neurons in contact [21]. For this depolarization to be possible, taste cells have receptor proteins or cell surface receptors in their membranes, which can be of two kinds:

(a) Channel or ionotropic receptors. They are known by the acronym TRP, which stands for transient receptor potential. In turn, according to their molecular specificity, they are subclassified into different groups: TRPc, TRPm, TRPp, TRPv, among others [29].
(b) G protein-associated or metabotropic receptors [30]. They are known by the acronym GPCR (G protein-coupled receptor, GPCRs for the plural) [31].

Based on the receptor protein, we classify taste cells as ionotropic, which are those in which the protein per se is an ion channel, and metabotropic, in which the receptor is associated with a G protein [2]. Both taste receptor proteins are mounted on the microvilli, acting as molecular antennae that listen to the chemical environment. Upon binding to molecules contained in food, the receptors trigger a signaling cascade within the cells, the end result of which is manifested in the opening and closing of other intracellular ion channels [21], activating synapses and thus causing excitation of nerve fibers [20]

4.1. *Channel or Ionotropic Receptors*

Channel receptors, which are poreiform proteins and are an ion channel per se, correspond to a large family of receptors, called TRP, whose function involves from insect sense organs to that of humans, including the functions of calcium and magnesium homeostasis, vasoregulation, gastrointestinal motility and hepatic development, among many others [24]. From the phylogenetic point of view, they are considered more primitive and less complex.

TRP channels are thus an ancient sensory apparatus of the cell and have been adapted to respond to all kinds of stimuli, both from inside and outside the cell. It is even considered that almost all cells have these channel receptors. They are thus the forefront of our sensory systems, responding to temperature, touch, pain, osmolarity, pheromones, taste, and other stimuli. The known functions are diverse. Yeasts use a TRP channel to sense and respond to hypertonicity. Nematodes use TRP channels at the tips of neuronal dendrites to sense and avoid noxious chemicals. Male mice use a pheromone-sensing TRP channel to distinguish males from females. Humans use TRP channels to appreciate flavors and to discriminate heat and cold [29]. Nearly all mammalian TRP channel genes are now known [32].

Epithelial sodium channels (ENaCs) were the first to be recognized in taste physiology [33]. Indeed, this new class of channels, the epithelial sodium channel (ENaC)/degenerin gene family, was discovered in the 1990s. Different investigations confirmed the existence of these channels in the African frog *Xenopus laevis*, in the mollusk *Helix aspersa*, and in the nematode *Caenorhabditis elegans*, with great genetic sequence homology between them and also coinciding with the recently described ENaCs in mammals and humans [34].

ENaCs were initially recognized for their specific response to amiloride, a potassium-sparing diuretic approved in 1967 for the treatment of arterial hypertension and heart failure, because they played a crucial role in the uptake of sodium (Na^+) in the distal part of the renal tubule, which was the target of aldosterone action. Hence, they were named epithelial sodium channels (ENaCs). Their homology with the degenerin channel of the nematode *C. elegans* led to the current classification of the epithelial sodium channel (ENaC)/degenerin gene family [34].

We now know that in humans, ENaCs are found in epithelial cells of the kidney, lung, respiratory tract, male and female reproductive tracts, sweat and salivary glands, placenta, colon, and some other organs. In these epithelia, ENaCs allow the flow of Na^+ ions from the extracellular fluid into the epithelial cell. As Na^+ is one of the major electrolytes in the extracellular fluid, the change in osmolarity initiated by Na^+ flux is accompanied by a flux of water accompanying Na^+ ions. Thus, the ENaC has a central role in extra- and intracellular fluid volume regulation, electrolyte homeostasis, blood pressure, airway clearance, germ cell transport, fertilization, implantation, and cell migration [33].

Observations that amiloride and other ENaC blockers alter taste responses to sodium salts led to the hypothesis that the ENaC was involved in salt taste reception. Finally, one study in mice showed that the ENaC responds to detecting sodium taste [35] and is primarily responsible for the salty taste.

New research showed that also other TRP channels are involved in thermosensation, mechanosensation, odor, and taste. For example, TRPm5 was found to be abundantly expressed in taste receptor cells, where it is involved in the perception of sweet, sour, and bitter tastes [36]. The TRPp3 channel receptor was also identified to be associated with the perception of sour taste [37], and two members of the PKD-like TRP ion channel may function as sour taste receptors [38]. For their part, Zhang et al. demonstrated that an ion channel called Otopetrin-1, a proton-selective channel normally involved in the sensation of gravity in the vestibular system, is essential for the perception of sourness in the gustative system [5].

In summary, ion channels or Transient Receptor Potential (TRP) channels are involved in taste physiology: (a) epithelial Na^+ channels (ENaC) are mainly responsible for a salty taste, (b) TRPm5 channels are involved in the perception of sweet, bitter, and sour tastes, and (c) acid-sensitive ion channels (ASICs), PKD-like TRP channels, and an ion channel called Otopetrin-1 are responsible for sour taste (see Figure 2).

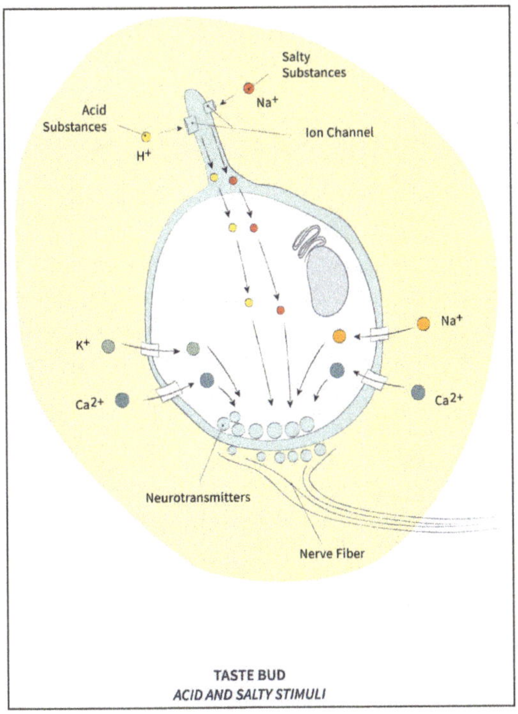

Figure 2. Scheme of the cellular mechanism for the transduction of sour and salty tastes.

4.2. G Protein-Coupled Receptors and G Protein

G protein-coupled receptors (GPCRs) are the largest known family of membrane receptors in eukaryotes, consisting of more than 800 members. These receptors recognize a wide range of extracellular stimuli such as photons, hormones, neurotransmitters, tastes, and odors to induce intracellular signaling pathways [31]. Because of their structure, forming seven transmembrane α-helices, they are also called receptors of the seven transmembrane domains [39]. More than 100 members of this family have been described in mammalian cells [30], and they constitute the third largest gene family in humans [40]. More than 50% of commercially available drugs directly or indirectly target GPCRs, highlighting their importance in various biological and therapeutic mechanisms [31].

The American Robert Lefkowitz, since the 1960s, has postulated the existence of receptors that formed part of the cell signaling system, based on his studies on alpha- and beta-adrenergic receptors. In 1980, Lefkowitz and his colleagues De Lean and Stadel proposed the so-called "ternary complex model", which involved the interaction of the receptor with a third component, which generated a receptor with high affinity for the ligand. It was later discovered that this third component was an intracellular G protein. Shortly thereafter, with fellow American Brian Kobilka, they succeeded in isolating the gene, making it clear that the beta-adrenergic receptor was part of a large family of receptors that had common features in terms of their structure and the way they functioned. In 2011, Kobilka, with his own research group, succeeded in obtaining the structure of the beta-adrenergic receptor bound to a G protein by X-ray crystallography [41]. Finally, both researchers received the Nobel Prize in Chemistry in 2012 for "their studies on G protein-coupled receptors" [40].

The researchers Alfred Gilman and Martin Rodbell, when studying cell stimulation by epinephrine, found that, upon binding to the receptor, the hormone did not stimulate enzymes directly, but did so through proteins coupled to the receptor, which were responsible for the activation of guanine triphosphate (GTP), which is why they called them G proteins. These stimulate adenylyl cyclase, which in turn produce cyclic adenosine monophosphate (cAMP) as a second messenger [42]. Thus, upon discovering the role of these proteins in cellular signal transduction, they received the Nobel Prize in 1994 [39].

In relation to the physiology of taste, in 1992, researchers McLaughlin and McKinnon collaborated with Margolskee to identify a protein they named gustducin, given its molecular similarity to transducin, another retinal cell protein that helps transform or transduce the light signal reaching the retina into an electrical impulse constitutive of vision. Gustducin and transducin are G proteins that are bound to the inner side of their respective surface receptors. When a genuine taste molecule binds to a receptor taste cell, with the specificity of a key in its lock, the gustducin subunits (α, β and γ) separate and catalyze biochemical reactions that result in the opening or closing of ion channels [21]. Gustducin has also been detected in nasal mucosal and stomach cells [20].

Two groups of researchers, the first led by Charles Zuker at the Howard Hughes Institute of Medicine at the University of California at San Diego and Nicholas Ryba at the National Dental and Craniofacial Institute, and the second led by Linda Buck at Harvard Medical School, identified in 1996 in mice and humans the true bitter taste receptors that activate gustducin. Both teams found that bitter taste receptors (T2Rs for plural and T2R for singular) belonged to a family of similar receptors consisting of perhaps 40 to 80 members [21].

Very soon, the receptors that recognize sweet substances and the umami receptor were also sought, and it was discovered that they were proteins that shared similar amino acid sequences and were named sweet taste receptors (T1R) [43]. The genomic library research failed to find additional members, so it was finally determined that two G protein-coupled receptors were involved in taste physiology: T1R, responsible for identifying a sweet taste and perhaps umami, and T2R, responsible for identifying a bitter taste [44].

The next and almost simultaneous task was to identify the encoding genes for these receptor proteins that were finally discovered in 2000, based on analyses of recently published human genome sequences in the genome regions related to bitter taste repotentiation in humans and mice [45]. Adler et al. examined a region of human chromosome 5 linked to the perception of a bitter compound, 6-n-propyl-2-thiouracil (PROP) [46], and by 2006 the genetic map of the T1R and T2R receptors was fully established [47].

As we have seen, different routes have been taken to obtain knowledge of the membrane receptors necessary to understand the chemosensory physiology of taste, in particular, the receptors GPCR (and their specific G protein, gustducin) and TRP. There is already a consensus that the somewhat more complex sweet, umami, and bitter tastes are mediated by GPCR (T1R and T2R) that in turn stimulate the protein gustducin [47], whereas the somewhat simpler salty and sour tastes are mediated by TRP [36].

4.3. Taste in the Central Nervous System

The neuronal transmission of taste perception reaches the central nervous system by means of nerve bundles and fascicles through the cranial nerves, activating the Nucleus of the Solitary Tract in the brain stem, responsible for the initial processing of information. Following the central route, information reaches the Parabrachial Nucleus, a more complex structure that integrates various aspects of sensory information. From there, information reaches the Thalamus, the third structure activated in the taste pathway, where the essential coding of the five basic tastes is integrated with other sensory stimuli, such as smell and texture. Finally, the information reaches the taste cortex, located at the boundary between the anterior insula and the frontal operculum of the cerebral cortex [48], a multimodal area capable of integrating all aspects of information, since its neurons not only respond to taste but also to temperature, touch, pain, and the state of the viscera (see Figure 3). The response orchestrated by groups of neurons in this cortex, called "ensembles", enables processing and integrating all the characteristics contained in a food and comparing them with the previously stored information associated with that taste. In this way, a specific combined code is achieved that will allow the subsequent recognition of that flavor within a wide range of combinations [27].

One area of intense research is how taste cues are encoded by the nervous system. The principles of sensory coding from the retina to the visual cortex were elucidated decades ago. We have a thorough understanding of the tonotopic and computational maps of the auditory system. Lateral inhibition and somatosensory receptive fields are well defined. Knowledge about taste is lacking and we still do not understand how the brain distinguishes sweet, sour, salty, etc. If taste does not follow a simple label code, how are taste signals transmitted and decoded? Studies currently underway shed light on the possibility that taste is encoded in the time domain, i.e., by the frequency and pattern of action potentials in the hindbrain and cortical neurons. Other laboratories are exploring higher-order cortical processing using functional magnetic resonance imaging to address the interplay between taste detection, preference, and appetite regulation [23].

It is now known that neurons in the different areas of the taste pathway can modify their chemical and electrical activity and their conformation, depending on the type of experience associated with taste. Thus, the taste cortex neurons are highly "plastic", i.e., they adapt rapidly and change their response as the hedonic value is transformed during the consumption of a new taste, but also during the consumption of a familiar taste, which allows for the constant updating of taste memory over days, months, or years later. Thanks to this plasticity, we can initially recognize that something is bitter in order to learn that it is not harmful and, subsequently, this now familiar taste can become pleasant with a highly pleasurable value. Classic examples are beer, wines, and some strong cheeses, which once tasted and once the initial aversion is overcome, usually provoke a pleasurable increase in their consumption. It is true that every time we consume a particular food, we can recognize it specifically, even though its hedonic connotation changes from time to time. In other words, the ability to recognize taste modalities remains intact in our brain; foods always interact with the same receptors in the mouth, but these end up activating different patterns of neurons depending on the history of experiences we have with that taste [27].

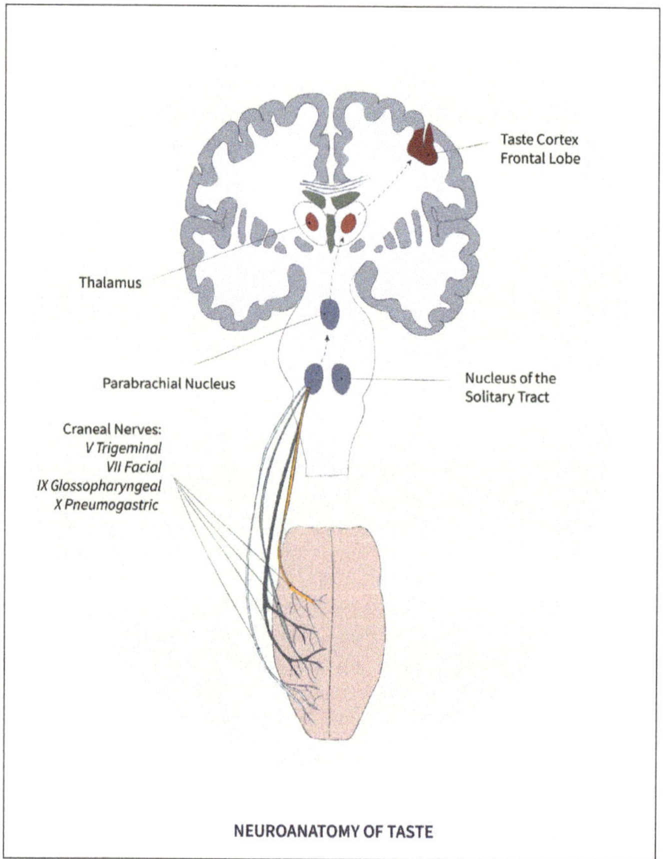

Figure 3. Scheme of the physiological pathway of flavors.

5. The Bitter Taste

It is produced almost entirely by organic substances, rather than ionic chemical elements. Initially it was thought that only two types of substances produced this taste: alkaloids and long-chain nitrogen-containing organic substances [26]. But in reality, thousands of compounds are perceived as bitter by humans. There is no reliable inventory in nature of bitter molecules but tens of thousands are estimated because, for naturally occurring bitter compounds alone, about 10% of plant species can synthesize toxic secondary metabolites and 2500 plant species alone contain cyanogenic glycosides, most of which are bitter. Bitter compounds are not only numerous but also structurally diverse. They include, among others, fatty acids, peptides, amino acids, amines, amides, azacycloalkanes, N-heterocyclic compounds, ureas, thioureas, carbamides, esters, lactones, carbonyl compounds, phenols, crown ethers, terpenoids, secoiridoids, alkaloids, glycosides, flavonoids, steroids, halogenated or acetylated sugars, and metal ions [49]. Of these, quinine is used as the standard reference for expressing a bitter taste [26].

Many bitter substances are of genuine plant origin, but others are derived from animals or are generated during food processing, aging, or decomposition. Culinary Maillard reaction and fermentation processes are also rich sources of bitter compounds, while chemical synthesis has provided unique bitter chemotypes [49].

As already mentioned, it is almost unanimous and universally accepted that the perception of bitter taste prevents the consumption of toxins from plants, decaying foods, and drugs, consistently producing rejection or aversion responses [4]. Such a claim has been made since the end of the last century and persists to this day:

> "The primitive function of this taste quality would seem to be to provoke the rejection of toxic substances." [50]

> "Bitter taste perception provides animals with critical protection against ingestion of poisonous compounds." [45]

> "Taste is a different matter, especially where bitter compounds are concerned. Virtually every naturally occurring toxin tastes bitter, 'so bitterness clearly evolved with the sole purpose of warning you against the ingestion of toxic substances,' says Zuker. The important thing is to recognize and reject anything bitter, not to get hung up on distinctions among different compounds. Indeed, experimental evidence indicates that humans are unable to discriminate one bitter substance from another."[51]

> "Bitter taste effectively warns us not to ingest potentially harmful compounds. One of the most interesting challenges in taste research is to understand how evolution shaped bitter taste receptors to accomplish this task." [20]

> "The universal character of the rejection provoked by intensely bitter molecules demonstrates the close connection between taste and disgust. Toxic compounds, such as strychnine and other alkaloids common among plants, often exhibit a strong bitter taste. In fact, many plants have evolved such compounds to protect themselves from herbivores. All animals generally reject substances with a sour or bitter taste." [21]

> "Human bitter taste receptors of the TAS2R gene family play a crucial role as warning sensors against the ingestion of toxic food compounds." [52].

> "In contrast to the sweet and umami taste, the bitter taste is a signal that prevents animals from ingesting toxic substances." [53]

> "Taste receptors are located on the epithelial surface throughout the alimentary canal to identify nutrients and potential toxins. In the oral cavity, the role of taste is to encourage or discourage ingestion." [54]

Of course, many bitter substances have a noticeable harmful effect. Reports of plants that are toxic to humans are extensive. However, there is no complete inventory to recognize which contain bitter principles or whether their toxicity is caused by these principles [55]. Most of the poisons used by humans for hunting animals [56], or for intentional poisoning of enemies or suicide, come from bitter plants. Classic examples from history are strychnine (*Strychnos nux vomica*), hemlock (*Conium maculatum*), and aconite (*Aconitum napellus*).

However, many foods, medicines, and additives are bitter or emit bitter tones, which makes their acceptance and consumption difficult. Indeed, the most popular stimulant beverages with caffeine are bitter because of their methylxanthine content. Also, cruciferous vegetables such as broccoli, cauliflower, cabbage, and watercress contain isothiocynates [4]. In many other foods, a certain bitter taste is perceived: olive oil due to compounds derived from oleuropein and ligstroside (from unripe olive fruits); carrots, rich in phenolic acids; most citrus fruits such as oranges, lemons, and grapefruit, as they contain compounds such as naringin and limonin; soy sauce due to the presence of aglycones; grape juices and wines due to the presence of tannins that give them their peculiar flavor; beer, made from the fermentation of malt, where the so-called isohumulones are produced; and most distilled alcoholic beverages, because they contain the compound called 6-n-propylthiouracil (PROP), responsible for their bitterness [57].

On the other hand, many common pharmaceutical compounds have a bitter taste, including antimalarials such as quinine and chloroquine, antibiotics such as erythromycin and floxacins [58], and psychotropic drugs such as haloperidol and procainamide [59]. In fact, most drugs are considered to have a bitter taste [60]. Some of the additives used for food preservation, which are often effective and inexpensive, also produce some unpleasant bitter taste. Generally speaking, chemical compounds that are within the group exhibiting antioxidant potential such as polyphenols, anthocyanins, and carotenoids are responsible for bitter taste [57].

For this reason, one of the purposes of food and pharmaceutical industries is to eliminate or diminish the bitter taste of these beverages, foods, medicines, and additives, either to facilitate their consumption or to avoid the undesirable effects that bitter substances tend to produce. Perhaps the simplest and most traditional formula has been the addition of sugar or sweeteners. In almost all cultures, culinary traditions usually add minimal amounts of seasonings and flavorings to provoke a harmonious balance of flavors, thus achieving, among other intentions, a reduction in the bitter taste. In recent years, the production of attractive foods has been widely explored by nutritional science to avoid unpleasant flavors, including bitterness, astringency, and pungency in various foods [57]. There is also a demand to improve the taste quality of pet and farm animal foods and to develop non-lethal wildlife repellents, e.g., non-toxic chemicals with off-flavors [43]. More recently, with the knowledge of the structure of bitter receptors, the development of bitter blockers is supposed to help mask the bitter taste of drugs [58].

However, although a bitter taste is usually unpleasant and repulsive when it is strong, it is bearable when it is weak [20]. Although bitter foods or beverages are unattractive, in some cases, the bitter taste forms an essential part of the desirable characteristics in that food. Indeed, this is the case with beer, extra virgin olive oil, wines, and some distilled spirits. Another example within beverages is tonic water containing quinine, which is considered a bitter substance tolerable at low concentrations [57]. Therefore, not all bitter compounds are toxic, as they can also be found in high concentrations and with health benefits in foods of vegetal origin [61].

As has been seen, just like with the sweet taste, there is no common chemical structure in the chemicals involved in the perception of bitter taste [21]. Thus, according to Villegas et al., a bitter taste cannot be predicted solely by the structure of the compound molecule. It depends on the size of that molecule, the functional group present, the position of the sugar if present, the decrease in hydrophobicity, and the molecular stereochemistry [57]. A very important characteristic of the bitter sensation is that it can be elicited by very small concentrations of substances, compared to the other tastes [50].

In a way, the discovery of specific receptors for the transduction of bitter taste in recent years has triggered an explosion of research that has not yet come to an end. Despite similar findings for sweet, umami, salty, and sour tastes, the scientific literature is more abundant in publications referring to T2R. Identified in 1996 [21], associated shortly after with T1R receptors, responsible for sweet and umami tastes [44], the genes encoding these receptor proteins were finally discovered in 2000 [45], and by 2006, the genetic map of the T1R and T2R receptors was fully established [47]. Recent genetic studies mention that the ability of humans to detect this taste is determined by a locus on chromosome 5 and possibly chromosome 7 [57]. However, it is known that some bitter compounds can also interact with proton channels [26] and with TRP [43], in particular the TRPm5 channel abundantly present in taste receptor cells [36].

Between 24 and 29 T2R receptors have been identified [62], which raises the question of how the wide range of bitter compounds is that can be detected by such a limited number of sensors [49]. Some suggest that while they all respond to bitter compounds, they cannot necessarily distinguish them from each other, so they would act more like universal bitter sensors [53]. Others, on the contrary, suppose that the basis for discriminating between different bitter compounds lies in the overlap of these receptors on taste papillae, together with their genetic polymorphism, thus allowing humans and animals to detect the enormous range of bitter compounds [23].

However, as with sweet stimuli, because of their large molecular size, bitter substances do not enter the taste cell and bind to the T2Rs [43]. Thus, they activate the G protein gustducin, which is cleaved, and its subunits in turn activate a nearby enzyme that converts precursor molecules inside into what are known as second messengers [24], increasing the intracellular calcium concentration (Ca^{2+}), although the mechanism by which this signaling pathway generates the electrical response and the changes that lead to the release of the neurotransmitter that allows signal propagation through the nervous system remains unclear (see Figure 4). Recent studies propose that calcium release stimulates TRPm5 channel receptors to subsequently release ATP, thus suggesting that both T2R and TRP receptors are simultaneously involved in the final transduction of bitter taste [53]. It is unclear why dual signaling should be required for bitter taste and whether it is more than parallel amplification [20].

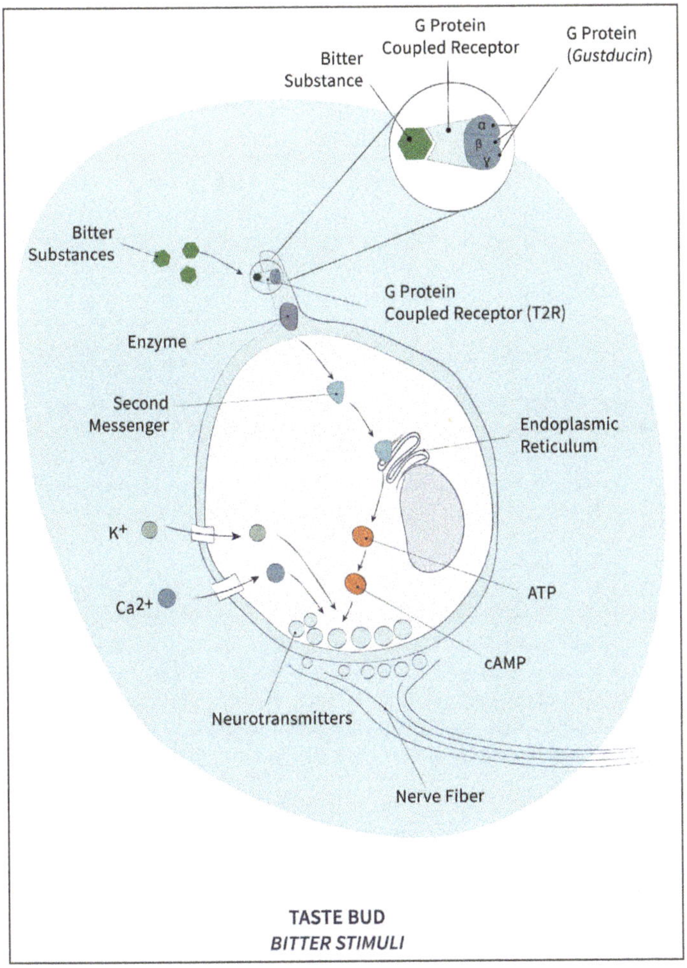

Figure 4. Scheme of the cellular mechanism for the transduction of bitter taste.

T2R expression was initially thought to be limited to the oral cavity but has recently been described in a number of other tissues, including the heart, intestine, nasal cavity, and lungs, and other cell types (smooth muscle, endothelial, epithelial, and inflammatory cells) [62]. The collection of gene expression omnibus indicates that T2Rs are expressed in additional human tissues, including the brain, skeletal muscle, endometrium, liver, and omental adipose tissue [59], although its role is still uncertain [61]. It is even remarkable that there are bitter compounds effective via the bloodstream. For example, by injecting a choline solution into the bloodstream of a subject, a bitter taste is suddenly perceived, a sensation which also disappears rapidly [50].

Some suggest that this broad expression of extraoral T2Rs would explain numerous side effects of current drugs, as most of them have a bitter taste [60]. This would imply that because of their bitter character, such drugs produce undesirable effects outside their therapeutic target, so the identification of T2R blockers (antagonists and inverse agonists) would help to eliminate these effects [58]. However, it also means that, in addition to their role in taste transduction, T2Rs in other pathways not only have a deleterious but also a physiological role [25].

The biology of bitter perception is still poorly supported. Neither the sensory receptor cells nor the receptor molecules have been physiologically or molecularly fully defined [45]. Given the amount of work that needs to be undertaken to understand the structure and function of these receptors, the next few years will be an interesting and exciting phase in T2R biology [31].

6. The Physiology of Taste and Health

The brain has the capacity to store information associated with what is consumed, which has a direct impact on the attitude and frequency with which certain foods are eaten for the benefit of our health [27]. Applied taste research is increasingly focused on the relationship between diet and health and on understanding the role of the sense of taste in encouraging or discouraging consumption [63].

Sensory information from taste cells is clear to help us detect and respond appropriately to our nutritional needs. The sweet taste of sugars, for example, enhances carbohydrate intake. These taste signals also trigger physiological responses, such as the release of insulin, which facilitates effective utilization of ingested nutrients. Faced with a lack of sodium, animals and humans seek sources of sodium in their intake. According to experimental results, humans and animals with dietary deficiencies tend to ingest foods high in vitamins and minerals [21]. It has also been established that pleasurable foods elevate dopamine levels, which may be crucial for food preferences and food intake control [4].

Current lifestyles are characterized by low physical activity and chronic poor nutrition which predisposes one to metabolic syndrome and its long-term consequences (hypertension, diabetes, and neurodegenerative diseases). The current trend for its treatment involves, among others, the increasing knowledge about the physiology of the sensory systems involved and eating habits. Prenatal experience may have a direct influence on adult food intake choices and could contribute to childhood obesity. Several studies suggest that early exposure to fruits and vegetables or foods high in energy, sugar, or fat have been linked to infants' preference to consume them. Thus, it may be useful to address early taste perception, how it influences eating behaviors, and to determine its repercussions on lifestyles and human health [4].

In addition, a critical gap in our understanding of taste is how taste mechanisms are related to mood, appetite, obesity, and satiety. The obvious link is that taste guides and largely determines food selection, with salty, sweet, and fatty tastes being the main players. A fascinating link between appetite and mood is that serotonin-enhancing drugs, commonly used to treat mood disorders and depression, have been shown to influence taste thresholds [23].

On the other hand, the available data provide some examples of the role of genetic variation in taste receptors in human nutrition and health. As a result, it may potentially predispose individuals to certain diseases. Thus, some taste receptor alleles may be risk factors for disease. Genotypes of these receptors may be useful as biomarkers to identify predispositions to some diseases and suggest interventions for their prevention [43].

PROP taster status has been found to be associated with a wide range of attributes/phenotypes, including increased perceived orosensory sensations, motion sickness, food preference, fat perception, body mass index, child height, alcohol consumption, and alcoholism [25]. Some studies have shown that supertasters and average tasters of PROP are more discriminating of fat content than nontasters of PROP, which influences their consumption. Indeed, one study showed that nontasters and medium tasters of PROP have a higher body mass index than supertasters in subjects with low dietary constraints. In addition, PROP taster status was found to be associated with stature and choice of eating in children. One study showed that girls with the PROP supertaster had significantly higher weight/height percentiles, whereas boys with the PROP supertaster had significantly lower weight/height percentiles compared with their counterparts. Thus, there is significant evidence of both association and lack of association between PROP taster status and dietary habits, food preferences, and body mass index, leading to the unanswered question of whether genetic variations are a deciding factor in a person's food habits and preferences [25].

On the other hand, genetic variation in taste receptors may be a biomarker of predisposition to alcoholism. Ethanol has bitter and sweet taste components. Variation in bitter and sweet taste response is associated with ethanol taste perception and beverage alcohol consumption. In mice, allelic variation in the sweet taste receptor gene TAS1R3 is associated with voluntary ethanol consumption. Although hedonic responses to sweet taste are considered one of the biomarkers of predisposition to alcoholism in humans, the genes responsible for this association are still unknown. An increased sensitivity to ethanol bitterness may protect against excessive alcohol consumption. According to this hypothesis, individuals carrying one or two sensitive alleles PAV (dominant haplotype) of the phenylthiocarbamide receptor gene, TAS2R38, had a lower annual consumption of alcoholic beverages than individuals homozygous for the insensitive allele AVI (recessive haplotype). Similarly, there is an association between the risk of alcohol dependence and TAS2R16 polymorphisms: an ancestral allele that is less sensitive to β-glucopyranosides in vitro is associated with an increased risk of alcohol dependence [43]. Other studies have confirmed that PROP taster status is linked to alcohol consumption and alcoholism as a result of the bitter taste it carries [25].

Many cruciferous vegetables are known to contain PROP-like compounds. These compounds are known as glucosinolates and are found in members of the *Brassica*, *Raphanus*, and *Nasturtium* genera, including radishes, cabbages, and watercress. Specific TAS2R38 genotypes are also associated with the perceived bitterness of these glucosinolate-producing plants. Glucosinolates can be toxic to the thyroid gland, so they must be detected before ingestion to prevent thyroid-related diseases. Also, a significant association was found between PROP taster status and vector-induced motion sickness. It was found that PROP nontasters experienced significantly higher degrees of motion sickness and nausea compared to average and super PROP tasters. The authors suggested that susceptibility to motion sickness and nausea has coevolved with nontasters to maintain protection against potential toxin consumption while allowing for the consumption of bitter compounds such as phytonutrients without initial rejection in the oral cavity. This suggests that the nontaster status of PROP is a positive evolutionary selection mechanism [25].

Taste aversion learning, whether natural or experimentally induced, can result from an association of substance and disease, even if there is a gap of several hours between the two. One of the side effects of radiation and chemotherapy treatments in cancer patients is loss of appetite. To a large extent, this is due more to conditioned taste aversions than to the gastrointestinal discomfort produced by these treatments [21].

7. Medicinal Bitters

A bitter taste has been shown to promote, at appropriate concentrations, salivation and increased appetite [50]. It has even been known that people who have increased perception to bitter tastes may have a greater overall acuity of the sense of taste and increased sensitivity to olfactory signals. In addition, it has been noted that many of the chemicals that impart a certain bitter taste to foods may be beneficial to health. Polyphenols, methylxanthines, isoflavones, and sulfonamides, present in cruciferous vegetables and carrots, have antioxidant effects and protect us from certain diseases [4]. Tannins present in grape wine may have a cardiovascular protective effect [64]. Xanthines contained in stimulant beverages, in addition to their stimulant effect, offer benefits at the cerebrovascular level and even serve to control migraines [65]. Therefore, despite not being entirely pleasant, their consumption is compensated by the health benefits of these unpleasant-tasting compounds [57].

On the other hand, an interesting chapter opens with the understanding of the role of T2Rs responsible for the detection of bitter taste, playing an important role in the maintenance of homeostasis and in the response to certain diseases [59]. Accumulating evidence suggests that T2R-mediated signaling contributes greatly to innate immunity in organ epithelia that are connected to the external environment [60]. A recent study confirmed that T2Rs in human airways detect secreted bacterial products, stimulating a secretion of antimicrobial peptides into the mucosa capable of inhibiting a variety of respiratory pathogens [66]. Another study showed that at the pulmonary level, T2R agonists increase the frequency of ciliary movements in epithelial cells, induce bronchial smooth muscle cells to relax, and modulate the production of pro-inflammatory mediators [62].

There is also increasing evidence of the effect of T2R activation at the gut level on epithelial cells and endocrine cells, promoting the secretion of hormones such as incretin (glucagon-like peptide-1), ghrelin, and other substances such as cholecystokinin and glucose-dependent insulinotropic polypeptide (GIP) [67], with obvious physiological and possible therapeutic effects. The existence of these "taste" mechanisms in the gut is perhaps not surprising, given the importance of sensing the chemical nature of light contents at all points along the gastrointestinal tract. However, the findings have generated new excitement in understanding how the gut participates in the sensing and control of appetite in general and digestive processes in particular [23].

Many foods and medicinal plants contain polyphenols, which are bitter-tasting substances which have shown therapeutic benefits. Recent studies confirm that polyphenols are ligands for extraoral T2Rs and this interaction in T2Rs at the brain level helps regulate appetite/satiety control, while T2Rs at the gut level contribute to the metabolism of adipose tissue and promote the secretion of gastrointestinal hormones such as ghrelin, which helps control blood glucose. "Together, these factors can contribute to understand the beneficial effects of polyphenol-rich diets but also might aid in identifying new pharmacological pathway targets for the treatment of diabetes and obesity." [9].

Deshmukh et al, summarized this as follows: "The plants containing bitters (bitter substances) are exclusively used due to their intensively bitter tastes, they increase the appetite and stimulates digestion by acting on the mucous membranes of the mouth. Also increases the flow bile, stimulate repair of gut wall lining and regulate the secretion of insulin and glucagon. They reflectively induce stimulation on the salivary gland and the secretion of gastric juice. The bitter taste recognizes at the very moment of excitation. The taste buds are situated at the root of the tongue and keep the bitter taste some time afterwards ('after-taste'). These are then sending the signal to the brain, which by reflexes than affect the swelling of the secreting mucous membranes. The bitters have therefore positive influence on the digestive processes, then it led to an improvement on appetite as well as an amelioration of the food intake. The bitter plants are generally showing antidiabetic and tonic action." [68].

It has even been claimed that any T2R could mediate unanticipated physiological changes in any T2R-expressing tissue exposed to significant concentrations of a bitter-tasting drug. T2Rs in respiratory and gastrointestinal tissues would be particularly available for ingestion or inhalation, but drugs absorbed into the bloodstream could reach T2Rs in almost any tissue in the body. This hypothesis, if confirmed, would have important implications for drug development and medical practice. Bitter-tasting phytochemicals, some of which are suspected to have biological activity, could similarly exert their therapeutic actions through extraoral T2Rs if target concentrations were sufficiently high [59].

As mentioned above, bitter-tasting molecular structures are not exclusive to a single type of secondary metabolite. Indeed, bitter principles are found in alkaloids, heterosides, essential oils, terpenes, isoprenoids, tannins, mucilages, alcohols, acids, and esters. For this reason, we must consider that more than the molecular structure, their bitter character activates their physiological and perhaps therapeutic function at oral and extraoral T2Rs. From a chemistry point of view, we still need a scientific explanation to determine exactly what happens at the molecular level to make some of these secondary metabolites bitter and others not. Table 2 shows some bitter compounds from food or medicinal plants with therapeutic effects.

Table 2. Bitter compounds of food or medicinal plants con therapeutic effect.

Bitter Compounds	Food or Medicinal Plants	Therapeutic Effect	Ref.
Polyphenols, methylxanthines, isoflavones, and sulfonamides	Cruciferous vegetables and carrots	Antioxidant effects and protect us from certain diseases	[4]
Tannins	Grape wine	Cardiovascular protective effect	[64]
Xanthines	Stimulant beverages (coffee, tea, chocolate, kola)	Benefits at the cerebrovascular level and control migraine	[65]
Polyphenols	Exist widely in plant and plant-based foods	Metabolism of adipose tissue and promotes the secretion of gastrointestinal hormones such as ghrelin, which helps control blood glucose	[9]
Thujone, sesquiterpene lactones: absinthin, anabsinthin, anabsin, and artabsin	Wormwood (*Artemisia absinthium*)	Anti-inflammatory, antioxidant, and antimicrobial effects, and it has been shown to influence GI tract and urinary system	[10]
Azadirachtin, meliacin, gedunin, nimbidin, nimbolides, salanin, nimbin, valassin, meliacin, limonoid	Neem (*Azadirachta indica*)	Antiplasmodial, antitrypanosomal, antioxidant, anti-cancer, antibacterial, antiviral, larvicidal, and fungicidal activities.	[12]
Phenolic components, Kuguaglycoside G, Momordicine	Bitter melon (*Momordica charantia*)	Antidiabetic, anti-obesity, anti-inflammatory, anti-cancer effects among others	[16]
Phellodendrine, Berberine	Amur cork tree (*Phellodendron amurense*)	Protect against airway inflammation, can reduce blood uric acid levels, reduce blood glucose levels, and slow the development of diabetic nephropathy	[17]
Sesquiterpene lactones: vernodalin, vernolide, hydroxyvernolide	Bitter leaf (*Vernonia amygdalina*)	Alleviate inflammation, pyrexia and nociception	[19]

Despite this novel evidence, phytochemical and pharmacological research focused on exploring the therapeutic role of medicinal plants is still in its incipient stages, not because of their chemical compounds per se but because these compounds have a bitter taste. Using a statistical inquiry, Grădinaru et al. offer a pioneering study on the relevance of phytochemical taste for anti-inflammatory and anti-cancer activity. Out of 624 phytochemicals, 461 were found to possess anti-cancer activity, and they found a robust statistical association between the bitter taste of these phytochemicals and their simultaneous anti-cancer and anti-inflammatory effects [69].

Finally, Dragoș et al. affirm: "The anti-inflammatory activity of plant-derived compounds is more strongly associated with their taste than with their chemical class. Bitter phytocompounds have a higher probability of playing an inflammation related role, exerting anti-inflammatory activity, by contrast to sour and sweet phytochemicals, which have a higher probability of being devoid thereof." [70].

8. Conclusions

For many years, the theory of taste physiology considered that the function of identifying bitter tastes was to detect and prevent the consumption of toxins from plants, decaying foods, and drugs. In my experience with indigenous peoples, I was surprised to learn that for them bitter medicinal plants have important medicinal, preventive, and therapeutic value. In reviewing recent scientific advances, we found that the T2R membrane receptors for bitter taste, G protein-associated or metabotropic receptors, are not only located in the oral mucosa but are also found in other organs and tissues of the human being, also fulfilling an important physiological and therapeutic role.

Indeed, several studies have confirmed their antioxidant effects, anti-inflammatory activity, appetite/satiety control, cardiovascular protection, increased frequency of ciliary movements in epithelial cells, maintenance of homeostasis, production of pro-inflammatory mediators and stimulation of antimicrobial peptide secretion, among others, with potential benefits for the prevention and treatment of many diseases.

Thus, an important chapter of research on bitter T2R receptors and new epistemological and research routes for medicinal plants has been opened. Perhaps the indigenous people are right. With this new knowledge, we will be able to understand the true biological basis through which bitter plants may act as "good medicine" [60].

Funding: This research was partially funded by the Centro de Estudios Médicos Interculturales.

Institutional Review Board Statement: Not applicable.

Informed Consent Statement: Not applicable.

Data Availability Statement: Data sharing is not applicable.

Acknowledgments: To the Ingano shaman Germán Mojomboy, the Tukano shaman Benedicto Mejía, and the deceased shamans Roberto Jacanamijoy, Laureano Becerra, José Becerra, and Bernardo Suárez, for their light and teachings on the value of their traditional medicine and medicinal plants. To Ana María Zuluaga for her contribution to the elaboration of the figures and the Graphical Abstract, and to Ana María Pacheco for her contribution to the English translation of this document.

Conflicts of Interest: The author declares no conflicts of interest.

References

1. Ikeda, K. New Seasonings. *Chem. Senses* **2002**, *27*, 847–849. [CrossRef] [PubMed]
2. Hernández, C.D.B. La bioquímica y fisiología del sabor. *Rev. Educ. Bioquim.* **2019**, *38*, 100–104.
3. Chandrashekar, J.; Hoon, M.A.; Ryba, N.J.P.; Zuker, C.S. The receptors and cells for mammalian taste. *Nature* **2006**, *444*, 288–294. [CrossRef] [PubMed]
4. Rubio-Navarro, L.; Torrero, C.; Regalado, M.; Salas, M. Desarrollo de la discriminación a los sabores. *Rev. Eneurobiología* **2013**, *4*, 3.
5. Zhang, J.; Jin, H.; Zhang, W.; Ding, C.; O'Keeffe, S.; Ye, M.; Zuker, C.S. Sour Sensing from the Tongue to the Brain. *Cell* **2019**, *179*, 392–402. [CrossRef] [PubMed]
6. Frings, S. The sour taste of a proton current. *Proc. Natl. Acad. Sci. USA* **2010**, *107*, 21955–21956. [CrossRef] [PubMed]
7. Zuluaga, G. *El Yoco: La Savia de la Selva*; Centro Editorial Universidad del Rosario: Bogotá, Colombia, 2004; 110p, ISBN 958-8225-14-0.
8. Zuluaga, G.; Amaya, C. Use of purgatives in traditional Colombian medicine. *Interciencia* **1991**, *16*, 322–328.
9. Trius-Soler, M.; Moreno, J.J. Bitter taste receptors: Key target to understand the effects of polyphenols on glucose and body weight homeostasis. Pathophysiological and pharmacological implications. Pathophysiological and pharmacological implications. *Biochem. Pharmacol.* **2024**, *in press*. [CrossRef]
10. Bach, B.; Cleroux, M.; Saillen, M.; Schönenberger, P.; Burgos, S.; Ducruet, J.; Vallat, A. A new chemical tool for absinthe producers, quantification of α/β-thujone and the bitter components in *Artemisia absinthium*. *Food Chem.* **2016**, *213*, 813–817. [CrossRef]
11. Neelamma, G.; Swamy, B.; Dhamodaran, P.; Vanitha, B. A Review on pharmacognostic and phytopharmacological perspective of artemisia vulgaris. *Eur. J. Pharm. Sci.* **2020**, *3*, 501–505.
12. Datta, A.; Grün, I.U.; Kwasniewski, M.T.; Fernando, L.N. Comparison of Two Adsorbent Based de-Bittering Procedures for Neem (*Azadirachta indica* A. Juss) Tea—Effect on Polyphenols, Anti-Oxidant Capacity, Color and Volatile Profile. *Plant Foods Hum. Nutr.* **2017**, *72*, 88–95. [CrossRef] [PubMed]
13. Meng, F.-C.; Wu, Z.-F.; Yin, Z.-Q.; Lin, L.-G.; Wang, R.; Zhang, Q.-W. *Coptidis rhizoma* and its main bioactive components: Recent advances in chemical investigation, quality evaluation and pharmacological activity. *Chin. Med.* **2018**, *13*, 13. [CrossRef] [PubMed]
14. Maňourová, A.; Leuner, O.; Tchoundjeu, Z.; Van Damme, P.; Verner, V.; Přibyl, O.; Lojka, B. Medicinal Potential, Utilization and Domestication Status of Bitter Kola (*Garcinia kola Heckel*) in West and Central Africa. *Forests* **2019**, *10*, 124. [CrossRef]
15. Hoel, H.; de Boer, H.J.; Kool, A.; Wangensteen, H. Analysis of bitter compounds in traditional preparations of *Gentiana purpurea* L. *Fitoterapia* **2024**, *175*, 105932. [CrossRef] [PubMed]
16. Bora, A.F.M.; Kouame, K.J.E.-P.; Li, X.; Liu, L.; Pan, Y. New insights into the bioactive polysaccharides, proteins, and triterpenoids isolated from bitter melon (*Momordica charantia*) and their relevance for nutraceutical and food application: A review. *Int. J. Biol. Macromol.* **2023**, *231*, 123173. [CrossRef] [PubMed]

17. Xu, K.; He, G.; Qin, J.; Cheng, X.; He, H.; Zhang, D.; Peng, W. High-efficient extraction of principal medicinal components from fresh *Phellodendron bark* (cortex phellodendri). *Saudi J. Biol. Sci.* **2018**, *25*, 811–815. [CrossRef] [PubMed]
18. Kubica, P.; Szopa, A.; Dominiak, J.; Luczkiewicz, M.; Ekiert, H. Verbena officinalis (*Common Vervain*)—A Review on the Investigations of This Medicinally Important Plant Species. *Planta Med.* **2020**, *86*, 1241–1257. [CrossRef] [PubMed]
19. Asante, D.-B.; Henneh, I.T.; Acheampong, D.O.; Kyei, F.; Adokoh, C.K.; Ofori, E.G.; Domey, N.K.; Adakudugu, E.; Tangella, L.P.; Ameyaw, E.O. Anti-inflammatory, anti-nociceptive and antipyretic activity of young and old leaves of *Vernonia amygdalina*. *Biomed. Pharmacother.* **2019**, *111*, 1187–1203. [CrossRef] [PubMed]
20. Lindemann, B. Receptors and transduction in taste. *Nature* **2001**, *413*, 219–225. [CrossRef]
21. Smith, D.; Margolskee, R. El sentido del gusto. *Investig. Y Cienc.* **2001**, *296*, 4–12.
22. Auvray, M.; Spence, C. The multisensory perception of flavor. *Conscious. Cogn.* **2008**, *17*, 1016–1031. [CrossRef] [PubMed]
23. Chaudhari, N.; Roper, S.D. The cell biology of taste. *J. Cell Biol.* **2010**, *190*, 285. [CrossRef] [PubMed]
24. Alvarez Gaviria, W. Cilia melanocytes and molecular bases of senses. *Acta Otorrinolaringol. Cir. Cabeza Cuello* **2007**, *35*, 45–57.
25. Bering, A. Genetic Analysis of Taste in Homo Sapiens. Brock University. 2012. Available online: http://hdl.handle.net/10464/4220 (accessed on 1 April 2024).
26. Morales, J.M.; María, E.; Sánchez, M.; Ángel, M.; García, C. FISIOLOGÍA DEL GUSTO. In *Libro Virtual de Formación en ORL*; 2009. Available online: https://seorl.net/PDF/Cavidad%20oral%20faringe%20esofago/069%20-%20FISIOLOG%C3%8DA%20DEL%20GUSTO.pdf (accessed on 1 April 2024).
27. Miranda, M.I. El Sabor de los Recuerdos: Formación de la Memoria Gustativa. Revista Digital Universitaria UNAM. 2011. Available online: https://www.ru.tic.unam.mx/handle/123456789/1864 (accessed on 30 May 2024).
28. Talavera, K.; Yasumatsu, K.; Voets, T.; Droogmans, G.; Shigemura, N.; Ninomiya, Y.; Margolskee, R.F.; Nilius, B. Heat activation of TRPM5 underlies thermal sensitivity of sweet taste. *Nature* **2005**, *438*, 1022–1025. [CrossRef] [PubMed]
29. Clapham, D.E. TRP channels as cellular sensors. *Nature* **2003**, *426*, 517–524. [CrossRef] [PubMed]
30. González Morán, M.G. Comunicación celular. Transducción de señales acopladas a proteínas G heterotriméricas. *Educ. Química* **2018**, *16*, 208. [CrossRef]
31. Jaggupilli, A.; Howard, R.; Upadhyaya, J.D.; Bhullar, R.P.; Chelikani, P. Bitter taste receptors: Novel insights into the biochemistry and pharmacology. *Int. J. Biochem. Cell Biol.* **2016**, *77*, 184–196. [CrossRef] [PubMed]
32. Ramsey, I.S.; Delling, M.; Clapham, D.E. An introduction to trp channels. *Annu. Rev. Physiol.* **2006**, *68*, 619–647. [CrossRef]
33. Pharmacology IU of B and C. Epithelial Sodium Channel (ENaC). Available online: https://www.guidetopharmacology.org/GRAC/FamilyDisplayForward?familyId=122 (accessed on 7 July 2020).
34. Kellenberger, S.; Schild, L. Epithelial Sodium Channel/Degenerin Family of Ion Channels: A Variety of Functions for a Shared Structure. *Physiol. Rev.* **2002**, *82*, 735–767. [CrossRef]
35. Abstracts from the Thirty-second Annual Meeting of the Association for Chemoreception Sciences. *Chem. Senses* **2010**, *35*, A1–A140. [CrossRef]
36. Kaske, S.; Krasteva, G.; König, P.; Kummer, W.; Hofmann, T.; Gudermann, T.; Chubanov, V. TRPM5, a taste-signaling transient receptor potential ion-channel, is a ubiquitous signaling component in chemosensory cells. *BMC Neurosci.* **2007**, *8*, 49. [CrossRef]
37. Nilius, B.; Owsianik, G. The transient receptor potential family of ion channels. *Genome Biol.* **2011**, *12*, 218. [CrossRef]
38. Ishimaru, Y.; Inada, H.; Kubota, M.; Zhuang, H.; Tominaga, M.; Matsunami, H. Transient receptor potential family members PKD1L3 and PKD2L1 form a candidate sour taste receptor. *Proc. Natl. Acad. Sci. USA* **2006**, *103*, 12569–12574. [CrossRef]
39. Jácome, A. Historia de los receptores. *Rev. Colomb. Endocrinol. Diabetes Y Metab.* **2017**, *4*, 47–50. [CrossRef]
40. García-Sáinz, J.A. El Premio Nobel de química 2012: Lefkowitz y Kobilka. *Educ. Quim.* **2013**, *24*, 79–81. [CrossRef]
41. Gonzales Gil, P. Receptores acoplados a proteínas G: Entendiendo cómo responde nuestro organismo a señales diversas. *Rev. Química* **2012**, *26*, 16–19.
42. Gilman, A. G Proteins: Transducers Of Receptor-Generated Signals. *Annu. Rev. Biochem.* **1987**, *56*, 615–649. [CrossRef] [PubMed]
43. Bachmanov, A.A.; Beauchamp, G.K. Taste Receptor Genes. *Annu. Rev. Nutr.* **2007**, *27*, 389–414. [CrossRef]
44. Hoon, M.A.; Adler, E.; Lindemeier, J.; Battey, J.F.; Ryba, N.J.P.; Zuker, C.S. Putative Mammalian Taste Receptors. *Cell* **1999**, *96*, 541–551. [CrossRef]
45. Chandrashekar, J.; Mueller, K.L.; Hoon, M.A.; Adler, E.; Feng, L.; Guo, W.; Zuker, C.S.; Ryba, N.J.P. T2Rs function as bitter taste receptors. *Cell* **2000**, *100*, 703–711. [CrossRef]
46. Adler, E.; Hoon, M.A.; Mueller, K.L.; Chandrashekar, J.; Ryba, N.J.P.; Zuker, C.S. A novel family of mammalian taste receptors. *Cell* **2000**, *100*, 693–702. [CrossRef] [PubMed]
47. Reed, D.R.; Tanaka, T.; McDaniel, A.H. Diverse tastes: Genetics of sweet and bitter perception. *Physiol. Behav.* **2006**, *88*, 215–226. [CrossRef] [PubMed]
48. Chávez, O.; Vega, G.; Sierra, A.; Ramírez, F.; Miramontes, Y.H. Fisiología del gusto. *Oral. Rev.* **2010**, *11*, 625–631.
49. Meyerhof, W.; Batram, C.; Kuhn, C.; Brockhoff, A.; Chudoba, E.; Bufe, B.; Appendino, G.; Behrens, M. The Molecular Receptive Ranges of Human TAS2R Bitter Taste Receptors. *Chem. Senses* **2010**, *35*, 157–170. [CrossRef] [PubMed]
50. Cometto-Muñiz, J. Caracteristicas de los componentes del sabor. *La. Aliment. Latinoam.* **1980**, *14*, 44–50.
51. Identification of Bitter-Taste Genes Provides Insight into the Organization of the Taste System. Available online: https://biology.ucsd.edu/about/news/article_031600.html (accessed on 27 July 2020).

52. Reichling, C.; Meyerhof, W.; Behrens, M. Functions of human bitter taste receptors depend on *N*-glycosylation. *J. Neurochem.* **2008**, *106*, 1138–1148. [CrossRef] [PubMed]
53. Fuentes, A.; Fresno, M.J.; Santander, H.; Valenzuela, S.; Felipe Gutiérrez, M.; Miralles, R.; Fuentes, A. Sensopercepción Gustativa: Una Revisión Gustatory Sensory Perception: A Review. *Int. J. Odontostomat* **2010**, *42*, 161–168. [CrossRef]
54. Hassan, L.; Newman, L.; Keast, R.; Danaher, J.; Biesiekierski, J.R. The effect of gastrointestinal bitter sensing on appetite regulation and energy intake: A systematic review. *Appetite* **2023**, *180*, 106336. [CrossRef]
55. Farzaei, M.H.; Bayrami, Z.; Farzaei, F.; Aneva, I.; Das, S.K.; Patra, J.K.; Das, G.; Abdollahi, M. Poisoning by Medical Plants. *Arch. Iran. Med.* **2020**, *23*, 117–127.
56. Pijoan, M. Venenos tribales. *Offarm* **2007**, *26*, 104–116.
57. Villegas, X.; Ruíz, H.; Bárcenas, M. Tecnologías de enmascaramiento de sabor amargo en alimentos. *Temas Sel. Ing. Aliment.* **2010**, *4*, 27–36.
58. Pydi, S.P.; Sobotkiewicz, T.; Billakanti, R.; Bhullar, R.P.; Loewen, M.C.; Chelikani, P. Amino acid derivatives as bitter taste receptor (T2R) blockers. *J. Biol. Chem.* **2014**, *289*, 25054–25066. [CrossRef] [PubMed]
59. Clark, A.A.; Liggett, S.B.; Munger, S.D. Extraoral bitter taste receptors as mediators of off-target drug effects. *FASEB J.* **2012**, *26*, 4827–4831. [CrossRef] [PubMed]
60. Lu, P.; Zhang, C.-H.; Lifshitz, L.M.; ZhuGe, R. Extraoral bitter taste receptors in health and disease. *J. Gen. Physiol.* **2017**, *149*, 181–197. [CrossRef] [PubMed]
61. Descamps-Solà, M.; Vilalta, A.; Jalsevac, F.; Blay, M.T.; Rodríguez-Gallego, E.; Pinent, M.; Beltrán-Debón, R.; Terra, X.; Ardévol, A. Bitter taste receptors along the gastrointestinal tract: Comparison between humans and rodents. *Front. Nutr.* **2023**, *10*, 1215889. [CrossRef] [PubMed]
62. Devillier, P.; Naline, E.; Grassin-Delyle, S. The pharmacology of bitter taste receptors and their role in human airways. *Pharmacol. Ther.* **2015**, *155*, 11–21. [CrossRef] [PubMed]
63. Hartley, I.E.; Liem, D.G.; Keast, R. Umami as an 'Alimentary' taste. A new perspective on taste classification. *Nutrients* **2019**, *11*, 182. [CrossRef]
64. Llerena, I.R.; Huerta, E.M. Vino y corazón. *Rev. Esp. Cardiol.* **2015**, *51*, 435–449. [CrossRef]
65. Hay, E.; Dhe, L. Tratamiento farmacológico de la migraña. *Rev. Fac. Med. (Méx.)* **2012**, *55*, 54–58.
66. Lee, R.J.; Kofonow, J.M.; Rosen, P.L.; Siebert, A.P.; Chen, B.; Doghramji, L.; Xiong, G.; Adappa, N.D.; Palmer, J.N.; Kennedy, D.W.; et al. Bitter and sweet taste receptors regulate human upper respiratory innate immunity. *J. Clin. Investig.* **2014**, *124*, 1393–1405. [CrossRef]
67. Santos-Hernández, M.; Reimann, F.; Gribble, F.M. Cellular mechanisms of incretin hormone secretion. *J. Mol. Endocrinol.* **2024**, *72*, e230112. [CrossRef]
68. Deshmukh, D.; Baghel, V.S.; Shastri, D.; Nandini, D.; Chauhan, N. Plant as bitter. *J. Adv. Pharm. Sci.* **2010**, *1*, 334–343.
69. Grădinaru, T.-C.; Gilca, M.; Vlad, A.; Dragoș, D. Relevance of Phytochemical Taste for Anti-Cancer Activity: A Statistical Inquiry. *Int. J. Mol. Sci.* **2023**, *24*, 16227. [CrossRef]
70. Dragoș, D.; Petran, M.; Gradinaru, T.-C.; Gilca, M. Phytochemicals and Inflammation: Is Bitter Better? *Plants* **2022**, *11*, 2991. [CrossRef]

pharmaceuticals

Review

Evaluating the Potential of *Plukenetia volubilis* Linneo (Sacha Inchi) in Alleviating Cardiovascular Disease Risk Factors: A Mini Review

Izzat Zulhilmi Abd Rahman [1], Nur Syahidah Nor Hisam [1,2], Amilia Aminuddin [1,*], Adila A. Hamid [1], Jaya Kumar [1] and Azizah Ugusman [1,*]

1 Department of Physiology, Faculty of Medicine, Universiti Kebangsaan Malaysia, Jalan Yaacob Latif, Kuala Lumpur 56000, Malaysia; izzat_zulhilmi@ukm.edu.my (I.Z.A.R.); p104164@siswa.ukm.edu.my (N.S.N.H.); adilahamid@ppukm.ukm.edu.my (A.A.H.); jayakumar@ukm.edu.my (J.K.)

2 Programme of Biomedical Science, Centre for Toxicology & Health Risk Studies, Faculty of Health Sciences, Universiti Kebangsaan Malaysia, Jalan Raja Muda Abdul Aziz, Kuala Lumpur 50300, Malaysia

* Correspondence: amilia@ppukm.ukm.edu.my (A.A.); dr.azizah@ppukm.ukm.edu.my (A.U.)

Abstract: *Plukenetia volubilis* Linneo or Sacha Inchi (SI), a traditional natural remedy indigenous to Peru and Brazil, has garnered global attention due to its exceptional nutritional composition. Its protective effects against various non-communicable diseases, notably cardiovascular disease (CVD), have become a subject of interest in recent research. This comprehensive review summarizes the existing evidence from 15 relevant articles concerning the impact of SI on common CVD risk factors, including dyslipidemia, obesity, diabetes, and hypertension. The relevant articles were derived from comprehensive searches on PubMed, Scopus, Google Scholar, and Web of Science using predefined criteria and keywords related to the topic. Overall, SI demonstrated positive effects in attenuating dyslipidemia, obesity, diabetes, and hypertension. The multifaceted mechanisms responsible for the protective effects of SI against these CVD risk factors are primarily attributed to its antioxidative and anti-inflammatory properties. While preclinical studies dominate the current scientific literature on SI, there are limited clinical trials to corroborate these findings. Therefore, future well-designed, large-scale randomized clinical trials are highly recommended to establish the efficacy of SI and determine its optimal dosage, potential drug and food interactions, and practical integration into preventive strategies and dietary interventions for the high-risk populations.

Keywords: antioxidant; cholesterol; diabetes; inflammation; obesity; *Plukenetia volubilis* Linneo; sacha inchi

1. Introduction

1.1. *Plukenetia volubilis Linneo*

Plukenetia volubilis Linneo, also known as sacha inchi (SI), Inca inchi, mountain peanut, and Inca nut is a perennial plant belonging to the Europhorbiaceae family. Native to the Peruvian and Northwestern Brazil jungle [1], the Europhorbiaceae family comprises 300 genera and 7500 species [2]. SI naturally thrives in the rainforests of the Americas, specifically at altitudes ranging from 200 to 1500 m [3]. However, it is now commercially cultivated in Asian countries such as Thailand, China, and Vietnam, as well as in Central and South America, because of its exceptional nutritional values [4]. SI has a long-standing traditional use for treating joint problems and relieving muscle pain [5], and providing skincare benefits such as moisturization, wound healing, insect bite treatment, and combating skin infections [6]. The various components of the entire SI plant, including seeds, kernels, and leaves, have significant economic potential for commercial exploitation [7].

The different parts of the SI plant contain various active compounds that contribute to its medicinal and nutritional properties. The seeds of SI are the most widely used part of the plant. They are a rich source of essential fatty acids, particularly omega-3 (ω-3) fatty acids such as α-linolenic acid (ALA). The seeds also contain omega-6 (ω-6) and omega-9 (ω-9) fatty acids [8]. In addition, they are abundant in tocopherols (α- and γ-tocopherols), flavonoids, phytosterols (stigmasterol, β-sitosterol, and campesterol), lignans, and phenyl alcohols [9]. SI oil is extracted from the seeds and is known for its exceptional nutritional profile. It is primarily composed of unsaturated fatty acids, including ω-3, ω-6, and ω-9 fatty acids. The oil is particularly high in ALA, which contributes to its ω-3 content. It also contains tocopherols, an antioxidant that helps protect the oil from oxidation [10]. SI oil has a favorable ratio of ω-3 to ω-6 fatty acids, making it a valuable addition to a healthy diet [11].

The leaves of the SI plant contain a variety of bioactive compounds, including phenolic compounds, flavonoids, and terpenoids. These compounds contribute to the antioxidative and anti-inflammatory properties of the leaves [7,12]. The leaves also contain chlorophyl, which provides a vibrant green color and has detoxifying properties [13]. Although less extensively studied, the roots of SI are shown to contain alkaloids, tannins, flavonoids, leptins, saponins, and other bioactive compounds [14]. The specific composition of the roots may vary and require further research to fully understand their nutritional and medicinal properties. Similarly, there is limited information on the SI shell composition. A small amount of lipid and a considerable amount of phenolic content in the shell has been reported [7]. The composition of SI plant parts can be influenced by factors such as growing conditions, environmental factors, and processing methods. These variations can affect the nutrient content and overall composition [15,16]. However, SI, in its various forms, offers a rich array of nutrients and bioactive compounds that contribute to its potential health benefits, including the potential to reduce risk factors associated with cardiovascular diseases (CVD).

1.2. Cardiovascular Diseases

CVD are chronic conditions affecting the heart and blood vessels, such as coronary artery disease (CAD), hypertension, stroke, and peripheral artery disease. They progress slowly and often remain asymptomatic for an extended period of time [17,18]. CVD remains the leading cause of death worldwide, accounting for 32% of global mortality in 2019, resulting in an estimated 17.9 million deaths [19]. This number is projected to rise to approximately 23 million by 2030 [20]. Furthermore, CVD has significant economic and social consequences. CVD have a negative effect on the patients' well-being, influencing their job performance and effectiveness, and resulting in significant financial setbacks, which can be interpreted as a reduction in human capital [21,22].

The economic loss due to workplace absenteeism due to chronic disease-related functional limitations among the working-age population is estimated to be approximately 4.95 billion per year [23]. According to the American Heart Association, the total expenses related to CVD in the United States in 2019 were estimated to be approximately USD 351.2 billion. This includes costs related to hospitalization, medications, procedures, and other medical expenses associated with the diagnosis and treatment of CVD [24]. While recent studies indicate a significant decrease in the prevalence of CVD in developed countries due to major advancements in CVD prevention and treatment [25], there has been an increasing trend of CVD in developing nations [26]. This rise can be attributed to the higher prevalence of CVD risk factors such as diabetes, hypertension, hypercholesterolemia, overweight/obesity, and smoking, which contribute to the development of atherosclerosis, CAD, and stroke [27,28].

1.3. The Role of Oxidative Stress and Inflammation in CVD

There is a significant body of evidence linking CVD and its risk factors to oxidative stress and inflammation [29]. Oxidative stress refers to an imbalance between the production of reactive oxygen species (ROS) and the body's ability to neutralize them, leading to cellular damage. Inflammation, on the other hand, is the body's immune response to harmful stimuli, such as infection or injury. A wide array of evidence strongly supports the pivotal role of oxidative stress and inflammation in the pathogenesis of CVD by contributing to vascular endothelial dysfunction [30].

Oxidative stress and inflammation are the primary catalysts for vascular endothelial dysfunction. The development of endothelial dysfunction is characterized by a reduction in the synthesis and/or bioavailability of nitric oxide (NO) [31]. This impairment can be attributed to several oxidative enzyme systems, including NADPH oxidase, xanthine oxidase, uncoupled endothelial nitric oxide synthase (eNOS), cyclooxygenases, lipoxygenases, and myeloperoxidases, which produce superoxide anion and contribute to vascular oxidative stress. This, in turn, leads to the deactivation of NO and subsequent endothelial dysfunction [32,33].

Numerous traditional risk factors for CVD, such as smoking, hypercholesterolemia, hypertension, obesity, and diabetes, are closely associated with endothelial dysfunction. These risk factors foster chronic inflammation, resulting in an increase in vasoconstrictive and prothrombotic substances, a decrease in antithrombotic factors, and abnormal vasoreactivity, collectively increasing the risk of cardiovascular events [34]. Elevated levels of pro-inflammatory cytokines like tumor necrosis factor-alpha (TNF-α), interleukin-1beta (IL-1β), interleukin-6 (IL-6), and interferon gamma (IFN-γ) have been detected in vascular endothelial dysfunction, primarily due to the activation of the nuclear factor-kappa B (NF-κB) pathway [35]. NF-κB serves as a crucial transcription factor that promotes CVD by stimulating the transcription of pro-inflammatory, pro-adhesion, and pro-oxidant genes. The NF-κB pathway is activated by various stimuli, including inflammatory cytokines, ROS, lipids, and mechanical forces acting on the vascular endothelium [36].

Moreover, endothelial dysfunction serves as a precursor to atherosclerosis, which is a primary underlying cause of CVD. The mechanisms contributing to atherosclerosis include the activation of pro-inflammatory signaling pathways, cytokine expression, and increased oxidative stress [37,38]. Risk factors for CVD, such as dyslipidemia, hypertension, and diabetes, synergistically induce endothelial dysfunction, leading to endothelial inflammation, macrophage differentiation, foam cell formation, platelet adhesion, and thrombus formation in the atheroma. These processes result in arterial narrowing and an increased risk of heart attack and stroke [39].

Thus, oxidative stress, inflammation, and vascular endothelial dysfunction are interconnected and have significant implications in the development and progression of CVD. In the context of CVD, persistent inflammation creates a vicious cycle that drives the progression of CVD-related complications [40]. Hence, targeting oxidative stress and inflammatory pathways may provide opportunities for interventions aimed at reducing CVD burden and improving cardiovascular health.

1.4. The Potential of SI for Cardiovascular Health

Recently, the utilization of natural products for the management and prevention of CVD has gained significant attention. Natural products derived from plants and other natural sources possess various bioactive compounds with antioxidative and anti-inflammatory effects that have the potential to promote cardiovascular health [41]. Several recent reviews have explored the nutritional compositions, physicochemical characteristics, extraction techniques, biological activities, and potential uses of SI for human health [7,14,15,42]. Although there have been initial studies and reviews concentrating on the health benefits of SI, there is currently a lack of a comprehensive review that emphasizes the potential of SI in reducing risk factors for CVD. Furthermore, as new research continues to emerge, there is a pressing need for an updated synthesis of findings related to SI and its benefits in the context of CVD.

Given the global burden of CVD and the increasing interest in plant-based preventive and therapeutic solutions, comprehending the potential of SI could open the door to innovative dietary recommendations and potential therapeutic treatments. In the following sections, we explored the potentials of SI in addressing prevalent modifiable risk factors of

CVD, with a particular focus on its effects on dyslipidemia, obesity, diabetes, and hypertension. Considering the multifaceted and interconnected nature of these four common risk factors, addressing them has the potential to lead to substantial reductions in overall CVD risk [43]. Each section provides a comprehensive analysis, supported by the latest scientific evidence, and offers an in-depth perspective on the contribution of SI in mitigating risk factors associated with CVD.

2. Literature Search

The relevant literature on this topic was searched across four primary electronic databases, namely PubMed, Scopus, Google Scholar, and Web of Science, from 2010 to 2023 using the search string '*Plukenetia volubilis* Linneo, Sacha Inchi' AND (antioxidant OR inflammation OR cholesterol OR obesity OR diabetes OR hypertension). Only original research articles aimed at elucidating the effects of SI on CVD risk factors, including hypertension, dyslipidemia, obesity, and diabetes in preclinical and clinical settings were included. The literature search yielded 15 relevant articles. In presenting the extracted data, the information was systematically organized into sections detailing the experimental model used, the preparation and dosage of SI, the outcomes, and the potential mechanisms of action. This structured approach ensured comprehensive coverage and clear characterization of the topic area.

3. Effects of SI on CVD Risk Factors

3.1. *Effects of SI on Dyslipidemia*

Within the spectrum of CVD risk factors, dyslipidemia has been identified as the most potent contributor [44]. Elevated serum levels of total cholesterol (TC), LDLc, and triglycerides (TG), or a decrease in serum high-density lipoprotein cholesterol (HDLc) levels are well-established risk factors for CVD [45]. The beneficial effects of SI on cholesterol levels have been confirmed in animal and clinical studies. Obese rats fed 2.5 mL of SI emulsion oil with different ω-3 content (0.2 g and 0.5 g ω-3/day) for eight weeks showed decreases in TC, TG, and LDLc levels, and increases in HDLc levels [46]. The treatment of patients with hypercholesterolemia with 5 or 10 mL of SI oil (contains 2 g and 4 g ω-3/day, respectively) for 16 weeks also caused a significant reduction in their total cholesterol and LDLc and increment in their HDLc levels [47].

SI oil is also helpful in preventing dyslipidemia in healthy individuals. Consumption of 10 or 15 mL of SI oil by healthy individuals for 16 weeks was found to significantly reduce their serum TC and LDLc levels and increase their HDLc levels [48]. In a randomized crossover clinical trial, the consumption of 15 mL SI oil alongside a high-fat meal reduced the postprandial increase in TC levels and the inflammatory marker interleukin- 6 (IL-6) in metabolically healthy men. However, no significant differences were observed in their HDLc and TG levels, which is most likely due to the short duration of the intervention [49]. In contrast, SI oil intake with a high-fat meal reduced the postprandial increase in IL-6 but failed to reverse the postprandial cholesterol increase in metabolically unhealthy men. This shows that the effect of SI on postprandial lipid levels following a high-fat meal depends on the individual's metabolic status [49].

SI exerts antihyperlipidemic activity in vitro, mainly via enzymatic inhibitory reaction [50]. The 3-hydroxy-3-methylglutaryl-coenzyme A (HMG-CoA) reductase is a rate-controlling enzyme in the mevalonate pathway of cholesterol biosynthesis. HMG-CoA reductase inhibitors, such as statins, have long been used to efficiently treat hypercholesterolemia. However, its multisystemic adverse effects necessitate the discovery of plant-based HMG-CoA reductase inhibitors with minimal side effects [51,52]. An in vitro study showed that 125 μg/mL of SI nutshell hot water extract inhibited HMG-CoA reductase activity by 65% [53]. Contrary to the mechanism of action of statins, SI nutshell extract exhibits a precise and effective non-competitive inhibition pattern [53,54]. In addition, there was a 38.1% reduction in cholesterol esterase activity using a similar SI extract concentration [53]. The inhibition of cholesterol esterase activity interferes with cholesterol absorption and transport into enterocytes, which contributes to the lipid-lowering effect of SI [55]. However, SI baby nut and leaf hot water extracts and SI nut oil did not show any HMG-CoA reductase or cholesterol esterase inhibitory effects [53].

Recent studies have identified a close relationship between the gut microbiome and dyslipidemia [56,57]. High dietary fat induces dysbiosis of the gut microbiota, resulting in lipid dysmetabolism [58]. SI oil consumption reversed gut microbiota dysbiosis in high-fat diet (HFD)-fed rats, thus improving their TC, TG, and LDLc levels [59]. One of the mechanisms is through the influence of the gut microbiota metabolome on bile acid composition. Bile acids regulate hepatic lipid metabolism by facilitating lipid absorption [60,61]. HFD altered gut microbiota metabolome and bile acid composition in the small intestine, leading to elevated levels of taurocholic acid (TCA), taurochenodeoxycholic acid (TCDCA), cholic acid, and glycocholic acid, which contribute to lipid dysmetabolism and hyperlipidemia. Supplementation with 0.5–1.5 mL/kg SI oil for eight weeks reversed the changes in gut microbiota metabolome and bile acid composition, and improved lipid dysmetabolism in HFD-fed rats [59]. Table 1 and Figure 1 summarize the current knowledge on the protective effects of SI on lipid metabolism and dyslipidemia.

Table 1. Effects of SI on lipid metabolism and dyslipidemia.

SI Preparation	Dose	Experimental Model	Outcomes	Reference
SI oil	5 or 10 mL for 16 weeks	Healthy adults	↓ TC and LDLc ↑ HDLc	[48]
SI oil	15 mL	Metabolically healthy and unhealthy men given high-fat meal	↓ postprandial TC and IL-6 in metabolically healthy men ↓ postprandial IL-6 in metabolically unhealthy men	[49]
SI oil	5 or 10 mL (contains 2 g or 4 g ω-3/day) for 16 weeks	Hypercholesterolemic patients	↓ TC and LDLc ↑ HDLc	[47]
SI emulsion oil	2.5 mL (contains 0.2 g or 0.5 g ω-3/day) for 8 weeks	Obese rats	↓ TC, TG, and LDLc ↑ HDLc	[46]
SI oil	0.5–1.5 mL/kg for 8 weeks	Obese rats	↓ TC, TG, and LDLc Reverse gut microbiota dysbiosis and metabolome Improve bile acid compositions	[59]
SI nutshell, baby nut and leaf hot water extracts SI nut oil	125 μg/mL	In vitro enzyme inhibitory assays	Only SI nutshell hot water extract ↓ HMG-CoA reductase and cholesterol esterase activities	[53]

Abbreviations: ↑, increase; ↓, decrease; HDLc, high-density lipoprotein cholesterol; HMG-CoA, 3-hydroxy-3-methylglutaryl-coenzyme; IL-6, interleukin-6; LDLc, low-density lipoprotein cholesterol; TC, total cholesterol.

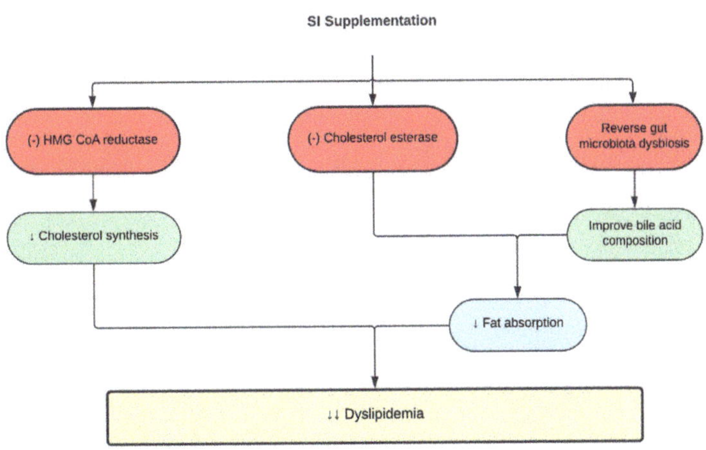

Figure 1. Protective effects of SI on dyslipidemia. (-), inhibit; ↓, decrease; HMG-CoA, 3-hydroxy-3-methylglutaryl-coenzyme A.

3.2. Effects of SI on Obesity

CVD is associated with obesity and high visceral fat deposition [62]. SI exerts anti-obesity effects in vivo. High-fat diet (HFD)-fed Sprague Dawley rats supplemented with 0.5–1.5 mL/kg SI oil for eight weeks showed significant reduction in their adipocyte size, hepatic steatosis, and inflammation. This is associated with increased hepatic lipase expression following SI oil supplementation [59]. Hepatic lipase is an essential lipolytic enzyme that facilitates lipoprotein uptake in the de novo lipid synthesis pathway [63]. Furthermore, SI oil suppressed the production of *lysophosphatidylcholine* (LysoPC) and lysophosphatidylethanolamine (LysoPE) [59], which have been identified as pro-inflammatory phospholipids found in patients with hyperlipidemia and HFD-induced obesity [64]. In addition, SI oil decreased the expression of hepatic phosphatidylglycerol phosphate synthase 1 (PGS1) in HFD-fed rats [59]. PGS1 catalyzes the production of phosphatidylglycerol, which is a potent inhibitor of lipolysis [65]. Therefore, the inhibition of PGS1 by SI oil reduced phosphatidylglycerol production and improved lipolysis [59].

Pancreatic lipase has been identified as a key enzyme in systemic lipid digestion and absorption [66]. Its inhibition has gained significant interest as an efficient method to reduce obesity [67]. Interestingly, SI meal-derived peptides, a by-product generated from SI oil, exhibited strong pancreatic lipase inhibitory activity, hypothetically by competitive binding to the pancreatic lipase catalytic sites [68]. Pancreatic lipase inhibitory peptides were previously demonstrated to reduce the amount of intracellular fat accumulations by neutralizing ROS production in oleic acid-induced HepG2 cells [68]. Meanwhile, the SI protein isolate showed high antioxidative activity, which might contribute to its pancreatic lipase inhibitory effect [69]. A similar lipase inhibition pattern was also observed with SI husk aqueous ethanol extract [70]. The lipase inhibitory effect of SI may be attributed to the synergistic actions of its various phenolic and active peptide compounds [70].

Obesity leads to complications such as dyslipidemia and CVD through mechanisms involving oxidative stress, low-grade inflammation, and cellular hypoxia [71]. Oxidative stress promotes lipid and protein oxidation [72], as evidenced by the production of the end-products; malondialdehyde (MDA) and advanced protein oxidation products (AOPP) [73–75]. Treatment of obese rats with the emulsion of SI oil (2.5 mL, contains 0.25 g and 0.5 g ω-3/day) reduced MDA and AOPP levels in the rat serum [46]. SI oil emulsion also enhanced antioxidant capacity by stimulating the activity of the antioxidant enzyme catalase [46,76]. Furthermore, SI oil emulsion attenuated inflammation in obese rats, as evidenced by reduced levels of the proinflammatory cytokines IL-6 and tumor necrosis factor-α (TNF-α) [46]. Collectively, the findings showed that the antioxidative and anti-inflammatory activities of SI contribute to its anti-obesity effect.

The pro-inflammatory state in obesity is associated with changes in adipokine release by adipose tissues, such as leptin and adiponectin [77,78]. Leptin regulates body fat composition by augmenting energy expenditure and inhibiting appetite [79]. However, leptin resistance and hyperleptinemia in obesity promote hunger, increase food consumption, and induce inflammation [80]. Meanwhile, adiponectin is an anti-inflammatory adipokine, and its level is reduced in obesity [81]. Interestingly, the emulsion of SI oil reduced leptin levels and increased adiponectin levels in obese rats [46]. Increased adiponectin levels are also responsible for the hypolipidemic effect of SI, as adiponectin activates lipoprotein lipase to degrade circulating TG [82]. The positive effects of SI oil on leptin and adiponectin levels were mediated via increased expression of peroxisome proliferator-activated receptor alpha (PPAR-α), which is a crucial transcription factor that regulates fatty acid metabolism and oxidative stress [76]. Table 2 and Figure 2 summarize the current knowledge on the protective effects of SI on obesity. Exploring the impact of SI supplementation on body mass index, body fat composition, and basal metabolic rate in individuals with obesity presents an intriguing opportunity since there has been no prior research delving into this subject.

Table 2. Effects of SI on obesity.

SI Preparation	Dose	Experimental Model	Outcomes	Reference
SI oil emulsion	2.5 mL (contains 0.25 g and 0.5 g ω-3/day) for 8 weeks	Obese rats	↓ MDA and AOPP ↑ catalase activity ↓ IL-6 and TNF-α ↓ leptin ↑ adiponectin ↑ PPAR-α	[46]
SI oil	0.5–1.5 mL/kg for 8 weeks	Obese rats	↓ mean adipocyte size ↓ hepatic steatosis, hepatic lipase activity and inflammation ↓ PGS1 expression ↑ lipolysis	[59]
SI meal-derived peptides	0.1–0.5 mM	In vitro enzyme inhibitory assay Oleic acid-induced HepG2 cells	↓ pancreatic lipase activity ↓ intracellular fat accumulation and ROS levels in HepG2 cells	[68]
SI husk aqueous ethanol extract	0.4 mg/mL	In vitro enzyme inhibitory assay	↓ lipase activity	[70]

Abbreviations: ↑, increase; ↓, decrease; AOPP, advanced protein oxidation products; IL-6, interleukin-6; MDA, malondialdehyde; PPAR-α, peroxisome proliferator-activated receptor alpha; PGS1, phosphatidylglycerol phosphate synthase 1; TNF-α, tumor necrosis factor alpha.

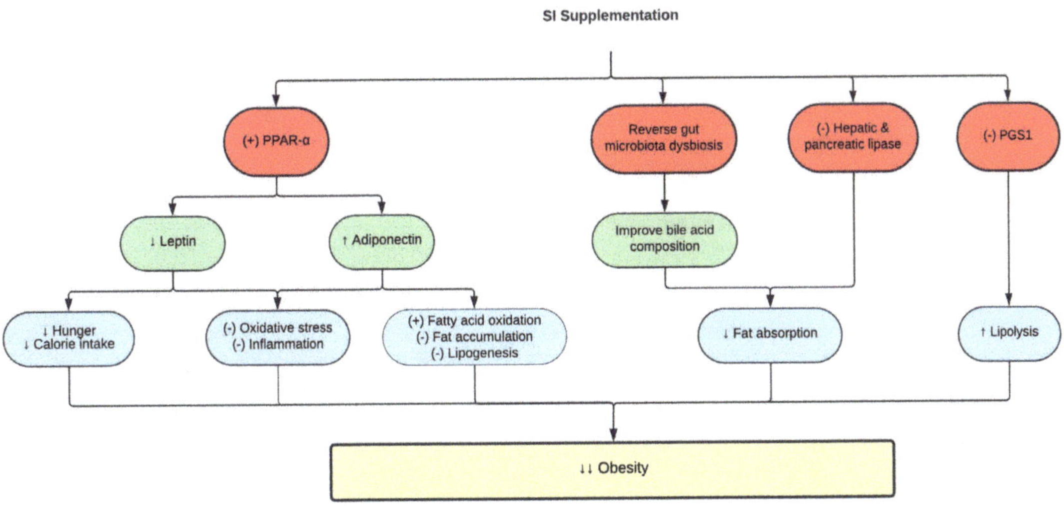

Figure 2. Protective effects of SI on obesity. (-), inhibit; (+), stimulate; ↑, increase; ↓, decrease; PGS1, phosphatidylglycerol phosphate synthase 1; PPAR-α, peroxisome proliferator-activated receptor alpha.

3.3. *Effects of SI on Glucose Metabolism and Diabetes*

Hyperglycemia is the hallmark of diabetes mellitus, which is also a risk factor for CVD [83]. The inhibition of α-glucosidase, α-amylase, and dipeptidyl peptidase (DPP-IV) is a common method used to assess the potential antidiabetic properties of natural products. α-glucosidase inhibitors block enzymes such as glucoamylase, sucrase, maltase, and isomaltase found at the brush border of the intestinal epithelium. This inhibition prevents the absorption of carbohydrates in the small intestine, reducing postprandial hyperglycemia [84]. On the other hand, α-amylase inhibitors hinder the breakdown of α-(1–4)-d-glucosidic linkages in starch, thereby decreasing carbohydrate digestion and absorption in the gastrointestinal tract and consequently lowering blood glucose levels [85]. DPP-IV inhibitors block the degradation of incretin hormones, specifically glucagon-like peptide-1 (GLP-1) and glucose-dependent insulinotropic polypeptide (GIP). Increased GLP-1 and GIP levels stimulate insulin release, inhibit glucagon secretion, and delay gastric emptying, thus improving postprandial glucose levels.

It has been reported that 0.035 mg/mL of SI husk and shell extracts exhibited strong α-glucosidase and α-amylase inhibitory activities [70]. Correspondingly, 25 μg/mL of SI essential oil exhibited robust α-amylase inhibition [86]. The potent α-glucosidase and α-amylase inhibitory effects are linked to the phenolic content in SI [87–90]. Furthermore, SI meal-derived peptides demonstrated potent DPP-IV inhibitory activity in vitro, which was further validated with increased glucose consumption by palmitic acid-induced insulin resistant HepG2 cells [91]. It is important to emphasize that α-amylase, α-glucosidase, and DPP-IV inhibitory assays serve as valuable screening tools to evaluate the antidiabetic potential of natural products. However, it is crucial to complement these results with further in vivo studies to validate their antidiabetic activity.

The most employed in vivo model for inducing diabetes in laboratory animals involves the chemical ablation of pancreatic β-cells using streptozotocin (STZ). STZ functions as a toxic glucose analog that selectively accumulates within pancreatic β-cells via the GLUT2 glucose transporters located on the plasma membrane. Once taken up by β-cells, STZ initiates oxidative stress and DNA alkylation, ultimately leading to pancreatic β-cell necrosis, reduced insulin production, and hyperglycemia [92–94]. Furthermore, it is important to note that GLUT2 transporters are not limited to pancreatic β-cells but are also found in the epithelial cells of the kidneys and hepatocytes. Therefore, the administration of STZ may lead to kidney and liver toxicity, in addition to its capacity to harm pancreatic β-cells [95]. A single, high dose of STZ injection induces pancreatic β-cell damage and diabetes in rats, mimicking type 1 diabetes [96]. A low dose of STZ injection combined with HFD to induce hyperglycemia and insulin resistance is a method to mimic type 2 diabetes in rats [97].

The treatment of type 2 diabetic rats with 0.5–2 mL/kg of SI oil for five weeks significantly reduced fasting blood glucose levels and improved insulin sensitivity indices and glucose tolerance in a dose-dependent manner [98]. Insulin plays a pivotal role in regulating glucose metabolism by activating the insulin receptor substrate (IRS)/phosphatidylinositol 3-kinase (PI3K)/protein kinase B (Akt) signaling pathway. The dysfunction of insulin receptors (IR) and subsequent impairment of downstream signaling are critical factors in the onset of insulin resistance [99]. This condition, which is characterized by the inability of cells to respond effectively to insulin, contributes to heightened hepatic gluconeogenesis and glycogenolysis. Ultimately, these processes culminate in elevated blood sugar levels, leading to hyperglycemia in individuals with diabetes [100]. SI enhances hepatic insulin sensitivity by downregulating IR-β and stimulating IRS-1 and Akt. Moreover, SI also inhibited the activities of glucose-6-phosphatase (G-6-Pase) and phosphoenolpyruvate carboxykinase-1 (PCK-1) in the liver of diabetic rats [98]. Reduced G-6-Pase and PCK-1 levels suppress hepatic gluconeogenesis and enhance glycogenesis, thereby reducing blood glucose levels [101]. The bioactive compounds present in SI, including ω-3 fatty acids, β-sitosterols, and flavonoids, contribute to its insulin sensitizing effect [98].

Extensive studies have shown the role of intestinal microflora in various stages of diabetes progression [102,103]. An intimate relationship exists between gut microbiota dysbiosis and diabetes [104–106]. Pathogenic bacteria in patients with diabetes were elevated in parallel with pro-inflammatory cytokines such as IL-6. These findings denote the involvement of gut microbiota dysbiosis and inflammation in the pathogenesis of diabetes. Interestingly, 400 mg/kg SI leaf water extract treatment for six weeks exerted prebiotic activity in type 1 diabetic rats by diversifying beneficial intestinal bacteria, primarily Akkermansia, Parabacteroides, Bacteroides, and Alloprevotella, while simultaneously suppressing diabetes-related bacteria, including Lactobacillus, Ruminococcaceae, Ruminiclostridium, and Oscillibacter [107]. The amelioration of gut microbiota dysbiosis with SI treatment led to a reduction in blood glucose levels, and improved glucose tolerance and insulin resistance in diabetic rats [107].

In a clinical trial, the addition of 15 mL SI oil to a high-fat breakfast attenuated postprandial hyperglycemia and improved insulin sensitivity in healthy individuals with higher baseline triglycerides and glycemic response. In addition, these individuals also showed increased sirtuin 1 (SIRT-1) gene expression in their peripheral blood mononuclear cells 4 h postprandially [108]. The SIRT-1 gene plays a pivotal role in glucose metabolism, and its expression is downregulated in people with obesity and insulin resistance [109,110]. Hence, SI oil improves glycemic control and insulin sensitivity by enhancing SIRT-1 expression. However, to date, there is no clinical trial involving SI supplementation in patients with diabetes.

Diabetes leads to target organ damage, and the liver is one of the target organs of diabetes complications [111]. SI oil supplementation protected the liver from diabetes-induced liver damage, as evidenced by reduced serum alanine transaminase and aspartate transaminase (AST) levels, and improved hepatic histopathological changes [98]. The underlying mechanisms of such findings were attributed to the antioxidative and anti-inflammatory effects of SI, as treatment with SI oil reduced the oxidative stress marker (MDA), enhanced the antioxidant enzyme activity (superoxide dismutase, catalase and glutathione peroxidase) and reduced the inflammatory markers (TNF-α and IL-6) in the liver of diabetic rats [98]. However, to date, no studies have investigated how SI impacts other diabetes-related target organ damage, such as those affecting the kidneys, heart, and blood vessels. A summary of the protective effects of SI on glucose metabolism and diabetes is shown in Table 3 and Figure 3.

Table 3. Effects of SI on blood glucose and diabetes.

SI Preparation	Dose	Experimental Model	Outcomes	Reference
SI oil	15 mL	Healthy adults given high-fat breakfast	↓ postprandial hyperglycemia ↑ insulin sensitivity ↑ SIRT-1 expression in healthy adults with higher baseline triglycerides and glycemic response	[108]
SI leaves water extract	400 mg/kg for 6 weeks	Type 1 diabetic rats	↓ FBS ↑ insulin sensitivity and glucose tolerance ↓ gut microbiota dysbiosis	[107]
SI oil	0.5–2 mL/kg for 5 weeks	Type 2 diabetic rats	↓ FBS ↑ insulin sensitivity indices and glucose tolerance ↑ IRS-1 and Akt ↓ IR-β ↓ G-6-Pase and PCK-1 activities ↑ hepatic glycogen content ↓ AST and ALT ↓ MDA ↑ SOD, CAT and GPX activities ↓TNF-α and IL-6	[98]
SI husk and shell aqueous ethanol extract	0.025 mg/mL	In vitro enzyme inhibitory assays	↓ α-glucosidase and α-amylase activities	[70]
SI essential oil	25 μg/mL	In vitro enzyme inhibitory assays	↓ α-amylase activity	[86]
SI meal-derived peptides	0.25–0.5 mM	In vitro enzyme inhibitory assay Palmitic acid-induced insulin resistant HepG2 cells	↓ DPP-IV activity ↑ glucose consumption by HepG2 cells	[91]

Abbreviations: ↑, increase; ↓, decrease; Akt, protein kinase B; ALT, alanine transaminase; AST, aspartate transaminase; CAT, catalase; DPP-IV, dipeptidyl peptidase IV; FBS, fasting blood sugar; G-6-Pase, glucose-6-phosphatase; GPX, glutathione peroxidase; IR-β, insulin receptor-β; IRS-1; insulin receptor substrate-1; IL-6, interleukin-6; MDA, malondialdehyde; PCK-1, phosphoenolpyruvate carboxykinase-1; SIRT-1, sirtuin-1; SOD, superoxide dismutase; TNF-α, tumor necrosis factor alpha.

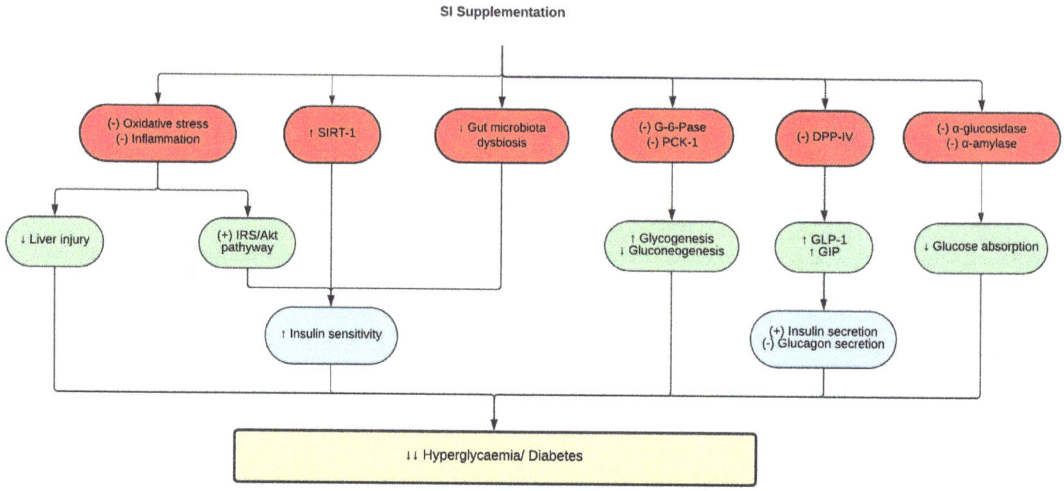

Figure 3. Protective effects of SI on glucose metabolism and diabetes. (-), inhibit; (+), stimulate; ↑, increase; ↓, decrease; Akt, protein kinase B; DPP-IV, dipeptidyl peptidase IV; G-6-Pase, glucose-6-phosphatase; GIP, glucose-dependent insulinotropic polypeptide; GLP-1, glucagon-like peptide-1; IRS, insulin receptor substrate; PCK-1, phosphoenolpyruvate carboxykinase-1; SIRT-1, sirtuin-1.

3.4. Effects of SI on Blood Pressure

Extensive evidence has consistently established a linear relationship between elevated blood pressure and the risk of CVD [112]. To date, few studies have been conducted to study the blood pressure-lowering effect of SI. Only one clinical trial was conducted to determine the effect of SI on blood pressure in human subjects. Gonzales et al. [48] revealed that clinically healthy adults who consumed 10 and 15 mL of SI oil for four months had reduced systolic and diastolic blood pressure. The reduction in blood pressure was suggested to be due to the LDL-lowering effect of SI oil. Increased LDL levels have been linked to the pathophysiology of hypertension [113–116]. However, there is no clinical trial involving SI supplementation in patients with hypertension.

The renin angiotensin aldosterone system regulates blood pressure and body fluid homeostasis. Overactivation of this system is implicated in the pathogenesis of hypertension; hence, angiotensin-converting enzyme (ACE) inhibitors are commonly prescribed to treat hypertension [117]. In vitro evaluation using 0.013 mg/mL SI husk and shell extracts demonstrated ACE inhibitory activities [70]. Similarly, SI protein hydrolysates showed strong ACE inhibitory activity at a concentration of 98 μg/mL [118]. This ACE inhibitory effect is correlated with the high phenolic content in SI, especially in the shell [70,119].

Individuals with hypertension may have faulty renal handling of calcium, particularly due to upregulation of the calcium signaling pathway. This leads to increased expression of L-type calcium channels (LTCC) that allow a massive calcium ion influx into the vascular smooth muscle cells, causing vasoconstriction and increasing the blood pressure. In addition, sodium retention and plasma volume expansion have been identified as precursor of hypertension [120]. The Na^+/K^+-ATPase pump is essential for maintaining the electrochemical gradient of sodium across the cell membrane. In hypertension, the expression of Na^+/K^+-ATPase is decreased, which contributes to sodium retention and plasma volume expansion [121]. SI shell extract (SISE) exerts its antihypertensive effect in spontaneous hypertensive rats (SHR) and high-salt-diet-fed Wistar-Kyoto (WKY) rats by restoring the expression of LTCC and Na^+/K^+-ATPase, thus maintaining calcium and sodium homeostasis [122].

Oxidative stress and chronic inflammation are involved in the pathogenesis of hypertension [123]. NO produced by eNOS is an important vasoactive molecule that modulates vascular functions and blood pressure. Continuous release of superoxide exceeding the endogenous antioxidant capacity reduces NO bioavailability [124–126]. Reduced NO levels lead to endothelial dysfunction, impaired vasodilation, and elevated blood pressure [127]. SISE decreased the blood pressure of SHR and WKY rats fed a high-salt diet by reducing oxidative stress and inflammation, and increasing the expression of eNOS and NO. Concurrently, the level of 5-methyltetrahydrofolate (5-MTHF), an active form of di- and tetrahydrofolic acid, was found to be increased with SISE treatment [122]. 5-MTHF maintains NO bioavailability by suppressing superoxide production [128].

Multiple studies have linked abnormal gut microbiota to the pathogenesis of hypertension [129,130]. Gut microbiome dysbiosis or imbalance of Firmicutes/Bacteroidetes (F/B) ratio is often correlated with various pathological conditions, including hypertension [131,132]. The gut microbiota of patients and animals with hypertension also showed reduced levels of beneficial bacteria such as Roseburia, and increased levels of harmful bacteria such as Prevotella [133]. One of the mechanisms underlying the antihypertensive effect of SISE is through reshaping of the gut microbiota and metabolome, in which SISE improved the prevalence of Roseburia and dihydrofolic acid levels in the gut and normalized the F/B ratio [122]. A summary of the effects of SI on blood pressure and hypertension is shown in Table 4 and Figure 4.

Table 4. Effects of SI on blood pressure and hypertension.

SI Preparation	Dose	Experimental Model	Outcomes	Reference
SI oil	10 or 15 mL for 4 months	Healthy adults	↓ SBP and DBP ↓ LDLc	[48]
SI shell extract	400 mg/kg for 51 days	SHR and WKY rats on high-salt diet	↓ SBP ↓ LTCC expression ↑ Na+/K+-ATPase expression Restored calcium and sodium homeostasis ↓ MDA ↑ SOD and GSH ↑ eNOS expression ↑ NO ↑ 5-MTHF Reshaped gut microbiota and metabolome, ↑ prevalence of Roseburia and dihydrofolic acid Normalized F/B ratio	[122]
SI protein hydrolysates	98 μg/mL	In vitro enzyme inhibitory assay	↓ ACE activity	[118]
SI husk and shell aqueous ethanol extract	0.013 mg/mL	In vitro enzyme inhibitory assay	↓ ACE activity	[70]

Abbreviations: ↑, increase; ↓, decrease; 5-MTHF, 5-methyltetrahydrofolate; ACE, angiotensin-converting enzyme; DBP, diastolic blood pressure; eNOS, endothelial nitric oxide synthase; F/B, Firmicutes/Bacteroidetes; GSH, glutathione; LDLc, low-density lipoprotein cholesterol; LTCC, L-type calcium channels; MDA, malondialdehyde; NO, nitric oxide; SBP, systolic blood pressure; SOD, superoxide dismutase.

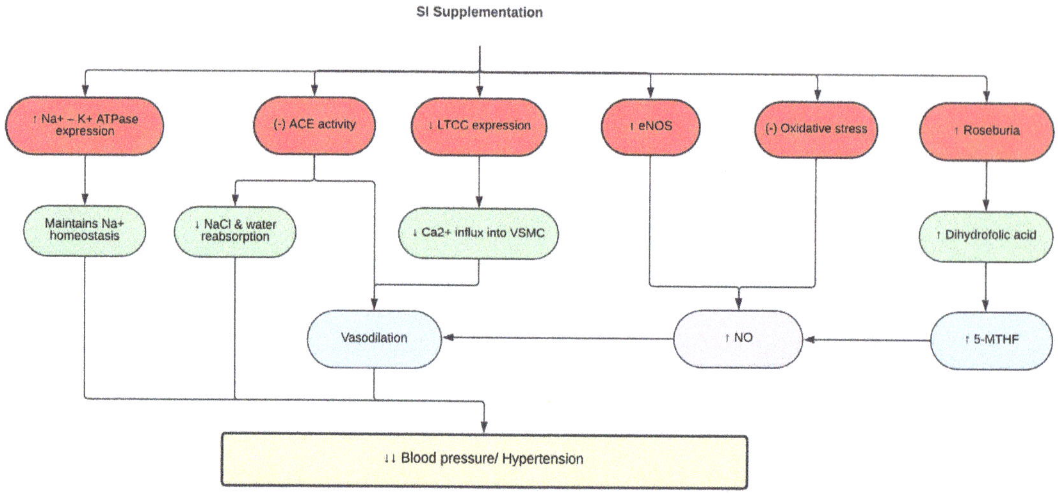

Figure 4. Protective effects of SI on blood pressure. (-), inhibit; ↑, increase; ↓, decrease; 5-MTHF, 5-methyltetrahydrofolate; ACE, angiotensin-converting enzyme; Ca^{2+}, calcium ions; eNOS, endothelial nitric oxide synthase; K^+, potassium ions; LTCC, L-type calcium channels; Na^+, sodium ions; NaCl, sodium chloride; NO, nitric oxide; VSMC, vascular smooth muscle cells.

4. Safety of SI

Food plants that are frequently consumed by humans often contain significant secondary metabolites, which can be harmful if consumed in excess [134]. While not always harmful, specific antinutritional components can lead to adverse effects by interfering with the digestion and absorption of essential macro- and micronutrients [135]. A study reported that raw SI seed consumption induced mild to severe toxicity in humans, which was attributed to the phytotoxin content, namely alkaloids, lectins, and saponins, in raw SI seeds [14]. Srichamnong et al. discovered a very mild toxic effect of fresh SI seeds on hepatic stellate cells [136]. Phytotoxins are relatively unstable under heat [136]; therefore, roasting the raw parts of the SI plant before consumption is essential to avoid any potential health risks.

Conversely, no morbidity or mortality was observed in acute (2000 mg/kg) and subchronic (50, 250, and 500 mg/kg for 90 days) toxicity studies and genotoxicity evaluation of rats and mice fed with SI seed powder [137]. Similarly, another oral toxicity study in rats and mice demonstrated that the consumption of 0.5 mL/kg of SI oil for 60 days was harmless, and the median lethal dose of 50 (LD50) was estimated to be more than 37 g/kg body weight [138]. Meanwhile, the consumption of 10 and 15 mL of SI oil for 16 weeks by healthy human subjects did not alter their hepatic and kidney functions, inflammatory biomarkers, and hemoglobin levels [48].

Despite its good safety profile, there was a rare, isolated case of occupational allergic rhinoconjunctivitis and bronchial asthma related to exposure to SI seeds [139]. Even though there were no more related cases documented, further investigation on SI allergenicity is warranted. Nausea is the most common side effect associated with SI oil consumption, which is most likely due to its unpleasant taste [48]. It is advisable to consume SI oil with food or salad for better taste. Moreover, other complaints related to gastrointestinal discomfort [48] have been reported, consistent with the previously documented minor side effects of fish oil containing ω-3 fatty acids [140]. Based on the available information, the adverse events reported by the subjects were not major and were unlikely to have a significant impact on their overall health. However, further studies are necessary to understand any potential chronic toxicity effects of SI. Furthermore, conducting a study to explore the potential combination of SI with other medications to mitigate its toxic or synergistic effects is a valuable endeavor. These discoveries would also be beneficial in considering SI as a viable dietary supplement.

5. Strength, Limitations, and Future Directions

This comprehensive review provides a holistic and multifaceted understanding of SI and its therapeutic potential in addressing major CVD risk factors including dyslipidemia, obesity, diabetes, and hypertension. However, a limitation of this review is the scarcity of large-scale clinical trials on SI. Most of the findings are based on preclinical research or small-scale clinical trials. While these provide valuable insights, they may not always be directly applicable to broader, more diverse populations. Therefore, large-scale randomized clinical trials are imperative to establish the efficacy and safety of SI in mitigating CVD risk factors. Moreover, the potential for chronic toxicity of SI deserves thorough exploration. As with many natural products, prolonged SI usage may have adverse effects that remain to be fully understood. Chronic toxicity studies will not only ensure the safety of SI for long-term consumption, but also provide insights into its optimal dosage and usage patterns.

Additionally, considering the complex treatment regimen that patients with CVD frequently adhere to, understanding how SI interacts with other medications is vital. Uncovering any synergistic or antagonistic effects it may have when combined with other drugs can have significant clinical implications. This knowledge would assist healthcare professionals in prescribing SI, ensuring its seamless integration with existing treatment plans while preventing unfavorable interactions. Furthermore, mechanistic studies will aid in unraveling the underlying molecular pathways responsible for the cardiovascular benefits of SI. Investigations into optimal dosages, potential interactions with drugs and food, and applications in clinical settings will pave the way for the practical integration of SI into preventive strategies and dietary interventions for the high-risk population.

6. Conclusions

This review emphasizes the significant potential of SI as a natural remedy for mitigating CVD risk factors. The presence of beneficial fatty acids, antioxidants, and anti-inflammatory compounds in SI underscores its capacity to positively impact lipid profiles, blood glucose levels, adipogenesis, and blood pressure regulation. These encouraging effects position SI as a viable dietary supplement and complementary therapy in the battle against CVD. However, most of the data are obtained from preclinical studies. Consequently, it is highly recommended that large-scale randomized clinical trials be conducted in the future to establish the efficacy of SI.

Author Contributions: Conceptualization, A.U., A.A.H. and A.A.; data curation, I.Z.A.R. and N.S.N.H.; writing—original draft preparation, I.Z.A.R. and N.S.N.H.; writing—review and editing, A.U., A.A.H., J.K. and A.A.; supervision, A.U.; project administration, A.U., A.A.H. and A.A.; funding acquisition, A.U. All authors have read and agreed to the published version of the manuscript.

Funding: This research was funded by Geran Universiti Penyelidikan, Universiti Kebangsaan Malaysia (GUP-2022-041).

Institutional Review Board Statement: Not applicable.

Informed Consent Statement: Not applicable.

Data Availability Statement: Data sharing is not applicable.

Conflicts of Interest: The authors declare no conflict of interest.

References

1. del-Castillo, Á.M.R.; Gonzalez-Aspajo, G.; de Fátima Sánchez-Márquez, M.; Kodahl, N. Ethnobotanical Knowledge in the Peruvian Amazon of the Neglected and Underutilized Crop Sacha Inchi (*Plukenetia volubilis* L.). *Econ. Bot.* **2019**, *73*, 281–287. [CrossRef]
2. Silalahi, M. Sacha Inchi (*Plukenetia volubilis* L.): Its Potential as Foodstuff and Traditional Medicine. *GSC Biol. Pharm. Sci.* **2022**, *18*, 213–218. [CrossRef]

3. Flores, S.; Flores, A.; Calderón, C.; Obregón, D. Synthesis and Characterization of Sacha Inchi (*Plukenetia volubilis* L.) Oil-Based Alkyd Resin. *Prog. Org. Coat.* **2019**, *136*, 105289. [CrossRef]
4. Gutiérrez, L.-F.; Quiñones-Segura, Y.; Sanchez-Reinoso, Z.; Díaz, D.L.; Abril, J.I. Physicochemical Properties of Oils Extracted from γ-Irradiated Sacha Inchi (*Plukenetia volubilis* L.) Seeds. *Food Chem.* **2017**, *237*, 581–587. [CrossRef] [PubMed]
5. Fanali, C.; Dugo, L.; Cacciola, F.; Beccaria, M.; Grasso, S.; Dachà, M.; Dugo, P.; Mondello, L. Chemical Characterization of Sacha Inchi (*Plukenetia volubilis* L.) Oil. *J. Agric. Food Chem.* **2011**, *59*, 13043–13049. [CrossRef] [PubMed]
6. Hanssen, H.P.; Schmitz-Hübsch, M. Sacha Inchi (*Plukenetia volubilis* L.) Nut Oil and Its Therapeutic and Nutritional Uses. In *Nuts and Seeds in Health and Disease Prevention*; Elsevier: Amsterdam, The Netherlands, 2011; pp. 991–994. ISBN 9780123756886.
7. Wang, S.; Zhu, F.; Kakuda, Y. Sacha Inchi (*Plukenetia volubilis* L.): Nutritional Composition, Biological Activity, and Uses. *Food Chem.* **2018**, *265*, 316–328. [CrossRef] [PubMed]
8. Goyal, A.; Tanwar, B.; Kumar Sihag, M.; Sharma, V. Sacha Inchi (*Plukenetia volubilis* L.): An Emerging Source of Nutrients, Omega-3 Fatty Acid and Phytochemicals. *Food Chem.* **2022**, *373*, 131459. [CrossRef]
9. Ramos-Escudero, F.; Muñoz, A.M.; Ramos Escudero, M.; Viñas-Ospino, A.; Morales, M.T.; Asuero, A.G. Characterization of Commercial Sacha Inchi Oil According to Its Composition: Tocopherols, Fatty Acids, Sterols, Triterpene and Aliphatic Alcohols. *J. Food Sci. Technol.* **2019**, *56*, 4503–4515. [CrossRef]
10. Mai, H.C.; Nguyen, D.C.; Thuong Nhan, N.P.; Bach, L.G. Physico-Chemical Properties of Sacha Inchi (*Plukenetia volubilis* L.) Seed Oil from Vietnam. *Asian J. Chem.* **2020**, *32*, 335–338. [CrossRef]
11. Simopoulos, A.P. The Importance of the Omega-6/Omega-3 Fatty Acid Ratio in Cardiovascular Disease and Other Chronic Diseases. *Exp. Biol. Med.* **2008**, *233*, 674–688. [CrossRef]
12. Nascimento, A.K.L.; Melo-Silveira, R.F.; Dantas-Santos, N.; Fernandes, J.M.; Zucolotto, S.M.; Rocha, H.A.O.; Scortecci, K.C. Antioxidant and Antiproliferative Activities of Leaf Extracts from *Plukenetia volubilis* Linneo (Euphorbiaceae). *Evid.-Based Complement. Altern. Med.* **2013**, *2013*, 950272. [CrossRef]
13. Mishra, V.K.; Kumar Bachheti, R.; Husen, A.; Mishra, V.K.; Bacheti, R.K. Medicinal Uses of Chlorophyll: A Critical Overview. In *Chlorophyll: Structure, Function and Medicinal Uses*; Nova Science Publishers, Inc.: Hauppauge, NY, USA, 2011; pp. 177–196.
14. Torres Sánchez, E.G.; Hernández-Ledesma, B.; Gutiérrez, L.-F. Sacha Inchi Oil Press-Cake: Physicochemical Characteristics, Food-Related Applications and Biological Activity. *Food Rev. Int.* **2023**, *39*, 148–159. [CrossRef]
15. Cárdenas, D.M.; Rave, L.J.G.; Soto, J.A. Biological Activity of Sacha Inchi (*Plukenetia volubilis* Linneo) and Potential Uses in Human Health: A Review. *Food Technol. Biotechnol.* **2021**, *59*, 253–266. [CrossRef]
16. Kittibunchakul, S.; Hudthagosol, C.; Sanporkha, P.; Sapwarobol, S.; Suttisansanee, U.; Sahasakul, Y. Effects of Maturity and Thermal Treatment on Phenolic Profiles and In Vitro Health-Related Properties of Sacha Inchi Leaves. *Plants* **2022**, *11*, 1515. [CrossRef]
17. Pagidipati, N.J.; Gaziano, T.A. Estimating Deaths from Cardiovascular Disease: A Review of Global Methodologies of Mortality Measurement. *Circulation* **2013**, *127*, 749–756. [CrossRef] [PubMed]
18. Francula-Zaninovic, S.; Nola, I.A. Management of Measurable Variable Cardiovascular Disease' Risk Factors. *Curr. Cardiol. Rev.* **2018**, *14*, 153–163. [CrossRef] [PubMed]
19. Roth, G.A.; Mensah, G.A.; Johnson, C.O.; Addolorato, G.; Ammirati, E.; Baddour, L.M.; Barengo, N.C.; Beaton, A.Z.; Benjamin, E.J.; Benziger, C.P.; et al. Global Burden of Cardiovascular Diseases and Risk Factors, 1990–2019. *J. Am. Coll. Cardiol.* **2020**, *76*, 2982–3021. [CrossRef] [PubMed]
20. Virani, S.S.; Alonso, A.; Benjamin, E.J.; Bittencourt, M.S.; Callaway, C.W.; Carson, A.P.; Chamberlain, A.M.; Chang, A.R.; Cheng, S.; Delling, F.N.; et al. Heart Disease and Stroke Statistics—2020 Update: A Report From the American Heart Association. *Circulation* **2020**, *141*, e139–e596. [CrossRef]
21. Ekinci, G. Economic Impacts of Cardiovascular Diseases: An Econometric Evaluation in Turkey. *Iran J. Public Health* **2023**, *52*, 118. [CrossRef] [PubMed]
22. Gulyamova, S.T.; Abdul Aziz, S.F.; Omar, N.H.; Mohd, R.H. Workplace-Related Socioeconomic Issues Associated with Job Performance and Productivity among Employees with Various Impairments: A Systematic Literature Review. *Soc. Sci.* **2023**, *12*, 275. [CrossRef]
23. Vuong, T.D.; Wei, F.; Beverly, C.J. Absenteeism Due to Functional Limitations Caused by Seven Common Chronic Diseases in US Workers. *J. Occup. Environ. Med.* **2015**, *57*, 779–784. [CrossRef] [PubMed]
24. Benjamin, E.J.; Muntner, P.; Alonso, A.; Bittencourt, M.S.; Callaway, C.W.; Carson, A.P.; Chamberlain, A.M.; Chang, A.R.; Cheng, S.; Das, S.R.; et al. Heart Disease and Stroke Statistics—2019 Update: A Report From the American Heart Association. *Circulation* **2019**, *139*, e56–e528. [CrossRef]
25. Karam, C.; Beauchet, A.; Czernichow, S.; de Roquefeuil, F.; Bourez, A.; Mansencal, N.; Dubourg, O. Trends in Cardiovascular Disease Risk Factor Prevalence and Estimated 10-Year Cardiovascular Risk Scores in a Large Untreated French Urban Population: The CARVAR 92 Study. *PLoS ONE* **2015**, *10*, e0124817. [CrossRef]
26. Celermajer, D.S.; Chow, C.K.; Marijon, E.; Anstey, N.M.; Woo, K.S. Cardiovascular Disease in the Developing World. *J. Am. Coll. Cardiol.* **2012**, *60*, 1207–1216. [CrossRef]
27. Chan, Y.Y.; Sahril, N.; Rezali, M.S.; Kuang Kuay, L.; Baharudin, A.; Abd Razak, M.A.; Azlan Kassim, M.S.; Mohd Yusoff, M.F.; Omar, M.A.; Ahmad, N.A. Self-Reported Modifiable Risk Factors of Cardiovascular Disease among Older Adults in Malaysia: A Cross-Sectional Study of Prevalence and Clustering. *Int. J. Environ. Res. Public Health* **2021**, *18*, 7941. [CrossRef]

28. Frąk, W.; Wojtasińska, A.; Lisińska, W.; Młynarska, E.; Franczyk, B.; Rysz, J. Pathophysiology of Cardiovascular Diseases: New Insights into Molecular Mechanisms of Atherosclerosis, Arterial Hypertension, and Coronary Artery Disease. *Biomedicines* **2022**, *10*, 1938. [CrossRef] [PubMed]
29. Cervantes Gracia, K.; Llanas-Cornejo, D.; Husi, H. CVD and Oxidative Stress. *J. Clin. Med.* **2017**, *6*, 22. [CrossRef] [PubMed]
30. de Almeida, A.J.P.O.; de Almeida Rezende, M.S.; Dantas, S.H.; de Lima Silva, S.; de Oliveira, J.C.P.L.; de Lourdes Assunção Araújo de Azevedo, F.; Alves, R.M.F.R.; de Menezes, G.M.S.; dos Santos, P.F.; Gonçalves, T.A.F.; et al. Unveiling the Role of Inflammation and Oxidative Stress on Age-Related Cardiovascular Diseases. *Oxidative Med. Cell. Longev.* **2020**, *2020*, 1954398. [CrossRef] [PubMed]
31. Higashi, Y. Roles of Oxidative Stress and Inflammation in Vascular Endothelial Dysfunction-Related Disease. *Antioxidants* **2022**, *11*, 1958. [CrossRef]
32. Daiber, A.; Di Lisa, F.; Oelze, M.; Kröller-Schön, S.; Steven, S.; Schulz, E.; Münzel, T. Crosstalk of Mitochondria with NADPH Oxidase via Reactive Oxygen and Nitrogen Species Signalling and Its Role for Vascular Function. *Br. J. Pharmacol.* **2017**, *174*, 1670–1689. [CrossRef]
33. Li, H.; Horke, S.; Förstermann, U. Vascular Oxidative Stress, Nitric Oxide and Atherosclerosis. *Atherosclerosis* **2014**, *237*, 208–219. [CrossRef]
34. Medina-Leyte, D.J.; Zepeda-García, O.; Domínguez-Pérez, M.; González-Garrido, A.; Villarreal-Molina, T.; Jacobo-Albavera, L. Endothelial Dysfunction, Inflammation and Coronary Artery Disease: Potential Biomarkers and Promising Therapeutical Approaches. *Int. J. Mol. Sci.* **2021**, *22*, 3850. [CrossRef]
35. Fiordelisi, A.; Iaccarino, G.; Morisco, C.; Coscioni, E.; Sorriento, D. NFkappaB Is a Key Player in the Crosstalk between Inflammation and Cardiovascular Diseases. *Int. J. Mol. Sci.* **2019**, *20*, 1599. [CrossRef] [PubMed]
36. Sun, S. The Noncanonical NF-κB Pathway. *Immunol. Rev.* **2012**, *246*, 125–140. [CrossRef]
37. Groenen, A.G.; Halmos, B.; Tall, A.R.; Westerterp, M. Cholesterol Efflux Pathways, Inflammation, and Atherosclerosis. *Crit. Rev. Biochem. Mol. Biol.* **2021**, *56*, 426–439. [CrossRef] [PubMed]
38. Soehnlein, O.; Libby, P. Targeting Inflammation in Atherosclerosis—From Experimental Insights to the Clinic. *Nat. Rev. Drug Discov.* **2021**, *20*, 589–610. [CrossRef] [PubMed]
39. Jebari-Benslaiman, S.; Galicia-García, U.; Larrea-Sebal, A.; Olaetxea, J.R.; Alloza, I.; Vandenbroeck, K.; Benito-Vicente, A.; Martín, C. Pathophysiology of Atherosclerosis. *Int. J. Mol. Sci.* **2022**, *23*, 3346. [CrossRef]
40. Pizzino, G.; Irrera, N.; Cucinotta, M.; Pallio, G.; Mannino, F.; Arcoraci, V.; Squadrito, F.; Altavilla, D.; Bitto, A. Oxidative Stress: Harms and Benefits for Human Health. *Oxidative Med. Cell. Longev.* **2017**, *2017*, 8416763. [CrossRef]
41. Samtiya, M.; Aluko, R.E.; Dhewa, T.; Moreno-Rojas, J.M. Potential Health Benefits of Plant Food-Derived Bioactive Components: An Overview. *Foods* **2021**, *10*, 839. [CrossRef]
42. Norhazlindah, M.F.; Jahurul, M.H.A.; Norliza, M.; Shihabul, A.; Islam, S.; Nyam, K.L.; Zaidul, I.S.M. Techniques for Extraction, Characterization, and Application of Oil from Sacha Inchi (*Plukenetia volubilis* L.) Seed: A Review. *J. Food Meas. Charact.* **2023**, *17*, 904–915. [CrossRef]
43. Hajar, R. Risk Factors for Coronary Artery Disease: Historical Perspectives. *Heart Views* **2017**, *18*, 109. [CrossRef]
44. Ibrahim, N.I.; Naina Mohamed, I. Interdependence of Anti-Inflammatory and Antioxidant Properties of Squalene–Implication for Cardiovascular Health. *Life* **2021**, *11*, 103. [CrossRef] [PubMed]
45. Hedayatnia, M.; Asadi, Z.; Zare-Feyzabadi, R.; Yaghooti-Khorasani, M.; Ghazizadeh, H.; Ghaffarian-Zirak, R.; Nosrati-Tirkani, A.; Mohammadi-Bajgiran, M.; Rohban, M.; Sadabadi, F.; et al. Dyslipidemia and Cardiovascular Disease Risk among the MASHAD Study Population. *Lipids Health Dis.* **2020**, *19*, 42. [CrossRef]
46. Ambulay, J.P.; Rojas, P.A.; Timoteo, O.S.; Barreto, T.V.; Colarossi, A. Effect of the Emulsion of Sacha Inchi (Plukenetia Huayabambana) Oil on Oxidative Stress and Inflammation in Rats Induced to Obesity. *J. Funct. Foods* **2020**, *64*, 103631. [CrossRef]
47. Garmendia, F.; Pando, R.; Ronceros, G. Effect of Sacha Inchi Oil (*Plukenetia volúbilis* L.) on the Lipid Profile of Patients with Hyperlipoproteinemia. *Rev. Peru. Med. Exp. Salud Publica* **2011**, *28*, 628–632.
48. Gonzales, G.F.; Gonzales, C. A Randomized, Double-Blind Placebo-Controlled Study on Acceptability, Safety and Efficacy of Oral Administration of Sacha Inchi Oil (*Plukenetia volubilis* L.) in Adult Human Subjects. *Food Chem. Toxicol.* **2014**, *65*, 168–176. [CrossRef] [PubMed]
49. Alayón, A.N.; Ortega Ávila, J.G.; Echeverri Jiménez, I. Metabolic Status Is Related to the Effects of Adding of Sacha Inchi (*Plukenetia volubilis* L.) Oil on Postprandial Inflammation and Lipid Profile: Randomized, Crossover Clinical Trial. *J Food Biochem* **2019**, *43*, e12703. [CrossRef]
50. Suwanangul, S.; Aluko, R.E.; Sangsawad, P.; Kreungngernd, D.; Ruttarattanamongkol, K. Antioxidant and Enzyme Inhibitory Properties of Sacha Inchi (*Plukenetia volubilis*) Protein Hydrolysate and Its Peptide Fractions. *J. Food Biochem.* **2022**, *46*, e14464. [CrossRef]
51. Bellosta, S.; Corsini, A. Statin Drug Interactions and Related Adverse Reactions: An Update. *Expert Opin. Drug Saf.* **2018**, *17*, 25–37. [CrossRef] [PubMed]
52. Vinci, P.; Panizon, E.; Tosoni, L.M.; Cerrato, C.; Pellicori, F.; Mearelli, F.; Biasinutto, C.; Fiotti, N.; Di Girolamo, F.G.; Biolo, G. Statin-Associated Myopathy: Emphasis on Mechanisms and Targeted Therapy. *Int. J. Mol. Sci.* **2021**, *22*, 11687. [CrossRef]
53. Prasongsub, W.; Pimsan, N.; Buranapattarachote, C.; Punturee, K. Anti-HMG-CoA Reductase and Antioxidant Activities of Sacha Inchi (*Plukenetia volubilis* L.) Nutshell Extract. *Thai-J. Cit. Index Cent. (TCI) ASEAN Cit. Index* **2021**, *54*, 18–26. [CrossRef]

54. da Costa, R.F.; Freire, V.N.; Bezerra, E.M.; Cavada, B.S.; Caetano, E.W.S.; de Lima Filho, J.L.; Albuquerque, E.L. Explaining Statin Inhibition Effectiveness of HMG-CoA Reductase by Quantum Biochemistry Computations. *Phys. Chem. Chem. Phys.* **2012**, *14*, 1389–1398. [CrossRef] [PubMed]
55. Asmaa, B.H.; Ream, N. In Vitro Screening of the Pancreatic Cholesterol Esterase Inhibitory Activity of Some Medicinal Plants Grown in Syria. *Int. J. Pharmacogn. Phytochem. Res.* **2016**, *8*, 1432–1436. Available online: www.ijppr.com (accessed on 18 September 2023).
56. Liu, Z.; Chen, Z.; Guo, H.; He, D.; Zhao, H.; Wang, Z.; Zhang, W.; Liao, L.; Zhang, C.; Ni, L. The Modulatory Effect of Infusions of Green Tea, Oolong Tea, and Black Tea on Gut Microbiota in High-Fat-Induced Obese Mice. *Food Funct.* **2016**, *7*, 4869–4879. [CrossRef]
57. Just, S.; Mondot, S.; Ecker, J.; Wegner, K.; Rath, E.; Gau, L.; Streidl, T.; Hery-Arnaud, G.; Schmidt, S.; Lesker, T.R.; et al. The Gut Microbiota Drives the Impact of Bile Acids and Fat Source in Diet on Mouse Metabolism. *Microbiome* **2018**, *6*, 134. [CrossRef] [PubMed]
58. Yang, Y.; Zhang, Y.; Xu, Y.; Luo, T.; Ge, Y.; Jiang, Y.; Shi, Y.; Sun, J.; Le, G. Dietary Methionine Restriction Improves the Gut Microbiota and Reduces Intestinal Permeability and Inflammation in High-Fat-Fed Mice. *Food Funct.* **2019**, *10*, 5952–5968. [CrossRef]
59. Li, P.; Huang, J.; Xiao, N.; Cai, X.; Yang, Y.; Deng, J.; Zhang, L.H.; Du, B. Sacha Inchi Oil Alleviates Gut Microbiota Dysbiosis and Improves Hepatic Lipid Dysmetabolism in High-Fat Diet-Fed Rats. *Food Funct.* **2020**, *11*, 5827–5841. [CrossRef]
60. Nie, Q.; Xing, M.; Chen, H.; Hu, J.; Nie, S. Metabolomics and Lipidomics Profiling Reveals Hypocholesterolemic and Hypolipidemic Effects of Arabinoxylan on Type 2 Diabetic Rats. *J. Agric. Food Chem.* **2019**, *67*, 10614–10623. [CrossRef]
61. Wahlström, A.; Sayin, S.I.; Marschall, H.-U.; Bäckhed, F. Intestinal Crosstalk between Bile Acids and Microbiota and Its Impact on Host Metabolism. *Cell Metab.* **2016**, *24*, 41–50. [CrossRef] [PubMed]
62. Shuster, A.; Patlas, M.; Pinthus, J.H.; Mourtzakis, M. The Clinical Importance of Visceral Adiposity: A Critical Review of Methods for Visceral Adipose Tissue Analysis. *Br. J. Radiol.* **2012**, *85*, 1–10. [CrossRef]
63. Balla, T.; Sengupta, N.; Kim, Y.J. Lipid Synthesis and Transport Are Coupled to Regulate Membrane Lipid Dynamics in the Endoplasmic Reticulum. *Biochim. Et Biophys. Acta (BBA) Mol. Cell Biol. Lipids* **2020**, *1865*, 158461. [CrossRef]
64. Fang, L.; Harkewicz, R.; Hartvigsen, K.; Wiesner, P.; Choi, S.-H.; Almazan, F.; Pattison, J.; Deer, E.; Sayaphupha, T.; Dennis, E.A.; et al. Oxidized Cholesteryl Esters and Phospholipids in Zebrafish Larvae Fed a High Cholesterol Diet. *J. Biol. Chem.* **2010**, *285*, 32343–32351. [CrossRef]
65. Kayser, B.D.; Lhomme, M.; Prifti, E.; Da Cunha, C.; Marquet, F.; Chain, F.; Naas, I.; Pelloux, V.; Dao, M.; Kontush, A.; et al. Phosphatidylglycerols Are Induced by Gut Dysbiosis and Inflammation, and Favorably Modulate Adipose Tissue Remodeling in Obesity. *FASEB J.* **2019**, *33*, 4741–4754. [CrossRef]
66. Mukherjee, M. Human Digestive and Metabolic Lipases—A Brief Review. *J. Mol. Catal. B Enzym.* **2003**, *22*, 369–376. [CrossRef]
67. Liu, L.; Wang, Y.; Peng, C.; Wang, J. Optimization of the Preparation of Fish Protein Anti-Obesity Hydrolysates Using Response Surface Methodology. *Int. J. Mol. Sci.* **2013**, *14*, 3124–3139. [CrossRef] [PubMed]
68. Wang, K.; Liu, X.; Zhang, X. Isolation and Identification of Lipid-Lowering Peptides from Sacha Inchi Meal. *Int. J. Mol. Sci.* **2023**, *24*, 1529. [CrossRef]
69. Suwanangul, S.; Sangsawad, P.; Alashi, M.A.; Aluko, R.E.; Tochampa, W.; Chittrakorn, S.; Ruttarattanamongkol, K. Antioxidant Activities of Sacha Inchi (*Plukenetia volubilis* L.) Protein Isolate and Its Hydrolysates Produced with Different Proteases. *Maejo Int. J. Sci. Technol.* **2021**, *15*, 48–60.
70. Kittibunchakul, S.; Hudthagosol, C.; Sanporkha, P.; Sapwarobol, S.; Temviriyanukul, P.; Suttisansanee, U. Evaluation of Sacha Inchi (*Plukenetia volubilis* L.) By-Products as Valuable and Sustainable Sources of Health Benefits. *Horticulturae* **2022**, *8*, 344. [CrossRef]
71. Ugusman, A.; Shahrin, S.A.S.; Azizan, N.H.; Pillai, S.B.; Krishnan, K.; Salamt, N.; Aminuddin, A.; Hamid, A.A.; Kumar, J.; Mokhtar, M.H. Role of Honey in Obesity Management: A Systematic Review. *Front. Nutr.* **2022**, *9*, 924097. [CrossRef] [PubMed]
72. Čolak, E.; Pap, D. The Role of Oxidative Stress in the Development of Obesity and Obesity-Related Metabolic Disorders. *J. Med. Biochem.* **2021**, *40*, 1–9. [CrossRef]
73. Savini, I.; Catani, M.; Evangelista, D.; Gasperi, V.; Avigliano, L. Obesity-Associated Oxidative Stress: Strategies Finalized to Improve Redox State. *Int. J. Mol. Sci.* **2013**, *14*, 10497–10538. [CrossRef] [PubMed]
74. Gianazza, E.; Brioschi, M.; Fernandez, A.M.; Banfi, C. Lipoxidation in Cardiovascular Diseases. *Redox Biol.* **2019**, *23*, 101119. [CrossRef]
75. Duryee, M.J.; Clemens, D.L.; Opperman, P.J.; Thiele, G.M.; Duryee, L.M.; Garvin, R.P.; Anderson, D.R. Malondialdehyde-Acetaldehyde Modified (MAA) Proteins Differentially Effect the Inflammatory Response in Macrophage, Endothelial Cells and Animal Models of Cardiovascular Disease. *Int. J. Mol. Sci.* **2021**, *22*, 12948. [CrossRef]
76. Rincón-Cervera, M.Á.; Valenzuela, R.; Hernandez-Rodas, M.C.; Barrera, C.; Espinosa, A.; Marambio, M.; Valenzuela, A. Vegetable Oils Rich in Alpha Linolenic Acid Increment Hepatic N-3 LCPUFA, Modulating the Fatty Acid Metabolism and Antioxidant Response in Rats. *Prostaglandins Leukot. Essent. Fat. Acids* **2016**, *111*, 25–35. [CrossRef]
77. Yan, K.; Deng, X.; Zhai, X.; Zhou, M.; Jia, X.; Luo, L.; Niu, M.; Zhu, H.; Qiang, H.; Zhou, Y. P38 Mitogen-Activated Protein Kinase and Liver X Receptor-α Mediate the Leptin Effect on Sterol Regulatory Element Binding Protein-1c Expression in Hepatic Stellate Cells. *Mol. Med.* **2012**, *18*, 10–18. [CrossRef] [PubMed]

78. de Faria, A.P.; Ritter, A.M.V.; Gasparetti, C.S.; Corrêa, N.B.; Brunelli, V.; Almeida, A.; Pires, N.F.; Modolo, R.; Moreno Junior, H. A Proposed Inflammatory Score of Circulating Cytokines/Adipokines Associated with Resistant Hypertension, but Dependent on Obesity Parameters. *Arq. Bras. Cardiol.* **2019**, *112*, 383–389. [CrossRef]
79. Klok, M.D.; Jakobsdottir, S.; Drent, M.L. The Role of Leptin and Ghrelin in the Regulation of Food Intake and Body Weight in Humans: A Review. *Obes. Rev.* **2007**, *8*, 21–34. [CrossRef] [PubMed]
80. Knight, Z.A.; Hannan, K.S.; Greenberg, M.L.; Friedman, J.M. Hyperleptinemia Is Required for the Development of Leptin Resistance. *PLoS ONE* **2010**, *5*, e11376. [CrossRef] [PubMed]
81. Almabrouk, T.A.M.; White, A.D.; Ugusman, A.B.; Skiba, D.S.; Katwan, O.J.; Alganga, H.; Guzik, T.J.; Touyz, R.M.; Salt, I.P.; Kennedy, S. High Fat Diet Attenuates the Anticontractile Activity of Aortic PVAT via a Mechanism Involving AMPK and Reduced Adiponectin Secretion. *Front. Physiol.* **2018**, *9*, 51. [CrossRef]
82. Yanai, H.; Yoshida, H. Beneficial Effects of Adiponectin on Glucose and Lipid Metabolism and Atherosclerotic Progression: Mechanisms and Perspectives. *Int. J. Mol. Sci.* **2019**, *20*, 1190. [CrossRef] [PubMed]
83. Othman, N.S.; Aminuddin, A.; Zainal Abidin, S.; Syafruddin, S.E.; Ahmad, M.F.; Mohd Mokhtar, N.; Kumar, J.; Hamid, A.A.; Ugusman, A. Profiling of Differentially Expressed MicroRNAs in Human Umbilical Vein Endothelial Cells Exposed to Hyperglycemia via RNA Sequencing. *Life* **2023**, *13*, 1296. [CrossRef] [PubMed]
84. Attjioui, M.; Ryan, S.; Ristic, A.K.; Higgins, T.; Goñi, O.; Gibney, E.R.; Tierney, J.; O'Connell, S. Comparison of Edible Brown Algae Extracts for the Inhibition of Intestinal Carbohydrate Digestive Enzymes Involved in Glucose Release from the Diet. *J. Nutr. Sci.* **2021**, *10*, e5. [CrossRef] [PubMed]
85. Ćorković, I.; Gašo-Sokač, D.; Pichler, A.; Šimunović, J.; Kopjar, M. Dietary Polyphenols as Natural Inhibitors of α-Amylase and α-Glucosidase. *Life* **2022**, *12*, 1692. [CrossRef] [PubMed]
86. You, Z.; Li, Y.; Zhang, K.; Zheng, X.; Wong, V.K.W.; Liu, W. Inhibitory Effect of Plant Essential Oils on α-Glucosidase. *Food Sci. Biotechnol.* **2022**, *31*, 1593–1602. [CrossRef] [PubMed]
87. Giuberti, G.; Rocchetti, G.; Lucini, L. Interactions between Phenolic Compounds, Amylolytic Enzymes and Starch: An Updated Overview. *Curr. Opin. Food Sci.* **2020**, *31*, 102–113. [CrossRef]
88. Taslimi, P.; Gulçin, İ. Antidiabetic Potential: In Vitro Inhibition Effects of Some Natural Phenolic Compounds on α-Glycosidase and α-Amylase Enzymes. *J. Biochem. Mol. Toxicol.* **2017**, *31*, e21956. [CrossRef] [PubMed]
89. Oboh, G.; Agunloye, O.M.; Adefegha, S.A.; Akinyemi, A.J.; Ademiluyi, A.O. Caffeic and Chlorogenic Acids Inhibit Key Enzymes Linked to Type 2 Diabetes (in Vitro): A Comparative Study. *J. Basic Clin. Physiol. Pharmacol.* **2015**, *26*, 165–170. [CrossRef] [PubMed]
90. TADERA, K.; MINAMI, Y.; TAKAMATSU, K.; MATSUOKA, T. Inhibition of ALPHA.-Glucosidase and ALPHA.-Amylase by Flavonoids. *J. Nutr. Sci. Vitaminol.* **2006**, *52*, 149–153. [CrossRef]
91. Zhang, A.; Wang, K.; Liu, X.; Zhang, X. Isolation and Identification of Dipeptidyl Peptidase-IV Inhibitory Peptides from Sacha Inchi Meal. *J. Sci. Food Agric.* **2023**, *103*, 2926–2938. [CrossRef]
92. Eleazu, C.O.; Eleazu, K.C.; Chukwuma, S.; Essien, U.N. Review of the Mechanism of Cell Death Resulting from Streptozotocin Challenge in Experimental Animals, Its Practical Use and Potential Risk to Humans. *J. Diabetes Metab. Disord.* **2013**, *12*, 60. [CrossRef]
93. Gheibi, S.; Kashfi, K.; Ghasemi, A. A Practical Guide for Induction of Type-2 Diabetes in Rat: Incorporating a High-Fat Diet and Streptozotocin. *Biomed. Pharmacother.* **2017**, *95*, 605–613. [CrossRef] [PubMed]
94. Szkudelski, T. The Mechanism of Alloxan and Streptozotocin Action in B Cells of the Rat Pancreas. *Physiol. Res.* **2001**, *50*, 537–546. [PubMed]
95. Zhu, B.T. Pathogenic Mechanism of Autoimmune Diabetes Mellitus in Humans: Potential Role of Streptozotocin-Induced Selective Autoimmunity against Human Islet β-Cells. *Cells* **2022**, *11*, 492. [CrossRef] [PubMed]
96. Furman, B.L. Streptozotocin-Induced Diabetic Models in Mice and Rats. *Curr. Protoc.* **2021**, *1*, e78. [CrossRef] [PubMed]
97. Mathias Akinlade, O.; Victor Owoyele, B.; Olufemi Soladoye, A. Streptozotocin-Induced Type 1 and 2 Diabetes in Rodents: A Model for Studying Diabetic Cardiac Autonomic Neuropathy. *Afr. Health Sci.* **2021**, *21*, 719–727. [CrossRef]
98. Rojanaverawong, W.; Wongmanee, N.; Hanchang, W. Sacha Inchi (*Plukenetia volubilis* L.) Oil Improves Hepatic Insulin Sensitivity and Glucose Metabolism through Insulin Signaling Pathway in a Rat Model of Type 2 Diabetes. *Prev. Nutr. Food Sci.* **2023**, *28*, 30–42. [CrossRef]
99. Li, M.; Chi, X.; Wang, Y.; Setrerrahmane, S.; Xie, W.; Xu, H. Trends in Insulin Resistance: Insights into Mechanisms and Therapeutic Strategy. *Signal Transduct. Target. Ther.* **2022**, *7*, 216. [CrossRef]
100. Jiang, S.; Young, J.; Wang, K.; Qian, Y.; Cai, L. Diabetic-induced Alterations in Hepatic Glucose and Lipid Metabolism: The Role of Type 1 and Type 2 Diabetes Mellitus (Review). *Mol. Med. Rep.* **2020**, *22*, 603–611. [CrossRef]
101. Hatting, M.; Tavares, C.D.J.; Sharabi, K.; Rines, A.K.; Puigserver, P. Insulin Regulation of Gluconeogenesis. *Ann. N. Y. Acad. Sci.* **2018**, *1411*, 21–35. [CrossRef]
102. Gurung, M.; Li, Z.; You, H.; Rodrigues, R.; Jump, D.B.; Morgun, A.; Shulzhenko, N. Role of Gut Microbiota in Type 2 Diabetes Pathophysiology. *EBioMedicine* **2020**, *51*, 102590. [CrossRef]
103. Yan, J.; Sheng, L.; Li, H. *Akkermansia muciniphila*: Is It the Holy Grail for Ameliorating Metabolic Diseases? *Gut Microbes* **2021**, *13*, 1984104. [CrossRef]

104. Bahar-Tokman, H.; Demirci, M.; Keskin, F.; Cagatay, P.; Taner, Z.; Ozturk-Bakar, Y.; Ozyazar, M.; Kiraz, N.; Kocazeybek, B. Firmicutes/Bacteroidetes Ratio in the Gut Microbiota and IL-1β, IL-6, IL-8, TLR2, TLR4, TLR5 Gene Expressions in Type 2 Diabetes. *Clin. Lab.* **2022**, *68*, 1903–1910. [CrossRef]
105. Fassatoui, M.; Lopez-Siles, M.; Díaz-Rizzolo, D.A.; Jmel, H.; Naouali, C.; Abdessalem, G.; Chikhaoui, A.; Nadal, B.; Jamoussi, H.; Abid, A.; et al. Gut Microbiota Imbalances in Tunisian Participants with Type 1 and Type 2 Diabetes Mellitus. *Biosci. Rep.* **2019**, *39*, BSR20182348. [CrossRef]
106. Demirci, M.; Bahar Tokman, H.; Taner, Z.; Keskin, F.E.; Çağatay, P.; Ozturk Bakar, Y.; Özyazar, M.; Kiraz, N.; Kocazeybek, B.S. Bacteroidetes and Firmicutes Levels in Gut Microbiota and Effects of Hosts TLR2/TLR4 Gene Expression Levels in Adult Type 1 Diabetes Patients in Istanbul, Turkey. *J. Diabetes Complicat.* **2020**, *34*, 107449. [CrossRef]
107. Lin, J.; Wen, J.; Xiao, N.; Cai, Y.T.; Xiao, J.; Dai, W.; Chen, J.P.; Zeng, K.W.; Liu, F.; Du, B.; et al. Anti-Diabetic and Gut Microbiota Modulation Effects of Sacha Inchi (*Plukenetia volubilis* L.) Leaf Extract in Streptozotocin-Induced Type 1 Diabetic Mice. *J. Sci. Food Agric.* **2022**, *102*, 4304–4312. [CrossRef]
108. Alayón, A.N.; Ortega Avila, J.G.; Echeverri Jiménez, I. Carbohydrate Metabolism and Gene Expression of Sirtuin 1 in Healthy Subjects after Sacha Inchi Oil Supplementation: A Randomized Trial. *Food Funct.* **2018**, *9*, 1570–1577. [CrossRef]
109. Ye, X.; Li, M.; Hou, T.; Gao, T.; Zhu, W.; Yang, Y. Sirtuins in Glucose and Lipid Metabolism. *Oncotarget* **2017**, *8*, 1845–1859. [CrossRef]
110. Zhou, S.; Tang, X.; Chen, H.-Z. Sirtuins and Insulin Resistance. *Front. Endocrinol.* **2018**, *9*, 748. [CrossRef]
111. Mohamed, J.; Nazratun Nafizah, A.H.; Zariyantey, A.H.; Budin, B.S. Mechanisms of Diabetes-Induced Liver Damage: The Role of Oxidative Stress and Inflammation. *Sultan Qaboos Univ. Med. J.* **2016**, *16*, e132–e141. [CrossRef]
112. Son, J.S.; Choi, S.; Lee, G.; Jeong, S.-M.; Kim, S.M.; Kim, K.; Yun, J.M.; Park, S.M. Blood Pressure Change from Normal to 2017 ACC/AHA Defined Stage 1 Hypertension and Cardiovascular Risk. *J. Clin. Med.* **2019**, *8*, 820. [CrossRef]
113. Losurdo, P.; Grillo, A.; Panizon, E.; Cappellari, G.G.; Fabris, B.; Bardelli, M.; Biolo, G.; Zanetti, M.; Carretta, R. Supplementation of Omega-3 Polyunsaturated Fatty Acids Prevents Increase in Arterial Stiffness After Experimental Menopause. *J. Cardiovasc. Pharmacol. Ther.* **2014**, *19*, 114–120. [CrossRef]
114. Spector, A.A.; Kim, H.-Y. Discovery of Essential Fatty Acids. *J. Lipid Res.* **2015**, *56*, 11–21. [CrossRef]
115. Bentsen, H. Dietary Polyunsaturated Fatty Acids, Brain Function and Mental Health. *Microb. Ecol. Health Dis.* **2017**, *28*, 1281916. [CrossRef]
116. Wang, H.; Li, Q.; Zhu, Y.; Zhang, X. Omega-3 Polyunsaturated Fatty Acids: Versatile Roles in Blood Pressure Regulation. *Antioxid. Redox Signal.* **2021**, *34*, 800–810. [CrossRef]
117. Ferrari, R. RAAS Inhibition and Mortality in Hypertension. *Glob. Cardiol. Sci. Pract.* **2013**, *2013*, 34. [CrossRef]
118. Chirinos, R.; Pedreschi, R.; Campos, D. Enzyme-Assisted Hydrolysates from Sacha Inchi (Plukenetia Volubilis) Protein with in Vitro Antioxidant and Antihypertensive Properties. *J. Food Process. Preserv.* **2020**, *44*, e14969. [CrossRef]
119. Bhullar, K.S.; Lassalle-Claux, G.; Touaibia, M.; Rupasinghe, H.P.V. Antihypertensive Effect of Caffeic Acid and Its Analogs through Dual Renin–Angiotensin–Aldosterone System Inhibition. *Eur. J. Pharmacol.* **2014**, *730*, 125–132. [CrossRef]
120. Blaustein, M.P.; Leenen, F.H.H.; Chen, L.; Golovina, V.A.; Hamlyn, J.M.; Pallone, T.L.; Van Huysse, J.W.; Zhang, J.; Wier, W.G. How NaCl Raises Blood Pressure: A New Paradigm for the Pathogenesis of Salt-Dependent Hypertension. *Am. J. Physiol.-Heart Circ. Physiol.* **2012**, *302*, H1031–H1049. [CrossRef]
121. Obradovic, M.; Sudar-Milovanovic, E.; Gluvic, Z.; Banjac, K.; Rizzo, M.; Isenovic, E.R. The Na+/K+-ATPase: A Potential Therapeutic Target in Cardiometabolic Diseases. *Front. Endocrinol.* **2023**, *14*, 1150171. [CrossRef]
122. Li, P.; Cai, X.; Xiao, N.; Ma, X.; Zeng, L.; Zhang, L.-H.; Xie, L.; Du, B. Sacha Inchi (*Plukenetia volubilis* L.) Shell Extract Alleviates Hypertension in Association with the Regulation of Gut Microbiota. *Food Funct.* **2020**, *11*, 8051–8067. [CrossRef]
123. Krzemińska, J.; Wronka, M.; Młynarska, E.; Franczyk, B.; Rysz, J. Arterial Hypertension—Oxidative Stress and Inflammation. *Antioxidants* **2022**, *11*, 172. [CrossRef]
124. Lamb, F.S.; Choi, H.; Miller, M.R.; Stark, R.J. TNFα and Reactive Oxygen Signaling in Vascular Smooth Muscle Cells in Hypertension and Atherosclerosis. *Am. J. Hypertens.* **2020**, *33*, 902–913. [CrossRef]
125. Rybalkin, S.D.; Rybalkina, I.G.; Fei, R.; Hofmann, F.; Beavo, J.A. Regulation of CGMP-Specific Phosphodiesterase (PDE5) Phosphorylation in Smooth Muscle Cells. *J. Biol. Chem.* **2002**, *277*, 3310–3317. [CrossRef]
126. Gudjoncik, A.; Guenancia, C.; Zeller, M.; Cottin, Y.; Vergely, C.; Rochette, L. Iron, Oxidative Stress, and Redox Signaling in the Cardiovascular System. *Mol. Nutr. Food Res.* **2014**, *58*, 1721–1738. [CrossRef]
127. Ugusman, A.; Kumar, J.; Aminuddin, A. Endothelial Function and Dysfunction: Impact of Sodium-Glucose Cotransporter 2 Inhibitors. *Pharmacol. Ther.* **2021**, *224*, 107832. [CrossRef]
128. Yuyun, M.F.; Ng, L.L.; Ng, G.A. Endothelial Dysfunction, Endothelial Nitric Oxide Bioavailability, Tetrahydrobiopterin, and 5-Methyltetrahydrofolate in Cardiovascular Disease. Where Are We with Therapy? *Microvasc. Res.* **2018**, *119*, 7–12. [CrossRef]
129. Al Samarraie, A.; Pichette, M.; Rousseau, G. Role of the Gut Microbiome in the Development of Atherosclerotic Cardiovascular Disease. *Int. J. Mol. Sci.* **2023**, *24*, 5420. [CrossRef]
130. Nesci, A.; Carnuccio, C.; Ruggieri, V.; D'Alessandro, A.; Di Giorgio, A.; Santoro, L.; Gasbarrini, A.; Santoliquido, A.; Ponziani, F.R. Gut Microbiota and Cardiovascular Disease: Evidence on the Metabolic and Inflammatory Background of a Complex Relationship. *Int. J. Mol. Sci.* **2023**, *24*, 9087. [CrossRef]

131. Abenavoli, L.; Scarpellini, E.; Colica, C.; Boccuto, L.; Salehi, B.; Sharifi-Rad, J.; Aiello, V.; Romano, B.; De Lorenzo, A.; Izzo, A.A.; et al. Gut Microbiota and Obesity: A Role for Probiotics. *Nutrients* **2019**, *11*, 2690. [CrossRef]
132. Stojanov, S.; Berlec, A.; Štrukelj, B. The Influence of Probiotics on the Firmicutes/Bacteroidetes Ratio in the Treatment of Obesity and Inflammatory Bowel Disease. *Microorganisms* **2020**, *8*, 1715. [CrossRef] [PubMed]
133. Yan, D.; Sun, Y.; Zhou, X.; Si, W.; Liu, J.; Li, M.; Wu, M. Regulatory Effect of Gut Microbes on Blood Pressure. *Anim. Models Exp. Med.* **2022**, *5*, 513–531. [CrossRef] [PubMed]
134. Mhd Rodzi, N.A.R.; Lee, L.K. Sacha Inchi (*Plukenetia volubilis* L.): Recent Insight on Phytochemistry, Pharmacology, Organoleptic, Safety and Toxicity Perspectives. *Heliyon* **2022**, *8*, e10572. [CrossRef] [PubMed]
135. Rousseau, S.; Kyomugasho, C.; Celus, M.; Hendrickx, M.E.G.; Grauwet, T. Barriers Impairing Mineral Bioaccessibility and Bioavailability in Plant-Based Foods and the Perspectives for Food Processing. *Crit. Rev. Food Sci. Nutr.* **2020**, *60*, 826–843. [CrossRef]
136. Srichamnong, W.; Ting, P.; Pitchakarn, P.; Nuchuchua, O.; Temviriyanukul, P. Safety Assessment of *Plukenetia volubilis* (Inca Peanut) Seeds, Leaves, and Their Products. *Food Sci. Nutr.* **2018**, *6*, 962–969. [CrossRef]
137. Rodeiro, I.; Remirez, D.; Flores, D. Sacha Inchi (*Plukenetia volubilis* L.) Powder: Acute Toxicity, 90 Days Oral Toxicity Study and Micronucleus Assay in Rodents. *J. Pharm. Pharmacogn. Res.* **2018**, *6*, 17–26.
138. Gorriti, A.; Arroyo, J.; Quispe, F.; Cisneros, B.; Condorhuamán, M.; Almora, Y.; Chumpitaz, V. Oral Toxicity at 60-Days of Sacha Inchi Oil (*Plukenetia volubilis* L.) and Linseed (*Linum usitatissimum* L.), and Determination of Lethal Dose 50 in Rodents. *Rev. Peru. Med. Exp. Salud Publica* **2010**, *27*, 352–360. [CrossRef]
139. Bueso, A.; Rodriguez-Perez, R.; Rodriguez, M.; Dionicio, J.; Perez-Pimiento, A.; Caballero, M.L. Occupational Allergic Rhinoconjunctivitis and Bronchial Asthma Induced by *Plukenetia volubilis* Seeds. *Occup. Environ. Med.* **2010**, *67*, 797–798. [CrossRef] [PubMed]
140. Malinowski, S.S.; Barber, K.E.; Kishk, O.A.; Mays, A.A.; Jones, S.R.; Turner, A.L.; Riche, D.M. Effect of Fish Oil Supplement Administration Method on Tolerability and Adherence: A Randomized Pilot Clinical Trial. *Pilot Feasibility Stud.* **2019**, *5*, 3. [CrossRef] [PubMed]

MDPI AG
Grosspeteranlage 5
4052 Basel
Switzerland
Tel.: +41 61 683 77 34

Pharmaceuticals Editorial Office
E-mail: pharmaceuticals@mdpi.com
www.mdpi.com/journal/pharmaceuticals

www.ingramcontent.com/pod-product-compliance
Lightning Source LLC
Chambersburg PA
CBHW040808250926
51850CB00007BA/1116
9783725861477